BMA

A Library

Clinical Imaging:

An Atlas of Differential Diagnosis

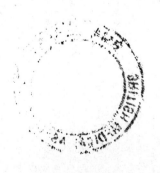

5th edition

Clinical Imaging:

An Atlas of Differential Diagnosis

Ronald L. Eisenberg, MD
Associate Professor Radiology
Harvard Medical School
Radiologist
Beth Israel Deaconess Medical Center
Boston, Massachusetts

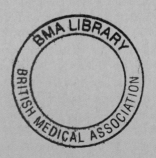
Wolters Kluwer | Lippincott Williams & Wilkins
Health
Philadelphia • Baltimore • New York • London
Buenos Aires • Hong Kong • Sydney • Tokyo

Acquisitions Editor: Brian Brown
Product Manager: Ryan Shaw
Vendor Manager: Alicia Jackson
Senior Manufacturing Manager: Benjamin Rivera
Senior Marketing Manager: Angela Panetta
Design Coordinator: Stephen Druding
Production Service: Spearhead Global, Inc.

© 2010 by LIPPINCOTT WILLIAMS & WILKINS, a WOLTERS KLUWER business
530 Walnut Street
Philadelphia, PA 19106 USA
LWW.com

Printed in China

Library of Congress Cataloging-in-Publication Data

Eisenberg, Ronald L.
    Clinical imaging : an atlas of differential diagnosis / Ronald L. Eisenberg. — 5th ed.
        p. ; cm.
    Includes bibliographical references and index.
    ISBN-13: 978-0-7817-8860-1 (alk. paper)
    ISBN-10: 0-7817-8860-9 (alk. paper)
    1.   Diagnostic imaging—Atlases. 2.   Diagnostic imaging—Handbooks, manuals, etc. 3.   Diagnosis, Differential—Atlases.
4.   Diagnosis, Differential—Handbooks, manuals, etc. I. Title.
    [DNLM: 1.   Diagnostic Imaging—Atlases. 2.   Diagnosis, Differential—Atlases. WN 17 E36c 2010]
    RC78.7.D53E36 2010
    616.07′54—dc22

                                                                                                    2009015308

Care has been taken to confirm the accuracy of the information presented and to describe generally accepted practices. However, the authors, editors, and publisher are not responsible for errors or omissions or for any consequences from application of the information in this book and make no warranty, expressed or implied, with respect to the currency, completeness, or accuracy of the contents of the publication. Application of the information in a particular situation remains the professional responsibility of the practitioner.

The authors, editors, and publisher have exerted every effort to ensure that drug selection and dosage set forth in this text are in accordance with current recommendations and practice at the time of publication. However, in view of ongoing research, changes in government regulations, and the constant flow of information relating to drug therapy and drug reactions, the reader is urged to check the package insert for each drug for any change in indications and dosage and for added warnings and precautions. This is particularly important when the recommended agent is a new or infrequently employed drug.

Some drugs and medical devices presented in the publication have Food and Drug Administration (FDA) clearance for limited use in restricted research settings. It is the responsibility of the health care provider to ascertain the FDA status of each drug or device planned for use in their clinical practice.

To purchase additional copies of this book, call our customer service department at (800) 638-3030 or fax orders to (301) 223-2320. International customers should call (301) 223-2300.

Visit Lippincott Williams & Wilkins on the Internet: at LWW.com. Lippincott Williams & Wilkins customer service representatives are available from 8:30 am to 6 pm, EST.

10 9 8 7 6 5 4 3 2 1

To Zina, Avlana, and Cherina

CONTENTS

PREFACE to the first edition

Pattern recognition leading to the development of differential diagnoses is the essence of radiology. Both the practicing radiologist faced with the reality of daily film reading and the senior resident taking the oral board examination are usually unaware of the underlying disease when they are presented with a specific finding for which they must suggest a differential diagnosis and a rational diagnostic approach. This book offers differential diagnoses for a broad spectrum of radiographic patterns, not only in conventional radiography but also in ultrasound and computed tomography. Added to these lists of differential possibilities are descriptions of the specific imaging findings to be expected for each diagnostic entity as well as differential points to aid the reader in arriving at a precise diagnosis. A wealth of illustrations is provided to point out the often subtle differences in appearance among conditions that can produce a similar overall radiographic pattern. Extensive cross referencing is provided to limit duplication and to permit the reader to find various radiographic manifestations of the same condition.

I must stress that this book in no way intends to supplant the current excellent textbooks in general radiology and imaging subspecialties. Rather, it is designed to complement these works by providing a handy reference for practicing radiologists and residents faced with the daily challenge of interpreting radiographic examinations.

PREFACE

The warm response from residents and practicing radiologists to the first four editions has been extremely gratifying. To reflect trends in diagnostic imaging, yet maintain the single-volume format, some sections on plain radiography have been eliminated to make room for new sections dealing with computed tomography and magnetic resonance imaging. Whenever appropriate, the lists of differential diagnoses from previous editions have been updated and new illustrations added.

I hope that this expanded volume will be even more successful than its predecessors in meeting the goal of providing a handy reference for practicing radiologists and residents faced with the increasingly complex daily challenge of interpreting radiographic examinations.

Localized Alveolar Pattern

Condition	Imaging Findings	Comments
Bacterial pneumonia		
Staphylococcus (Fig C 1-1)	Rapid development of extensive alveolar infiltrates, usually involving a whole lobe or even several lobes. Air bronchograms are infrequent because the acute inflammatory exudate fills the airways, leading to segmental collapse and a loss of volume.	Most frequently occurs in children, especially during the first year of life. In adults, usually affects hospitalized patients with lowered resistance or as a complication of a viral respiratory infection. A characteristic finding in childhood disease is the development of pneumatoceles, thin-walled cystic spaces in the parenchyma that typically disappear spontaneously within several weeks. Pleural effusion (or empyema) often occurs.
Streptococcus (see Fig C 17-3)	Indistinguishable from staphylococcal pneumonia. Homogeneous or patchy consolidation in a segmental distribution with a lower lobe predominance and often some loss of volume.	Uncommon condition that usually follows viral infections such as measles, pertussis, and epidemic influenza. Unlike staphylococcal infection, streptococcal pneumonia rarely causes the development of pneumatoceles. Early and rapid accumulation of empyema fluid was a characteristic feature before the advent of antibiotics.
Pneumococcus (Fig C 1-2)	Homogeneous consolidation that almost invariably abuts against a visceral pleural surface and almost always contains an air bronchogram.	Most commonly occurs in alcoholics and other compromised hosts. Cavitation and pleural reaction are rare. In children, may produce the so-called round or spherical pneumonia, in which a well-circumscribed spherical consolidation on both frontal and lateral views simulates a pulmonary or mediastinal mass (Fig C 1-3).

A

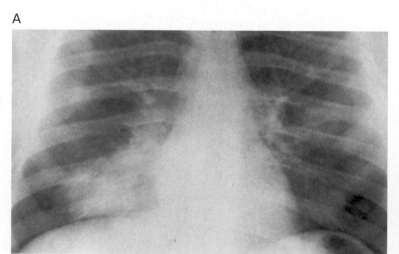

B

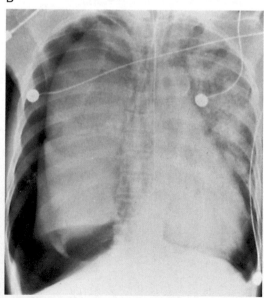

Fig C 1-1
Staphylococcal pneumonia. (A) Ill-defined bronchopneumonia at the right base. (B) In another patient, there is consolidation in the left upper lobe and entire right lung with a moderate right pneumothorax. The extensive consolidation presents further collapse of the right lung. The pneumothorax was due to the rupture of a pneumatocele, although no pneumatocele can be identified.

Condition	Imaging Findings	Comments
Klebsiella (Fig C 1-4)	Homogeneous parenchymal consolidation containing air bronchograms (simulates pneumococcal pneumonia). Primarily involves the right upper lobe. Typically induces a large inflammatory exudate, causing increased volume of the affected lobe and characteristic bulging of an adjacent interlobar fissure (see Fig C 15-1).	Most commonly develops in alcoholics and in elderly patients with chronic pulmonary disease. Unlike acute pneumococcal pneumonia, *Klebsiella* pneumonia causes frequent and rapid cavitation, and there is a much greater incidence of pleural effusion and empyema.

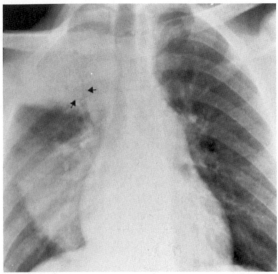

Fig C 1-2
Pneumococcal pneumonia. Homogeneous consolidation of the right upper lobe and the medial and posterior segments of the right lower lobe. Note the associated air bronchograms (arrows).

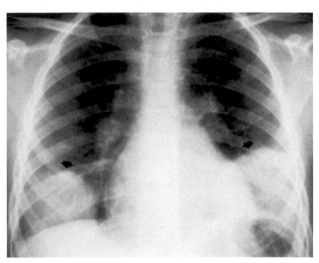

Fig C 1-3
"Spherical" pneumonia. Frontal view of the chest shows a rounded soft-tissue density in the posterolateral aspects of both lower lobes (arrows) with mild bilateral hilar prominence.[1]

A   B

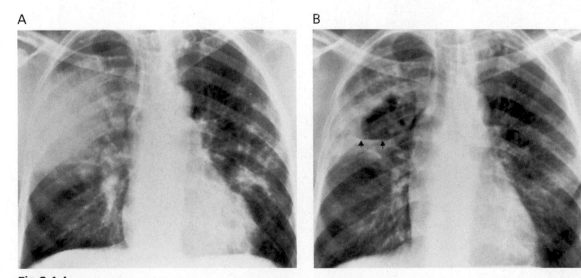

Fig C 1-4
***Klebsiella* pneumonia.** (A) Air-space consolidation involving much of the right upper lobe. (B) Progression of the necrotizing infection produces a large abscess cavity with an air-fluid level (arrows).

Condition	Imaging Findings	Comments
Other enteric gram-negative bacteria (Fig C 1-5)	Nonspecific, often inhomogeneous pattern of consolidation that most commonly affects the lower lobes. Cavitation is relatively common, and pleural effusion may occur.	*Escherichia coli, Serratia marcescens,* Enterobacteriaceae, *Proteus, Pseudomonas aeruginosa, Salmonella,* and *Brucella.* Most commonly develop in debilitated or immunocompromised patients.
Haemophilus influenzae (Fig C 1-6)	Nonspecific patchy pulmonary infiltrate that is often bilateral. May be unilateral lobar or segmental consolidation, simulating pneumococcal disease. Typically extensive pleural involvement that often appears out of proportion to the associated parenchymal infiltrate.	Serious infections primarily affect children under the age of 4 years and older patients who have undergone antibiotic therapy or who suffer from diseases that increase their general susceptibility to infection. This organism is the leading cause of epiglottitis (see Fig C 35-2), the second leading cause of childhood otitis media, and a common cause of childhood bacterial meningitis.
Haemophilus pertussis (whooping cough) (Fig C 1-7)	Various combinations of atelectasis, segmental pneumonia, and hilar lymph node enlargement. Coalescence of air-space consolidation contiguous to the heart produces a typical "shaggy heart" contour.	Although often considered to have been largely eradicated by immunization, immunity is apparently not lifelong, and pertussis has become a not uncommon cause of bronchitis in adults. Acute infection most frequently affects nonimmunized children younger than 2 years of age.
Tularemia (see Fig C 14-2)	Patchy consolidations that may be bilateral, multilobar, or both. Ipsilateral hilar adenopathy and pleural effusion occur in approximately half the cases.	Pneumonia represents hematogenous spread or inhalation of *Francisella tularensis,* which is usually transmitted to humans from infected animals (rodents, small mammals) or insect vectors.

A

B

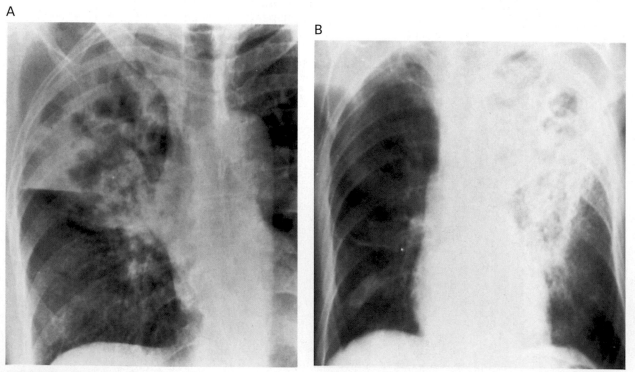

Fig C 1-5
Enteric gram-negative bacteria. (A) *Proteus.* (B) *Pseudomonas.*[2]

Condition	Imaging Findings	Comments
Yersinia pestis (see Figs C 2-13 and C 14-3)	Patchy segmental infiltration or dense lobar consolidation simulating pneumococcal pneumonia. Typically, there is enlargement of hilar and paratracheal lymph nodes and, often, pleural effusion.	The pneumonic type of plague causes severe pulmonary consolidation, necrosis, and hemorrhage and is usually fatal. This organism is still widespread among wild rodents.
Anthrax	Patchy parenchymal infiltrates that are usually associated with pleural effusion and mediastinal widening (lymph node enlargement and hemorrhagic mediastinitis).	Bacterial disease of cattle, sheep, and goats that primarily affects humans who inhale spores from infected animals or their products (eg, wool, hides).
Legionnaires' disease (Fig C 1-8)	Patchy or fluffy alveolar infiltrate that rapidly progresses to involve adjacent lobes and the contralateral side.	Acute gram-negative bacterial pneumonia that occurs in local outbreaks or as sporadic cases and may cause a fulminant, often fatal, pneumonia. Small pleural effusions are common, whereas cavitation and hilar adenopathy are unusual. Most patients respond well to erythromycin, though the radiographic resolution often lags behind the clinical response.

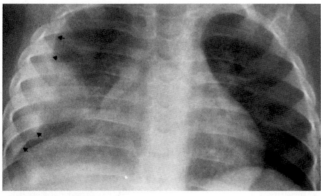

Fig C 1-6
***Haemophilus influenzae* pneumonia.** In addition to the ill-defined right lower lung consolidation, note the extensive pleural thickening or fibrinous exudate (arrows) that appears out of proportion to the associated parenchymal infiltrate.[3]

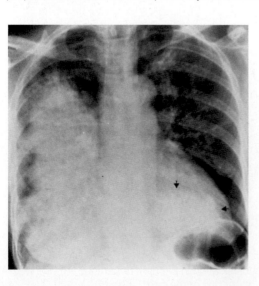

Fig C 1-7
***Haemophilus pertussis*.** Bilateral central parenchymal infiltrates and linear areas of atelectasis obscure the normally sharp cardiac border to produce the shaggy heart contour.

Fig C 1-8
Legionnaires' disease. There is extensive consolidation of much of the right lung, with a smaller area of infiltrate (arrows) at the left base.

Condition	Imaging Findings	Comments
Bacteroides (Fig C 1-9)	Patchy or confluent consolidation that is generally confined to the lower lobes. Cavitation and empyema are common.	Gram-negative anaerobic bacteria that are commonly found in the gastrointestinal and genital tracts. Pneumonia develops from aspiration of infected material or septic infarctions resulting from emboli arising in veins in the peritonsillar area or pelvis.
Fungal pneumonia Histoplasmosis (Fig C 1-10)	In the primary form, single or multiple areas of consolidation that are most often in the lower lung and associated with hilar lymph node enlargement.	Striking hilar adenopathy, which may cause bronchial compression, may develop without radiographic evidence of parenchymal disease. Although the findings simulate primary tuberculosis, pleural effusion rarely occurs with histoplasmosis.
Blastomycosis (Fig C 1-11)	Nonspecific patchy areas of air-space consolidation.	Cavitation and miliary nodules infrequently occur. Blastomycosis may appear as a solitary pulmonary mass that, when associated with unilateral lymph node enlargement, may mimic a bronchogenic carcinoma.

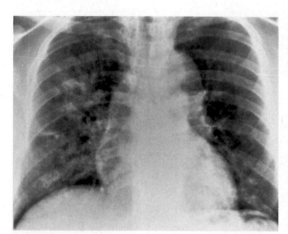

Fig C 1-9
***Bacteroides* pneumonia.** Patchy areas of consolidation primarily involve the middle and lower portions of the right lung.

A   B

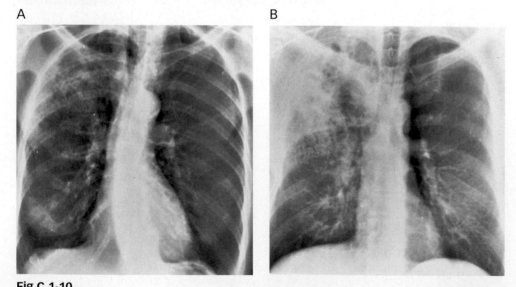

Fig C 1-10
Histoplasmosis. (A) Initial film demonstrates an ill-defined area of parenchymal consolidation in the right upper lobe. (B) One week later, there is a marked extension of the infiltrate, which now involves most of the upper half of the right lung.

Condition	Imaging Findings	Comments
Coccidioidomycosis (Fig C 1-12)	Pulmonary involvement usually begins as a fleeting area of patchy pneumonia that is often accompanied by ipsilateral hilar adenopathy and, less frequently, by pleural effusion.	Thin-walled cavities without surrounding reaction are suggestive of this organism (see Fig C 9-5).
Cryptococcosis (torulosis) (Fig C 1-13)	Segmental or lobar consolidation that most commonly occurs in the lower lobes.	More commonly produces a single, fairly well-circumscribed mass that is usually in the periphery of the lung and is often pleural based. Cavitation is relatively uncommon compared with its frequency in the other mycoses.
Actinomycosis/ nocardiosis (Figs C 1-14 and C 1-15)	Nonsegmental air-space consolidation (may resemble pneumonia or a tumor mass). Cavitation and empyema are common if not appropriately treated.	Extension of the infection into the pleura produces an empyema, which classically leads to osteomyelitis of the ribs and the formation of a sinus tract.

A

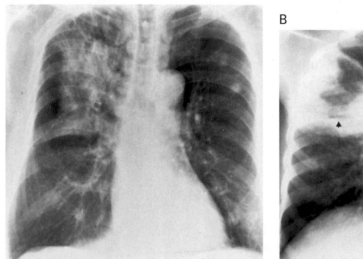

B

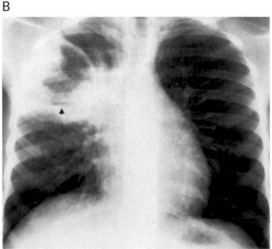

Fig C 1-11
Blastomycosis. (A) Patchy areas of air-space consolidation in the right upper lung associated with several nodules in the left upper lung. (B) In another patient, there is development of a right upper lobe cavity with thick walls and a faintly visible air-fluid level (arrow). There is an associated soft-tissue mass along the lateral wall of the cavity.[4]

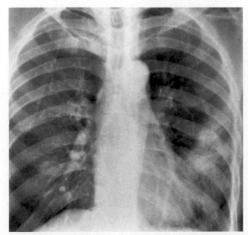

Fig C 1-12
Coccidioidomycosis pneumonia. Ill-defined area of patchy infiltrate in the left lower lung.

A

B

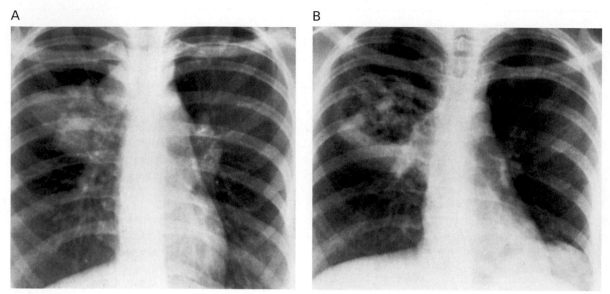

Fig C 1-13
Cryptococcosis. (A) Initial film demonstrates an air-space consolidation in the right upper lung. (B) With progression of the infection, the right upper lung pneumonia has cavitated, and a left lower lobe air-space consolidation has developed.

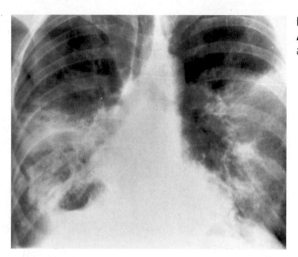

Fig C 1-14
Actinomycosis. Bilateral, nonsegmental air-space consolidation.

A

B

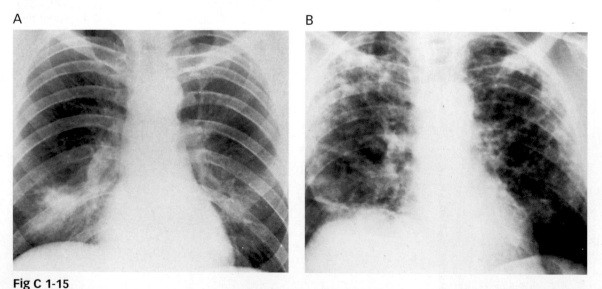

Fig C 1-15
Nocardiosis. (A) Initial chest radiograph demonstrates an area of nonspecific alveolar infiltrate in the right lower lobe. (B) Without appropriate therapy, infection spreads to involve both lungs diffusely with a patchy infiltrate and multiple small cavities.

Condition	Imaging Findings	Comments
Candidiasis	Patchy, segmental, homogeneous air-space consolidation.	Reflects hematogenous dissemination. Cavitation and hilar adenopathy may occur.
Aspergillosis (see Fig C 22-1)	Single or multiple areas of consolidation with poorly defined margins.	Almost always a secondary infection in which the fungus colonizes a damaged bronchial tree, pulmonary cyst, or cavity of a patient with underlying lung disease. The radiographic hallmark is a pulmonary mycetoma, a solid homogeneous rounded mass separated from the wall of the cavity by a crescent-shaped air space.
Mucormycosis (see Fig C 11-7)	Progressive severe pneumonia that is widespread and confluent and often cavitates.	Occurs in patients with diabetes or an underlying malignancy (leukemia, lymphoma). Usually originates in the nose and paranasal sinuses, where the infection may destroy the walls and create an appearance that simulates a malignant neoplasm.
Sporotrichosis (see Fig C 11-6)	Various nonspecific patterns (fibronodular infiltrates, cavitary nodular masses, chronic pneumonia). Hilar lymph node enlargement is common and may cause bronchial obstruction. Spread through the pleura into the chest wall may produce a sinus tract.	Chronic infection that is usually limited to the skin and the draining lymphatics. In rare instances, disseminated disease can involve the lungs and the skeletal system (extensive destructive arthritis with large-joint effusions).
Mycoplasma/viral infection (Figs C 1-16 and C 1-17)	Patchy air-space consolidation that is usually segmental and predominantly involves the lower lobes. Bilateral and multilobar involvement is common.	Initially, acute interstitial inflammation appears as a fine or coarse reticular pattern. Most infections are mild, though the radiographic signs are more extensive than might be expected from the physical examination.

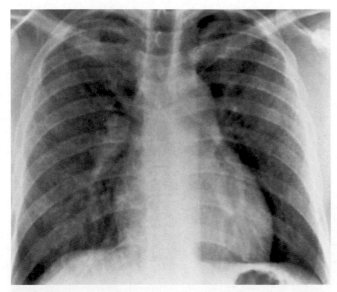

Fig C 1-16
***Mycoplasma* pneumonia.** Initial acute interstitial inflammation produces a diffuse fine reticular pattern.

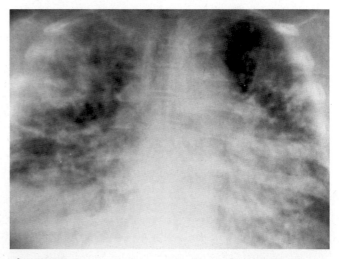

Fig C 1-17
Viral pneumonia. Diffuse peribronchial infiltrate with associated air-space consolidation obscures the heart border (shaggy heart sign). A patchy alveolar infiltrate is present in the right upper lung.

Condition	Imaging Findings	Comments
Mononucleosis	Nonspecific patchy air-space consolidation.	Generalized lymphadenopathy and splenomegaly are characteristic findings. Hilar lymph node enlargement, usually bilateral, can be demonstrated in approximately 15% of cases (see Fig C 11-1). Pneumonia is a rare complication.
Varicella	Extensive bilateral fluffy nodular infiltrate that tends to coalesce near the hilum and lung bases.	Healed varicella pneumonia classically appears as tiny miliary calcifications (see Fig C 17-5), scattered widely throughout both lungs, which develop several years after the acute infection.
Cytomegalovirus	In adults, rapid development of diffuse bilateral alveolar infiltrates that are most common in the outer third of the lungs.	Primarily involves patients with underlying reticuloendothelial disease or immunologic deficiencies, or those receiving immunosuppressive therapy (especially after renal transplantation). May be radiographically indistinguishable from *Pneumocystis carinii* pneumonia.
Rickettsial infection (Fig C 1-18)	Dense, homogeneous, segmental, or lobar consolidation simulating pneumococcal disease. Predominantly affects the lower lobes and may be bilateral.	Pneumonia develops in approximately half the patients with Q fever. Pleural effusion occurs in about one-third of the cases, whereas hilar involvement and small focal lesions are rare.
Parasitic pneumonia *Pneumocystis carinii* (Fig C 1-19; see Figs C 2-14 and C 4-19)	Initially, a hazy, perihilar granular infiltrate that spreads to the periphery and appears predominantly interstitial. In later stages, patchy areas of air-space consolidation with air bronchograms. Massive consolidation with virtually airless lungs may be a terminal appearance.	Common organism in immunosuppressed patients (especially those with AIDS and those treated for lymphoproliferative diseases or with renal transplants). Hilar adenopathy and significant pleural effusions are rare and should suggest an alternative diagnosis. Because the organism cannot be cultured and the disease it causes is usually fatal if untreated, an open-lung biopsy is often necessary if a sputum examination reveals no organisms in a patient suspected of having this disease.

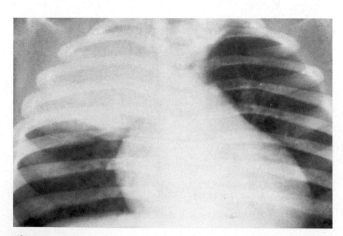

Fig C 1-18
Q fever. Right upper lobe air-space consolidation simulating pneumococcal pneumonia.

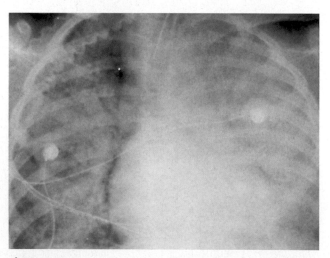

Fig C 1-19
***Pneumocystis carinii* pneumonia.** Severe, bilateral airspace consolidation with air bronchograms. The patient was undergoing immunosuppressive therapy for lymphoma and died shortly after this radiograph was made.

Condition	Imaging Findings	Comments
Amebiasis	Air-space consolidation in the right lower lobe that may be obscured by an extensive pleural effusion.	Usually arises from direct extension of hepatic infection through the right hemidiaphragm (occasionally may be of hematogenous origin).
Toxoplasmosis	Combined interstitial and alveolar disease, often with hilar lymph node enlargement.	Especially virulent organism in immunocompromised patients. Central nervous system involvement is common and may lead to a brain abscess.
Ascariasis (see Fig C 20-4)	Patchy or extensive areas of consolidation that are often bilateral.	Reflects an allergic response caused by larvae migrating through the lungs.
Cutaneous larva migrans (creeping eruption) (see Fig C 20-7)	Transient, migratory pulmonary infiltrates associated with lung and blood eosinophilia.	Pulmonary involvement develops in approximately half the patients about 1 week after the skin eruption caused by penetration and migration of the larvae of the dog and cat hookworm (*Ancylostoma braziliense*).
Strongyloidiasis (see Fig C 20-5)	Ill-defined patchy areas of air-space consolidation or fine miliary nodules.	Pulmonary manifestations occur during the stage of larval migration (in most patients, the chest radiograph remains normal).
Paragonimiasis (see Figs C 8-3 and C 11-9)	Patchy air-space consolidation that primarily involves the bases of the lungs. Characteristic finding is the "ring shadow," composed of a thin-walled cyst with a prominent crescent-shaped opacity along one side of its border.	Chronic infection of the lung caused by a trematode that is acquired by eating raw, or poorly cooked, infected crabs or crayfish. Although many patients with a heavy infestation are asymptomatic, others present with cough, pain, hemoptysis, and brownish sputum.
Tuberculosis Primary (Fig C 1-20)	In primary disease, a lobar or segmental air-space consolidation that is usually homogeneous, dense, and well defined. Associated enlargement of the hilar or mediastinal lymph nodes is very common (see Figs C 10-1 and C 10-2). Pleural effusion often occurs, especially in adults (see Fig C 33-1).	Primary tuberculosis may affect any lobe. The diagnosis cannot be excluded because the infection is not in the upper lobe. Although traditionally considered a disease of children and young adults, with the dramatic decrease in the prevalence of tuberculosis (especially in children and young adults), primary pulmonary disease can develop at any age.

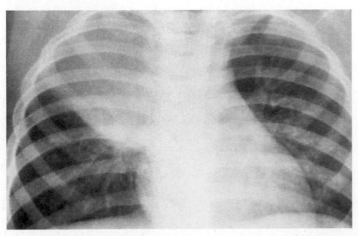

Fig C 1-20
Primary tuberculosis. Consolidation of the right upper lobe.

Condition	Imaging Findings	Comments
Secondary (reactivation)	Initially a nonspecific hazy, poorly marginated alveolar infiltrate that most commonly affects the upper lobes, especially the apical and posterior segments. Cavitation is common (see Fig C 9-3) and may result in bronchogenic spread characterized by multiple patchy infiltrates.	Bilateral (though often asymmetric) upper lobe disease is common and is almost diagnostic of reactivation tuberculosis. Because an apical lesion may be obscured by overlying clavicle or ribs, an apical lordotic view is often of value. Pleural effusion and lymph node enlargement are rare in secondary disease.
Atypical mycobacteria (see Fig C 11-4)	Often radiographically indistinguishable from primary tuberculosis, though pleural effusion and hilar adenopathy are much less common.	Often produces thin-walled cavities with minimal surrounding parenchymal disease. Patients with an atypical mycobacterial infection have a negative tuberculin test and do not respond to antituberculous therapy.
Postobstructive pneumonitis (Fig C 1-21)	Homogeneous increase in density corresponding exactly to a lobe or one or more segments, usually with a substantial loss of volume.	With slowly progressive, obstructive endobronchial processes such as bronchogenic carcinoma and bronchial adenoma, infection is frequent so that there may be only slight or moderate loss of volume. Pneumonitis, bronchiectasis, and abscesses that develop behind the obstruction are usually sufficient to counteract, at least partly, collapse induced by air absorption. The characteristic radiographic picture of "obstructive pneumonitis" should immediately suggest the presence of an obstructing endobronchial lesion. Nonneoplastic causes include mucoid impaction (hypersensitivity aspergillosis), aspirated foreign bodies, and the tracheobronchial form of amyloidosis.
Pulmonary infarct (Fig C 1-22)	Area of consolidation that most commonly involves the lower lobes and is often associated with pleural effusion and elevation of the ipsilateral hemidiaphragm. A highly characteristic, though uncommon, appearance is a pleural-based, wedge-shaped density that has a rounded apex (Hampton hump) and often occurs in the costophrenic sulcus. In many instances, an infarction produces a nonspecific parenchymal density that simulates an acute pneumonia.	Although it is often said that infarction invariably extends to a visceral pleural surface, this is of little diagnostic value, as most pneumonias have a similar appearance. The pattern of resolution of the consolidation is of value in distinguishing among acute inflammatory processes, pulmonary hemorrhage, edema, and frank necrosis. Pulmonary infarctions tend to shrink gradually while retaining the same general configuration seen on initial views (resorption of the perimeter of the infarct with preservation of the pleural base). In contrast, the resolution of pneumonia tends to be patchy and is characterized by a fading of the radiographic density throughout the entire involved area. Parenchymal hemorrhage and edema generally clear within 4 to 7 days; the resolution of necrotic lung tissue usually requires 3 weeks or more.

Condition	Imaging Findings	Comments
Pulmonary contusion Fig C 1-23 (see Figs C 6-14 and C 34-2)	Varies from irregular patchy areas of air-space consolidation to an extensive homogeneous density involving almost an entire lung.	Most common pulmonary complication of blunt chest trauma in which there is exudation of edema and blood into both the air spaces and the interstitium of the lung. In the absence of an appropriate clinical history of trauma or evidence of rib fractures, pulmonary contusion may be indistinguishable from pneumonia. Resolution typically occurs rapidly, with complete clearing within 2 weeks.

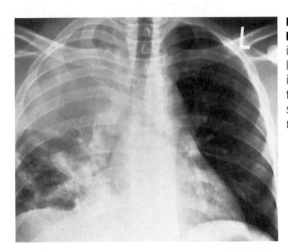

Fig C 1-21
Postobstructive pneumonitis. Homogeneous increased density involving the right upper lobe secondary to carcinoma of the lung. Patchy increased opacification at the right base is due to a combination of atelectasis and infiltrate secondary to extension of the tumor into neighboring bronchi.

A   B

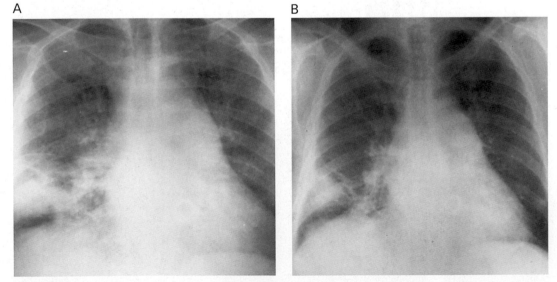

Fig C 1-22
Pulmonary infarction. (A) Chest film made 3 days after open-heart surgery demonstrates a very irregular opacity at the right base (pneumonia versus pulmonary embolization with infarction). (B) On a film made 5 days later, the consolidation is seen to have reduced in size yet to have retained the same general configuration as on the initial view. The diagnosis of pulmonary embolism was confirmed by a radionuclide lung scan.[5]

Condition	Imaging Findings	Comments
Lipoid pneumonia (Fig C 1-24)	Granular pattern of small, scattered alveolar densities that predominantly occur in the perihilar and lower lobe areas.	Caused by the aspiration of various vegetable, animal, or mineral oils into the lungs. As the oil is taken from the alveolar spaces by macrophages that pass into the interstitial space, a fine reticular pattern is produced. Infrequently appears as a granulomatous-lipoid mass that may be huge and may simulate bronchogenic carcinoma (see Fig C 6-15).
Lung torsion	Opacification of the affected lung develops if the torsion is not relieved and the vascular supply is compromised.	Rare complication of trauma that occurs almost invariably in children, presumably because of the easy compressibility of their thoracic cage. Torsion occurs through 180°, that the base of the lung comes to lie at the apex of the hemithorax and the apex at the base. The pulmonary opacification is due to exudation of blood into the air spaces and interstitial tissues.

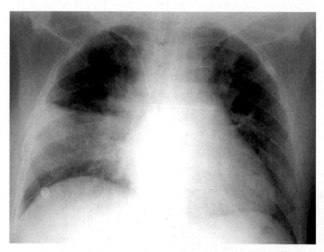

Fig C 1-23
Pulmonary hemorrhage. Consolidation of the middle lobe in a patient with AIDS-related Kaposi's sarcoma.[6]

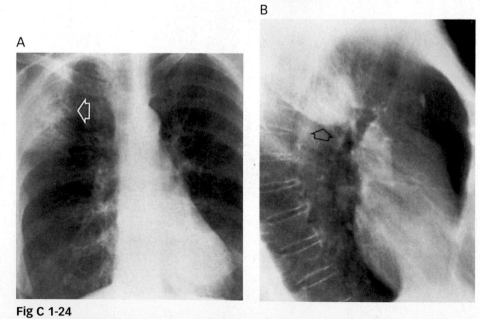

A

B

Fig C 1-24
Lipoid pneumonia. (A) Frontal and (B) lateral views demonstrate an air-space consolidation in the posterior segment of the right upper lobe (arrows). Note the prominence of interstitial reticular markings leading from the right hilum to the infiltrate.

Condition	Imaging Findings	Comments
Localized pulmonary edema (Fig C 1-25)	Nonsymmetric, atypical alveolar consolidation.	Most commonly occurs in patients with preexisting lung disease such as chronic emphysema. Unilateral pulmonary edema is most frequently related to dependency.
Bronchioloalveolar (alveolar cell) carcinoma (Fig C 1-26)	In the less common diffuse form, a pattern varying from poorly defined nodules scattered throughout both lungs to irregular pulmonary infiltrates, often with air bronchograms.	More frequently appears as a well-circumscribed, peripheral solitary nodule that often contains an air bronchogram (see Fig C 6-13) (never associated with solitary nodule caused by bronchogenic carcinoma or a granuloma). Although the margins of the tumor are usually well circumscribed, the mass may be poorly defined and simulate an area of focal pneumonia.

A
B

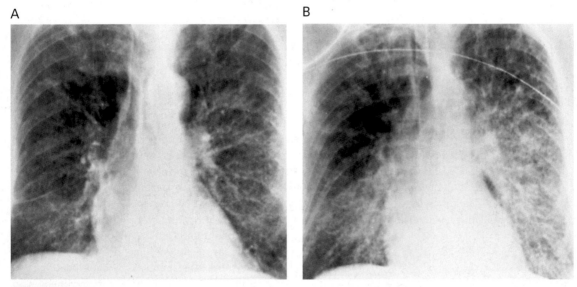

Fig C 1-25
Pulmonary edema in pulmonary emphysema. (A) Initial chest radiograph demonstrates a paucity of vascular markings in the right middle and upper zones along with increased interstitial markings elsewhere. (B) With the onset of congestive heart failure, there is patchy interstitial and alveolar edema that does not affect the segments in which the vascularity had been severely diminished.

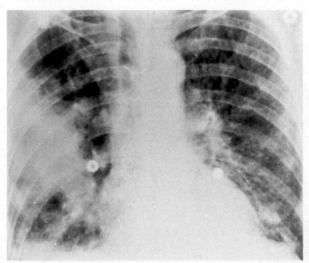

Fig C 1-26
Alveolar cell carcinoma. Patchy, ill-defined right-sided mass simulates an area of focal pneumonia.

Condition	Imaging Findings	Comments
Lymphoma	Patchy areas of parenchymal infiltrate that may coalesce to form a large homogeneous nonsegmental mass. Cavitation and pleural effusion may occur.	Pleuropulmonary involvement usually occurs by direct extension from mediastinal nodes along the lymphatics of the bronchovascular sheaths. At times, it may be difficult to distinguish a superimposed infection after radiation therapy or chemotherapy from the continued spread of lymphomatous tissue. However, any alveolar lung infiltrate in a patient with known lymphoma is more likely to represent an infectious than a lymphomatous process. Primary pulmonary lymphoma is rare and presents as a homogeneous mass that rarely obstructs the bronchial tree and thus almost invariably contains an air bronchogram. When most or all of a segment or lobe is involved, the appearance may simulate acute pneumonia.
Pseudolymphoma	Segmental consolidation extending outward from a hilum and containing an air bronchogram.	Rare benign condition that histologically closely resembles malignant lymphoma. Although apparently segmental, in most cases the consolidation stops short of the visceral pleura at the periphery of the lung.
Löffler's syndrome (idiopathic eosinophilic pneumonia) (see Fig C 18-1)	Transient, rapidly changing, nonsegmental areas of parenchymal consolidation associated with blood eosinophilia. The infiltrates are often located in the periphery of the lung, running more or less parallel to the lateral chest wall and simulating a pleural process.	A similar appearance can develop secondary to parasites (filariasis, ascariasis, cutaneous larva migrans), drug therapy (nitrofurantoin), and fungal infections (hypersensitivity bronchopulmonary aspergillosis). When caused by an identifiable extrinsic agent, the disease usually is acute and responds promptly to the removal of the offending organism or drug. When no obvious cause is detectable, the pulmonary consolidation and eosinophilia tend to be more prolonged and persistent, though there is usually a dramatic response to steroids.
Radiation pneumonitis (Fig C 1-27)	Patchy areas of irregular consolidation that are localized to the radiation port and are often associated with a considerable loss of volume.	Acute radiation pneumonitis is rarely detectable less than 1 month after the end of treatment and must be differentiated from bacterial pneumonia. The late or chronic stage of radiation damage is characterized by extensive fibrosis and loss of volume that may be difficult to distinguish from the lymphangitic spread of a malignant tumor.
Sarcoidosis (see Fig C 2-17)	Ill-defined densities that may be discrete or may coalesce into large areas of segmental consolidation. This pattern resembles an acute inflammatory process and may contain an air bronchogram.	Infrequent manifestation. More characteristic radiographic changes are a diffuse reticulonodular pattern and typical bilateral enlargement of hilar and paratracheal lymph nodes (see Figs C 11-6 and C 12-8).

Condition	Imaging Findings	Comments
Progressive massive fibrosis (pneumoconiosis) (see Figs C 8-9 and C 8-10)	Nonsegmental conglomerate masses that are usually bilateral and relatively symmetric and almost always restricted to the upper half of the lungs. They commonly develop in the mid-zone or periphery of the lung and tend to migrate later toward the hilum, leaving overinflated and emphysematous lung tissue between the consolidation and the pleural surface.	Caused by the confluence of numerous individual nodules in patients with advanced silicosis or coal-miner's pneumoconiosis. The conglomerate fibrotic lesions may cavitate as a result of central ischemic necrosis or tuberculous caseation.
Asbestosis/talcosis	In patients with extensive interstitial fibrosis, large conglomerate opacities may develop that are well or ill defined, are often multiple and nonsegmental, and predominantly involve the lower lung (in contrast to the upper lobe predominance of the conglomerate opacities in silicosis).	Pleural plaque formation, which may be massive and bizarre in shape, is characteristic of both conditions (see Figs C 32-4 and C 32-5). In asbestosis, there is often thin, curvilinear calcification of the diaphragmatic pleura, obscuration of the heart border (shaggy heart sign), and a high incidence of associated malignancy (bronchogenic carcinoma, mesothelioma).
Systemic lupus erythematosus	Nonspecific patchy infiltrate that is more commonly situated peripherally in the lung bases.	Often associated with bilateral pleural effusions and cardiac enlargement due to pericardial effusion (see Fig C 33-4).

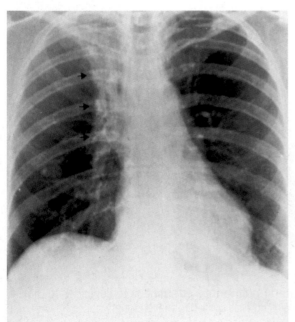

Fig C 1-27
Radiation pneumonitis. After postmastectomy radiation, a mass of fibrous tissue (arrows) extends from the right hilum to parallel the right border of the mediastinum.

Pulmonary Edema Pattern (Symmetric Bilateral Alveolar Pattern)

Condition	Comments
Cardiovascular disease causing pulmonary venous hypertension (Figs C 2-1 and C 2-2)	Most common cause of the pulmonary edema pattern. Usually associated with cardiomegaly (especially if the result of left ventricular failure); other cardiogenic causes include mitral valvular disease, left atrial myxoma, and the hypoplastic left heart syndromes. Noncardiogenic causes include disorders of the pulmonary veins (primary or secondary to mediastinal fibrosis or tumor), veno-occlusive disease, and anomalous pulmonary venous return. Unilateral pulmonary edema is probably most frequently related to dependency (Fig C 2-2). A patchy, asymmetric pattern may develop in patients with emphysema.
Renal failure/uremia (Fig C 2-3)	Causes include acute glomerulonephritis and chronic renal disease. Complex mechanism (left ventricular failure, decreased oncotic pressure, hypervolemia, increased capillary permeability). May produce a dense "butterfly" pattern.

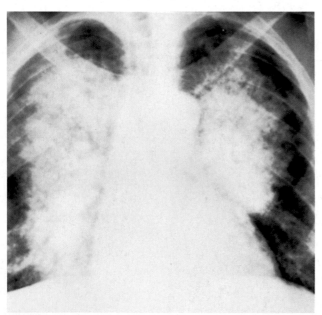

Fig C 2-1
Congestive heart failure. Diffuse bilateral symmetric infiltration of the central portion of the lungs along with relative sparing of the periphery produces the butterfly, or bat's wing, pattern. The margins of the edematous lung are sharply defined. The consolidation is fairly homogeneous and is associated with a well-defined air bronchogram on both sides.[7]

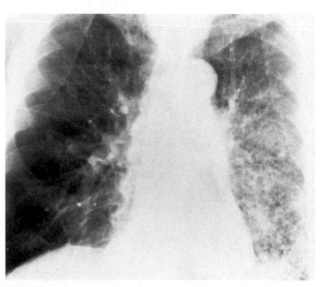

Fig C 2-2
Unilateral pulmonary edema due to dependency. Diffuse alveolar pattern is limited to the left lung.

Condition	Comments
Fluid overload/ overtransfusion (hypervolemia, hypoproteinemia) (Fig C 2-4)	A common cause of the pattern, particularly during the postoperative period and in elderly patients. Rapid clearing with appropriate treatment. The pulmonary edema pattern may also be the result of an incompatible blood transfusion.
Neurogenic/postictal (Fig C 2-5)	An often asymmetric pattern of pulmonary edema may develop after head trauma, seizures, or stroke. Related to increased intracranial pressure (typically disappears within several days after surgical relief). Normal heart size (if no underlying cardiac disease).

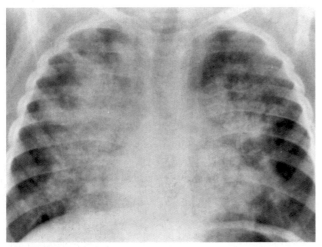

Fig C 2-3
Chronic renal failure. Typical perihilar alveolar densities producing the butterfly pattern of uremic lung. Unlike pulmonary edema due to congestive heart failure, in chronic renal failure the cardiac silhouette is of normal size.

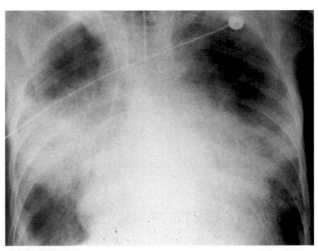

Fig C 2-4
Fluid overload. Pulmonary edema pattern developing in the postoperative period in an elderly patient. Note the endotracheal tube and pulmonary artery catheter.

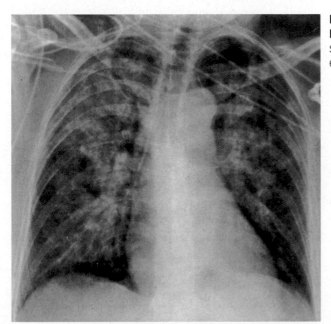

Fig C 2-5
Neurogenic pulmonary edema. Diffuse bilateral air-space consolidations with a heart of normal size and no evidence of pleural effusions or Kerley lines.[109]

Condition	Comments
Inhalation of noxious gases (Fig C 2-6)	Transient pulmonary edema pattern that develops within a few hours of exposure and clears within a few days (if not fatal). Causes include the inhalation of nitrogen dioxide (silo-filler's disease), sulfur dioxide, phosgene, chlorine, carbon monoxide, and hydrocarbon compounds.
Aspiration of gastric contents (Mendelson's syndrome)	Often an asymmetric pattern of pulmonary edema (depends on the position of the patient when aspiration occurred). Caused by vomiting related to anesthesia, seizure, or coma (alcohol or barbiturate poisoning, cerebrovascular accident). Grave prognosis unless immediate steroid and antibiotic therapy (then resolves in 7 to 10 days).
Near-drowning (Fig C 2-7)	No radiographic difference between fresh and saltwater aspiration. Complete resolution, usually in 7 to 10 days.
Aspiration of hypertonic contrast material	High osmotic force causes massive influx of fluid into the alveolar air spaces.
High altitude	Pulmonary edema pattern (often irregular and patchy) is a manifestation of mountain or altitude sickness. Rapid clearing after oxygen administration or return to sea level.
Transient tachypnea of newborn	Loss of definition of prominent vascular markings due to retained fetal lung fluid that clears rapidly in 1 to 4 days. Normal heart size. Predisposing factors include cesarean section, prematurity, breech delivery, and maternal diabetes.
Rapid re-expansion of lungs (post-thoracentesis)	Unilateral pulmonary edema pattern (unless both lungs re-expanded) that follows the rapid removal of large amounts of air or fluid from the pleural space.
Fat embolism (Fig C 2-8)	Develops 1 to 2 days after trauma (usually leg fractures). The radiographic resolution requires 7 days or longer. Absence of cardiomegaly, pulmonary venous hypertension, and interstitial edema differentiates this condition from cardiogenic edema.

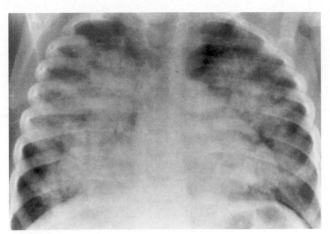

Fig C 2-6
Hydrocarbon poisoning. Diffuse pulmonary edema pattern, with the alveolar consolidation most prominent in the central portions of the lung.

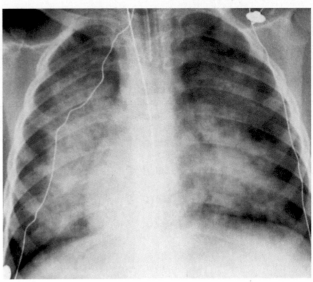

Fig C 2-7
Near-drowning. Diffuse pulmonary edema pattern.

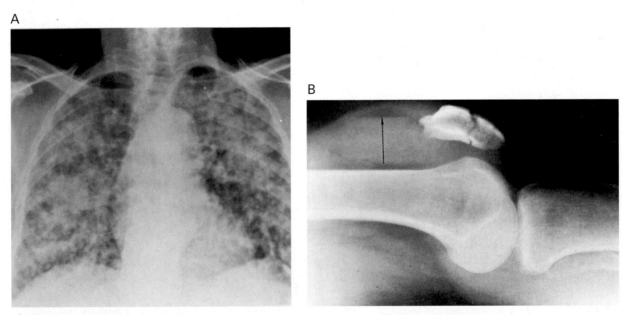

Fig C 2-8
Fat embolism. (A) Frontal chest radiograph made 3 days after a leg fracture demonstrates diffuse bilateral air-space consolidation due to alveolar hemorrhage and edema. Unlike cardiogenic pulmonary edema, the distribution in this patient is predominantly peripheral rather than central, and the heart is not enlarged. (B) Recumbent radiograph of the knee obtained with a horizontal beam demonstrates the characteristic fat-blood interface (arrow) in a large suprapatellar effusion. Marrow fat that enters torn peripheral vessels can be trapped by the pulmonary circulation and lead to diffuse alveolar consolidation.[8]

Condition	Comments
Amniotic fluid embolism (Fig C 2-9)	Diffuse air-space consolidation that is virtually indistinguishable from the appearance caused by other forms of acute pulmonary edema. The entrance of amniotic fluid containing particulate matter into the maternal circulation during spontaneous delivery or cesarean section can cause sudden and massive obstruction of the pulmonary vascular bed, leading to shock and often death. Because the condition is often rapidly fatal, radiographs are infrequently obtained; most of the rare nonfatal cases are incorrectly diagnosed.
Thoracic trauma (contused lung) (Fig C 2-10)	Alveolar edema pattern due to contusion or hemorrhage is the most common pulmonary complication of blunt chest trauma. The appearance is seldom symmetric (involvement is greater on the side of maximum impact). Unlike traumatic fat embolism, the radiographic changes of pulmonary contusion and hemorrhage are apparent soon after trauma and resolve rapidly (usually in 1 to 7 days).
Nontraumatic pulmonary hemorrhage (Figs C 2-11 and C 2-12)	Bilateral alveolar consolidation that may occur in patients with bleeding diatheses, idiopathic pulmonary hemosiderosis, Goodpasture's syndrome, polyarteritis nodosa, or Wegener's granulomatosis. There is usually clearing 2 to 3 days after a single bleeding episode, though reticular changes may persist much longer.

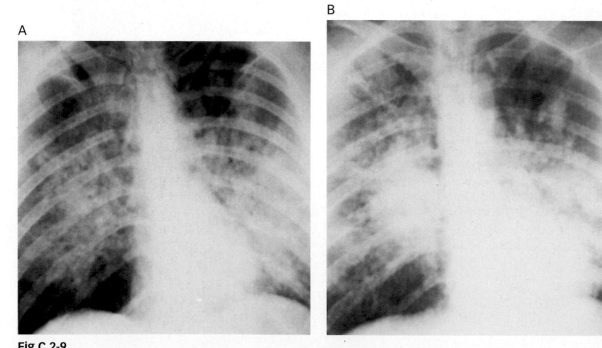

B

A

Fig C 2-9
Amniotic fluid embolism. (A) Initial film 6 hours after the onset of acute symptoms, showing heavy bilateral perihilar infiltrate. (B) Twelve hours later, the infiltrates have become more confluent in the perihilar zones.[9]

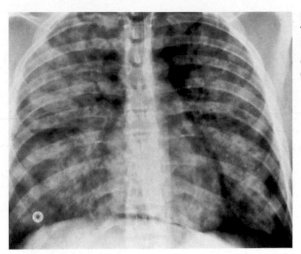

Fig C 2-10
Thoracic trauma. Continuous positive-pressure ventilation has caused diffuse interstitial emphysema, pneumothorax, and pneumoperitoneum to be superimposed on a pattern of diffuse alveolar opacities.

A

B

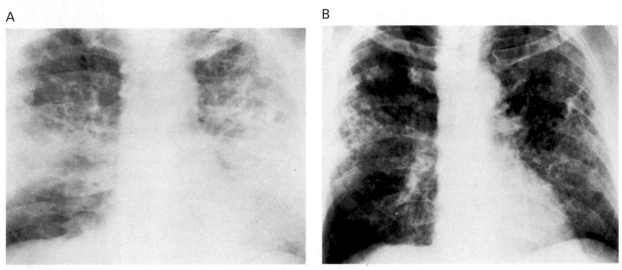

Fig C 2-11
Pulmonary hemorrhage. (A) Diffuse bilateral air-space consolidation developed in a patient receiving high-dose anticoagulant therapy. (B) With resolution of the hemorrhage, a reticular pattern is seen in the same distribution as the alveolar infiltrate.

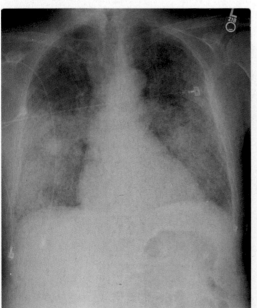

Fig C 2-12
Goodpasture's syndrome. Frontal chest film in a patient with massive pulmonary hemorrhage demonstrates extensive bilateral pulmonary consolidation, which is confluent in most areas. Note the normal heart size.

Condition	Comments
Acute radiation pneumonitis	Alveolar edema pattern is generally confined to the irradiated area. Rarely develops while the patient is receiving radiation therapy (radiographic changes are seldom apparent until at least 1 month after the end of treatment).
Narcotic abuse (Fig C 2-13)	Alveolar pulmonary edema pattern that may be unilateral due to gravitational influences. Most commonly a complication of heroin or methadone abuse. The radiographic findings may be delayed 6 to 10 hours after admission, and there is usually rapid resolution (1 to 2 days). The persistence of an edema pattern after 48 hours suggests aspiration or superimposed bacterial pneumonia.
Cocaine abuse (Fig C 2-14)	Both cardiogenic and noncardiogenic pulmonary edema have been reported in association with intravenous cocaine abuse and crack cocaine smoking and are common findings at autopsies of drug addicts. The pathogenesis of cocaine-induced pulmonary edema is complex and multifactorial. Myocardial ischemia and infarction, myocardial dysfunction, arrhythmia, and dilated cardiomyopathy may be contributing factors in cardiogenic edema. Damage to the pulmonary capillary endothelium with increased permeability may play a role in noncardiogenic edema.
Adult respiratory distress syndrome (ARDS) or "shock lung" (Fig C 2-15)	Bilateral pulmonary edema pattern that is typically delayed up to 12 hours after the clinical onset of respiratory failure. Severe, unexpected, life-threatening acute respiratory distress developing in a patient with no major underlying lung disease. Causes include sepsis, oxygen toxicity, disseminated intravascular coagulation, and cardiopulmonary bypass.

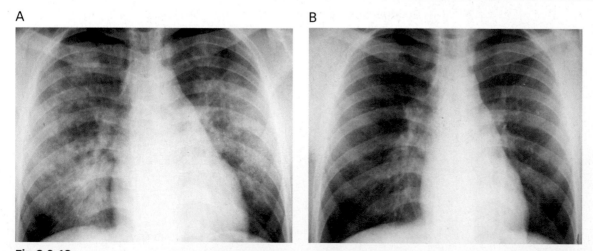

A

B

Fig C 2-13
Heroin abuse. (A) Initial radiograph obtained shortly after presentation to the emergency department reveals bilateral areas of increased opacity, a finding consistent with acute lung injury. (B) Follow-up study obtained two days later shows complete clearing of the areas of increased opacity. Such rapid clearing is common in heroin-induced lung injury.[10]

Condition	Comments
Pneumonia (Figs C 2-16 and C 2-17)	Bilateral alveolar infiltrates may develop after a broad spectrum of infections. The underlying organisms include bacteria, fungi, mycoplasma, viruses, malaria, and even worm infestation (almost invariably blood eosinophilia). In patients with AIDS, a butterfly pattern sparing the periphery of the lung is highly suggestive of *Pneumocystis carinii* pneumonia.

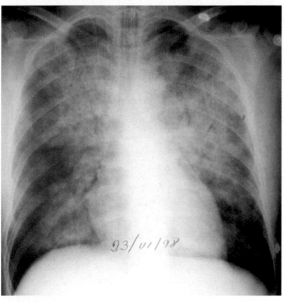

Fig C 2-14
Cocaine abuse. Extensive bilateral heterogeneous central and parahilar opacities representing cardiogenic pulmonary edema in a woman who presented with shortness of breath and chest pain after smoking crack cocaine.[11]

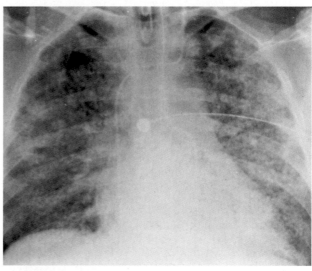

Fig C 2-15
Adult respiratory distress syndrome. Ill-defined areas of alveolar consolidation with some coalescence scattered throughout both lungs.

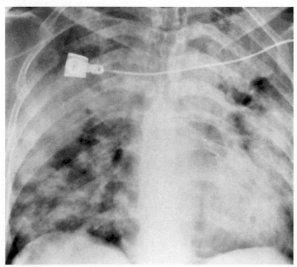

Fig C 2-16
Plague pneumonia. Diffuse air-space consolidation involves both lungs.

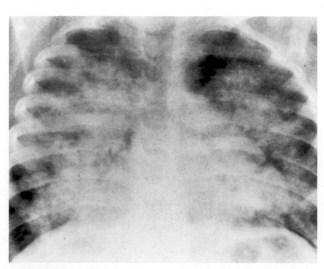

Fig C 2-17
***Pneumocystis carinii* pneumonia in acquired immuno-deficiency syndrome.** Diffuse bilateral pulmonary infiltrates.

Condition	Comments
Neoplasm	Symmetric bilateral alveolar infiltrates, usually associated with reticulonodular and linear densities, may develop in patients with alveolar cell carcinoma or lymphangitic metastases. Patients with lymphoma and leukemia may also develop bilateral alveolar infiltrates that predominantly involve the perihilar areas and lower lungs, though these findings are more often due to superimposed pneumonia, drug reaction, or hemorrhage than to the underlying malignancy itself.
Alveolar microlithiasis (Fig C 2-18)	Rare disease of unknown etiology characterized by the presence of a myriad of very fine micronodules of calcific density in the alveoli of the lungs of a usually asymptomatic person. Characteristic "black pleura" sign (due to contrast between the extreme density of the lung parenchyma on one side of the pleura and the ribs on the other side).
Alveolar proteinosis (Fig C 2-19)	Rare condition of unknown etiology characterized by the deposition in the air spaces of the lung of a somewhat granular material high in protein and lipid content. The bilateral and symmetric alveolar infiltrates are identical in distribution and character to those of pulmonary edema, though there is no evidence of cardiac enlargement or pulmonary venous hypertension. There is usually complete radiographic resolution, though it may occur asymmetrically and in a spotty fashion and may even be associated with the development of new foci of air-space consolidation in areas not previously affected.
Sarcoidosis (Fig C 2-20)	Infrequent manifestation (more commonly a diffuse reticulonodular pattern). Hilar and mediastinal lymph nodes are often enlarged.
Drug hypersensitivity/ allergy (penicillin)	Rapid development of an alveolar edema pattern.
Pulmonary embolism with infarction	Bilateral alveolar consolidation, primarily involving the lower zones, is a rare manifestation of extensive thromboembolism with infarction. Associated findings include enlarged central pulmonary arteries with rapid tapering, loss of lung volume (elevated hemidiaphragms), small pleural effusions, and a prominent azygos vein. The radiographic appearance is usually rather benign, considering the severity of the clinical symptoms.

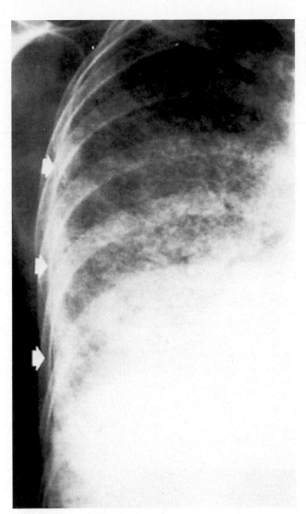

Fig C 2-18
Alveolar microlithiasis. Nearly uniform distribution of typical fine, sand-like mottling in the lungs. The tangential shadow of the pleura is displayed along the lateral wall of the chest as a dark lucent strip (arrows).[12]

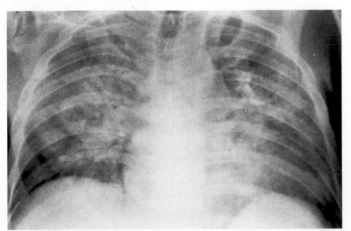

Fig C 2-19
Pulmonary alveolar proteinosis. Diffuse, bilateral air-space consolidation predominantly involves the central portions of the lung and simulates pulmonary edema. The patient was asymptomatic, and serial radiographs over several months showed little change.

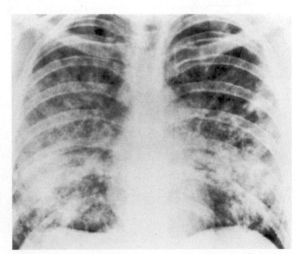

Fig C 2-20
Sarcoidosis. Diffuse reticular nodular and alveolar infiltrates.

Unilateral Pulmonary Edema Pattern

Condition	Comments
Ipsilateral pulmonary edema 　Rapid thoracentesis of 　large pleural effusion/ 　rapid evacuation of a 　pneumothorax 　(Fig C 3-1)	Typically occurs during the procedure or within 1 hour after it. Rapid re-expansion of the collapsed lung with a sudden increase in hydrostatic pressure and persistent high surface tension results in edema.
Prolonged lateral 　decubitus position 　(Fig C 3-2)	Gravity raises the hydrostatic pressure in the dependent lung, impairing circulation and affecting the production of surfactant. This mechanism may occur in some patients with methadone-induced edema who are found unconscious and lying on one side.
Pulmonary contusion 　(Fig C 3-3)	Direct damage to the pulmonary capillaries may cause not only intrapulmonary bleeding but also exudation of cells leading to edema. Blood products in the alveoli may also disrupt the surfactant system.

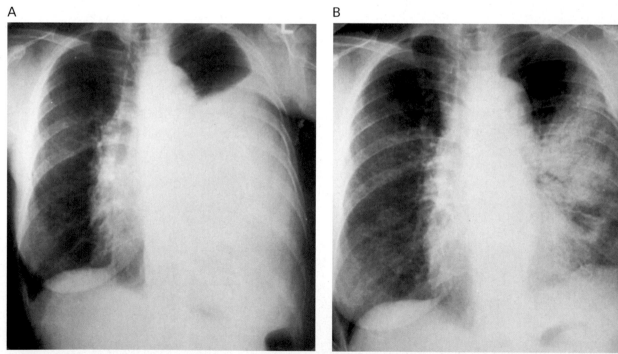

A　　　　　　　　　　　　　　　　B

Fig C 3-1
Rapid thoracentesis. (A) Initial radiograph of an elderly woman with metastatic adenocarcinoma of the breast and a massive left pleural effusion. (B) Repeat examination taken 2 hours after the rapid removal of 2500 mL of fluid shows a left-sided pulmonary edema. The segment of left lung not compressed by effusion remains free of edema. Over the next 6 days, the edema resolved spontaneously.[13]

Condition	Comments
Postoperative systemic-to-pulmonary artery shunts (congenital heart disease)	Dramatic and almost immediate reaction resulting from increased blood flow to the side with the anastomosis. The Waterston and Blalock-Taussig procedures produce right-sided edema; the Potts procedure results in left-sided edema. In either case, increased blood flow causes high hydrostatic pressure. This results in increased venous pressure combined with pulmonary capillary damage and decreased surfactant, producing high surface tension.

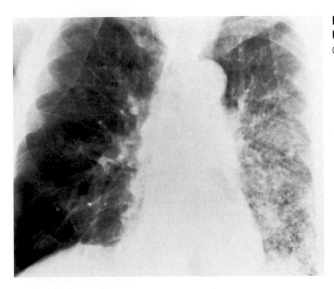

Fig C 3-2
Unilateral pulmonary edema due to dependency. The diffuse alveolar pattern is limited to the left lung.

A

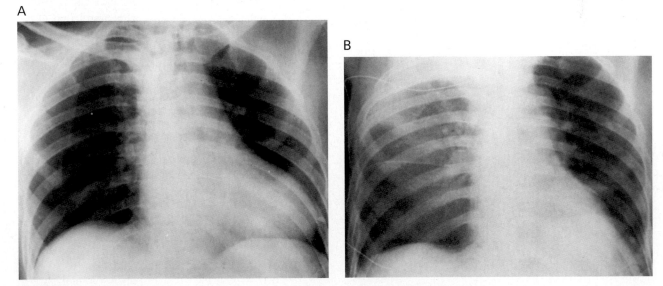

B

Fig C 3-3
Pulmonary contusion. (A) Admission chest radiograph shows several right rib fractures and an early right perihilar infiltrate. (B) Repeat examination shows right-sided post-traumatic pulmonary edema and capillary hemorrhage that developed the next day and persisted for a few weeks. An organized extrapleural hematoma is present in the right apex.[13]

Condition	Comments
Bronchial obstruction ("drowned lung")	Pulmonary edema in airless lung tissue peripheral to a totally obstructed bronchus is related to increased surface tension resulting from disruption of the alveolar lining layer caused by hypoxia due to loss of blood flow. This phenomenon usually clears within 1–24 hours after removal of the obstruction. Infection plays no role in this process.
Unilateral veno-occlusive disease	Congenital obstruction of pulmonary venous return or venous occlusion by primary or metastatic tumor causes edema, when the venous pressure rises higher than the colloid osmotic pressure of the blood.
Unilateral aspiration	Edema secondary to direct irritation of the alveolar lining layer with increased capillary permeability and an adverse effect on the surfactant system may develop unilaterally in patients after aspiration of freshwater or seawater, ethyl alcohol, kerosene, or gastric juices during anesthesia, a coma, or an epileptic seizure.
Central venous pressure catheter misdirected into a pulmonary artery	Rapid infusion of hypotonic saline stimulates neural reflexes and possibly a release of vasoactive substances resulting from a local decrease in colloid osmotic pressure.
Contralateral pulmonary edema Perfusion defects (Fig C 3-4)	Because an unperfused area cannot become edematous, contralateral pulmonary edema (ie, edema affecting only the normally perfused lung) can occur in such conditions as unilateral pulmonary emphysema with destruction of the capillary bed in the affected lung; congenital absence or hypoplasia of a pulmonary artery; Swyer-James syndrome; pulmonary thromboembolism involving an entire lung; and after lobectomy, in which the remaining lung becomes emphysematous on a compensatory basis and thus is underperfused.
Re-expansion of pneumothorax in a patient with left heart failure	Temporary compromise of perfusion of the previously collapsed lung due to increased pulmonary vascular resistance permits edema to occur only in the opposite lung.

A

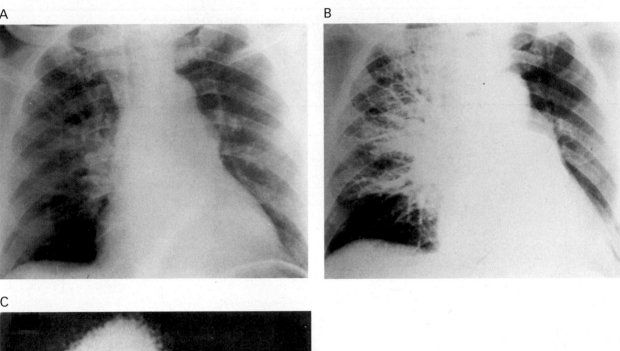

B

C

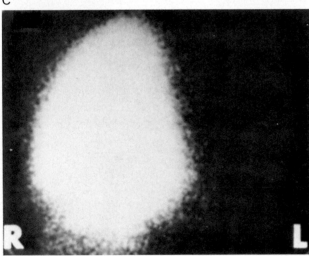

Fig C 3-4
Edema contralateral to pulmonary embolization. (A)
Chest radiograph in an acutely dyspneic older man shows
moderate cardiomegaly and early right-sided edema that
spares the base. (B) An angiogram obtained at the bedside
shows nonopacification of all left pulmonary branches and a
few segmental right lower lobe branches. (C) Radionuclide
scan shows complete lack of perfusion in the left lung and
poor perfusion of the right lower lobe.[13]

Diffuse Reticular or Reticulonodular Pattern

Condition	Comments
Lymphangitic metastases (Fig C 4-1)	More prominent in the lower lung zones and often associated with pleural effusion and enlargement of hilar or mediastinal lymph nodes. Most frequent primary tumor sites are the breast, stomach, thyroid, pancreas, larynx, cervix, and lung.
Lymphoma (Fig C 4-2)	Usually associated with hilar and mediastinal lymph node enlargement in Hodgkin's disease (often absent in non-Hodgkin's lymphoma). A similar pattern may occur in the terminal stages of leukemia.

A
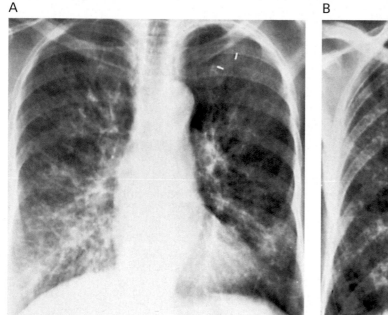

B
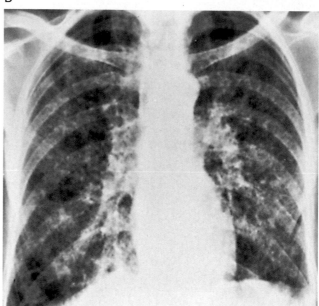

Fig C 4-1
Lymphangitic metastases. (A) Coarsened bronchovascular markings of irregular contour and poor definition primarily involve the right lower lung. Note the septal (Kerley) lines and the left mastectomy in this patient with carcinoma of the breast. (B) In this patient with metastatic carcinoma of the stomach, a superimposed nodular component representing hematogenous deposits produces a coarse reticulonodular pattern.

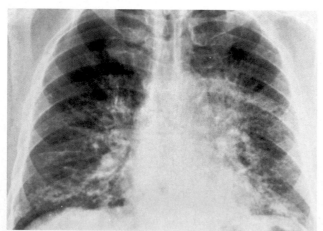

Fig C 4-2
Lymphoma. Diffuse reticular and reticulonodular changes, with striking prominence of the left hilar region.

Condition	Comments
Inorganic dust inhalation (pneumoconiosis)	
Silicosis (Fig C 4-3)	Often more prominent in the middle and upper lung zones. Frequent enlargement of hilar lymph nodes ("eggshell" calcification is infrequent but almost pathognomonic). Other radiographic patterns include well-circumscribed nodular opacities and progressive massive fibrosis. In Caplan's syndrome, silicosis is associated with rheumatoid arthritis and rheumatoid necrobiotic nodules (see Fig C 7-7).
Asbestosis (Fig C 4-4)	In the early stages, more prominent in the lower lung zones. The major radiographic abnormalities are pleural thickening, plaque formation, and calcification. A combination of parenchymal and pleural changes may partially obscure the heart border (shaggy heart sign). High incidence of mesothelioma (also bronchogenic and alveolar cell carcinoma).
Other inorganic dusts (Figs C 4-5 to C 4-7)	Numerous conditions such as talcosis, berylliosis, coal-workers' pneumoconiosis, aluminum (bauxite) pneumoconiosis, and radiopaque dust causing dense nodules (siderosis [iron], stannosis [tin], baritosis [barium], antimony, and rare-earth compounds). Also occurs from talc (magnesium silicate) in intravenous drug abusers.

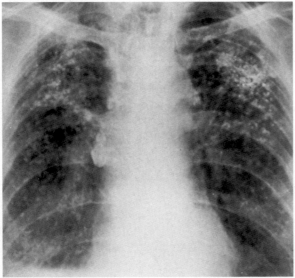

Fig C 4-3
Silicosis. Prominence of interstitial markings, upward retraction of the hila, and bilateral calcific densities that tend to conglomerate in the upper lobes.

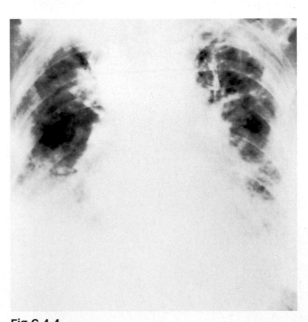

Fig C 4-4
Asbestosis. Severe disorganization of lung architecture with generalized coarse reticulation, which has become confluent in the right base and obliterates the right hemidiaphragm. There is marked pleural thickening, particularly in the apical and axillary regions. A spontaneous pneumothorax is on the left.[7]

Condition	Comments
Organic dust inhalation (Figs C 4-8 and C 4-9)	Late stage in such conditions as farmer's lung, bird-breeder's lung, silo-filler's disease (nitrogen dioxide), bagassosis (sugar cane), byssinosis (cotton), and mushroom-worker's lung.
Oxygen toxicity (Fig C 4-10)	Most commonly develops in infants undergoing long-term oxygen therapy for respiratory distress (has also been described in adults). Fibrosis, atelectasis, and focal areas of emphysema produce a "spongy" lung.

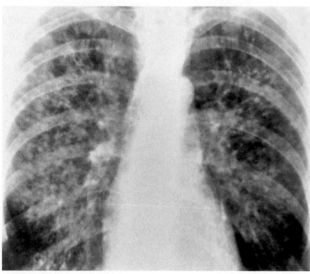

Fig C 4-5
Berylliosis. Diffuse reticulonodular pattern throughout both lungs, with relative sparing of the apices and bases.

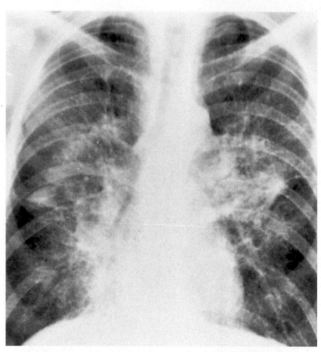

Fig C 4-6
Coal-workers' pneumoconiosis. Ill-defined masses of fibrous tissue in the perihilar region extend to the right base.

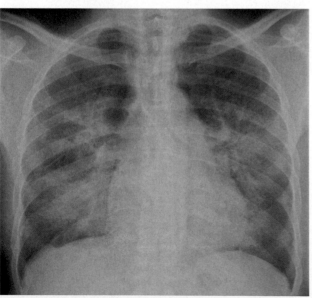

Fig C 4-7
Talc granulomatosis. File nodular opacities and areas of coalescence in an intravenous drug abuser.[11]

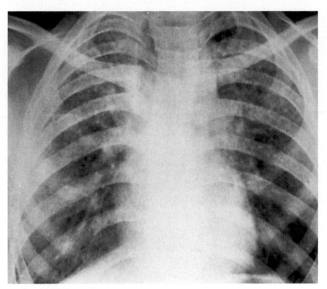

Fig C 4-8
Pigeon-breeder's lung. Diffuse reticulonodular infiltrate primarily involves the perihilar and upper lobe regions.

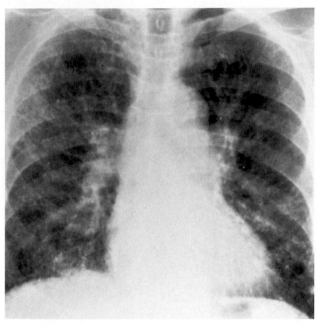

Fig C 4-9
Byssinosis. Prolonged exposure has resulted in irreversible pulmonary insufficiency and a diffuse reticular pattern.

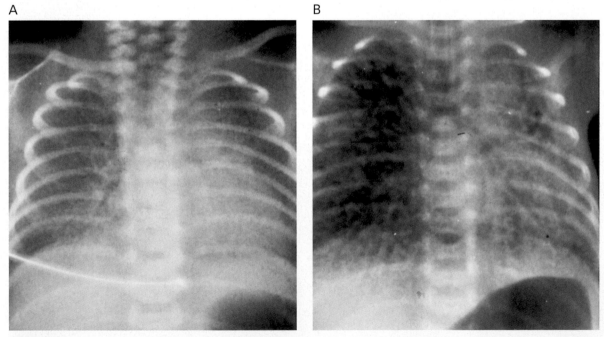

A

B

Fig C 4-10
Oxygen toxicity. (A) Initial chest radiograph of an infant demonstrates a typical granular parenchymal pattern with air bronchograms due to hyaline membrane disease. (B) After intensive oxygen therapy, multiple small round lucencies resembling bullae have developed, giving the lungs a sponge-like appearance.

Condition	Comments
Drug-induced pulmonary disease (Figs C 4-11 and C 4-12)	Allergic reaction to the drug with associated eosinophilia (nitrofurantoin) or toxic effect of a chemotherapeutic agent (busulfan, bleomycin, methotrexate).
Connective tissue disorders	
Scleroderma (see Fig C 5-5)	More prominent in the lung bases. Extrapulmonary findings include abnormal peristalsis of the esophagus and small bowel, erosion of the terminal tufts, and calcification in the fingertips.
Dermatomyositis/ polymyositis	More prominent in the lung bases. May have a coexisting primary malignancy elsewhere.
Rheumatoid disease (Fig C 4-13)	More prominent in the lung bases. Usually associated with evidence of rheumatoid arthritis.
Systemic lupus erythematosus	More prominent in the lung bases. Often has a coexisting pleural effusion.
Sjögren's syndrome	More prominent in the lung bases. Triad of keratoconjunctivitis sicca, xerostomia, and recurrent swelling of the parotid gland. Strong predominance in females. Changes in the joints resemble those of rheumatoid or psoriatic arthritis.
Chronic bronchitis (Fig C 4-14)	Coarse increase in interstitial markings ("dirty chest") that is often associated with emphysema and signs of pulmonary arterial hypertension.
"Small airways disease"	Inflammatory narrowing, mucous plugging, and fibrous obliteration of small airways of the lungs.

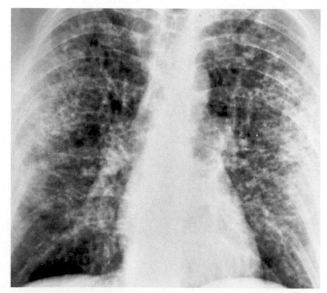

Fig C 4-11
Busulfan-induced lung disease. Severe coarse reticular pattern.

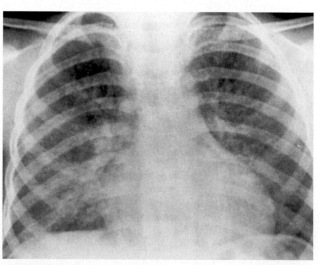

Fig C 4-12
Methotrexate-induced lung disease. Diffuse interstitial pattern with patches of alveolar consolidation in a child treated for myelogenous leukemia. After methotrexate therapy ended, there was rapid clinical and radiographic improvement.[14]

Condition	Comments
Acute bronchiolitis	More prominent in the lower lung zones and associated with severe overinflation of the lungs. Generally affects young children (under 3 years) and adults with pre-existing chronic respiratory disease. Bronchiolitis obliterans is the end stage of lower respiratory tract damage due to a variety of diseases.

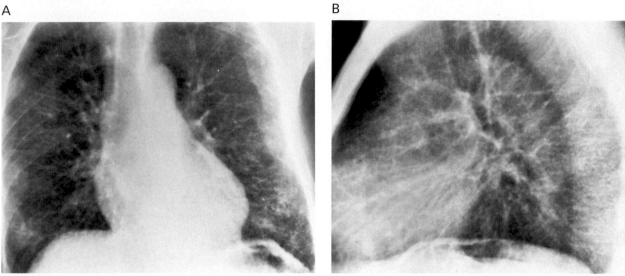

A   B

Fig C 4-13
Rheumatoid lung. (A) Frontal and (B) lateral views of the chest show diffuse thickening of the interstitial structures with prominent pleural thickening.

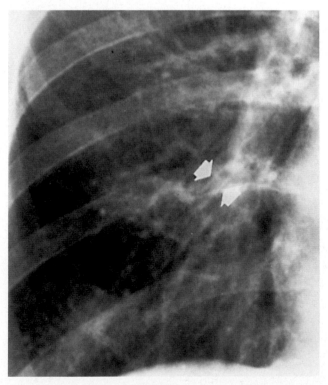

Fig C 4-14
Chronic bronchitis. Coned view of the right lower lung demonstrates a coarse increase in interstitial markings. The arrows point to the characteristic parallel-line shadows ("tramlines") outside the boundary of the pulmonary hilum.

Condition	Comments
Interstitial pulmonary edema (Fig C 4-15)	Loss of the normal sharp definition of pulmonary vascular markings (especially in the lower lung zones), perihilar haze, and thickening of the interlobular septa (Kerley-B lines). Also cardiomegaly and often redistribution of pulmonary blood flow from the lower to the upper lobes. Recurrent episodes of interstitial and alveolar edema and hemorrhage in patients with chronic left heart failure may result in the development of a coarse, often poorly defined reticular pattern that predominantly involves the middle and lower lung zones.
Infectious agents Tuberculosis (Fig C 4-16)	Localized or generalized prominence of interstitial structures reflects the healing phase in which tuberculous granulation tissue is replaced by fibrosis. The resulting scarring may result in considerable loss of volume.
Fungal infections (Fig C 4-17)	Localized or generalized prominence of interstitial structures may develop secondary to coccidioidomycosis, cryptococcosis, blastomycosis, and histoplasmosis.
Viral pneumonia (Fig C 4-18)	Generalized prominence of bronchovascular markings that may be a manifestation of various viral agents.

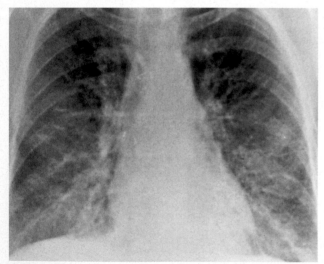

Fig C 4-15
Interstitial pulmonary edema. Edema fluid in the interstitial space causes a loss of the normal sharp definition of pulmonary vascular markings and a perihilar haze. At the bases, note the thin horizontal lines of increased density (Kerley-B lines) that represent fluid in the interlobular septa.

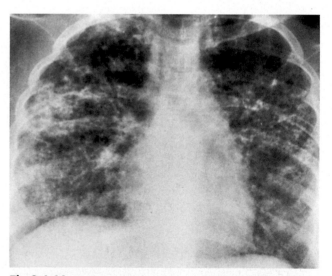

Fig C 4-16
Secondary tuberculosis. Diffuse interstitial fibrosis pattern.

Condition	Comments
Mycoplasma (Fig C 4-19)	More prominent in the lower lung zones. This appearance is less common than the localized form, in which a fine reticular infiltrate progresses rapidly to consolidation.

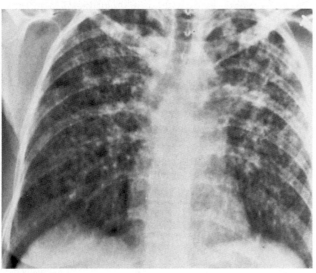

Fig C 4-17
Blastomycosis. Diffuse interstitial disease with upper lobe predominance. Note the volume loss in the upper lobe and the overdistention of the lower lobes along with the formation of bullae at the bases.[4]

A

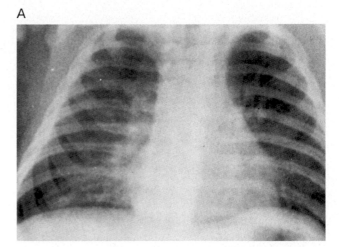

B

Fig C 4-18
Viral pneumonia. Diffuse interstitial infiltrates with perihilar haze in (A) a child and (B) an adult.

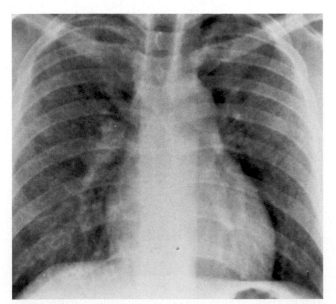

Fig C 4-19
Mycoplasma pneumoniae. Diffuse, fine reticular pattern represents acute interstitial inflammation. The radiographic pattern is indistinguishable from that of most viral pneumonias.

Condition	Comments
Pneumocystis carinii (Fig C 4-20)	More prominent in the perihilar areas. This pattern occurs in the early stages of the disease and is followed by patchy consolidations simulating pulmonary edema.
Schistosomiasis	Probably produced by migration of ova through vessel walls with subsequent reaction to these foreign bodies. Vascular obstruction may cause pulmonary hypertension (dilatation of central pulmonary arteries with rapid peripheral tapering).
Filariasis (see Fig C 18-6)	Tropical pulmonary eosinophilia. Patients with pulmonary disease usually do not have the characteristic cutaneous and lymphatic changes as in elephantiasis.
Toxoplasmosis	Early stage of the disease. Hilar lymph node enlargement is common.
Sarcoidosis (Figs C 4-21 and C 4-22)	Frequently associated with hilar and mediastinal lymph node enlargement, which often regresses spontaneously as the parenchymal disease develops.
Pulmonary Langerhans cell histiocytosis (Fig C 4-23)	More prominent in the upper lung zones. Most common cause of the coarse "honeycomb" pattern. Spontaneous pneumothorax is a frequent complication. Approximately one-third of patients are asymptomatic when initially diagnosed on a screening chest radiograph.

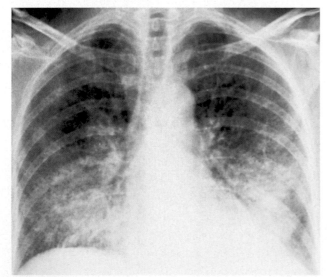

Fig C 4-20
Pneumocystis carinii. Diffuse reticular pattern in a patient with acute myelogenous leukemia. Note the early development of alveolar consolidations at the bases. A later film showed the typical pulmonary edema pattern.

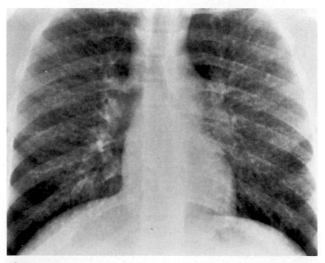

Fig C 4-21
Sarcoidosis. Diffuse reticulonodular pattern widely distributed throughout both lungs.

Condition	Comments
Cystic fibrosis (Fig C 4-24)	Coarse reticular pattern with overinflation of the lungs. Often segmental areas of consolidation or atelectasis due to pneumonia or bronchiectasis. Pulmonary fibrosis along the cardiac border may produce the shaggy heart appearance.

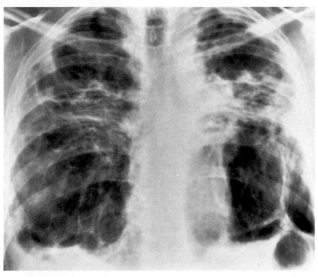

Fig C 4-22
Sarcoidosis. In end-stage disease, there is severe fibrous scarring, bleb formation, and emphysema.

A

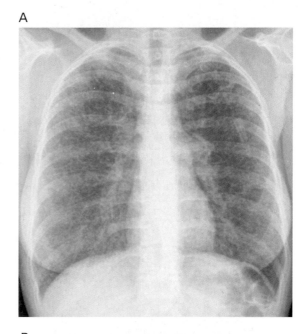

B

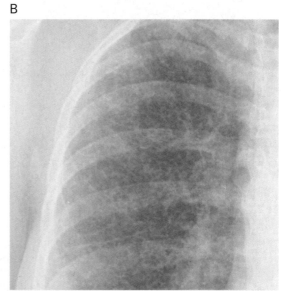

Fig C 4-23
Pulmonary Langerhans cell histiocytosis. (A) Frontal view shows widespread cystic changes in the lung and subsequent diffuse reticular opacities produced by the overlapping cysts. (B) Magnified view of the right upper lung shows the confluent superimposed lung cysts in detail.[15]

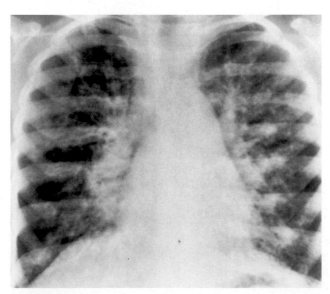

Fig C 4-24
Cystic fibrosis. Diffuse peribronchial thickening appears as a perihilar infiltrate associated with hyperexpansion and flattening of the hemidiaphragms.

Condition	Comments
Dysautonomia (familial autonomic dysfunction; Riley-Day syndrome) (Fig C 4-25)	Appearance identical to that of cystic fibrosis. Often associated with patchy areas of pneumonia and atelectasis. An autosomal recessive condition, found almost exclusively in Jews, which causes widespread neurologic abnormalities.
Usual interstitial pneumonia (UIP) (Fig C 4-26)	Most commonly seen in patients with idiopathic pulmonary fibrosis. In the early stages, more prominent in the lower lung zones. Progressive volume loss on sequential studies.
Desquamative interstitial pneumonia (DIP) (Fig C 4-27)	More prominent in the lower lung zones. Progressive loss of lung volume on sequential studies. Spontaneous pneumothorax and pleural effusion may occur.
Idiopathic pulmonary hemosiderosis/ Goodpasture's syndrome	Often more prominent in the perihilar areas and the middle and lower lung zones. Initially represents a transition stage from acute air-space hemorrhage to complete resolution. Persistence of the reticular pattern after several bleeding episodes indicates irreversible interstitial fibrosis. Repeated pulmonary hemorrhage results in anemia and pulmonary insufficiency (also renal disease in Goodpasture's syndrome).

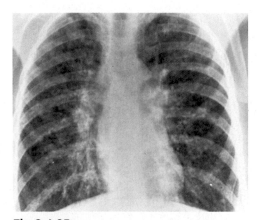

Fig C 4-25
Dysautonomia. Pattern identical to that of cystic fibrosis.

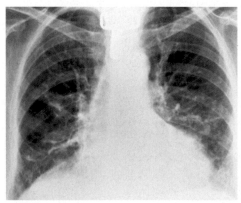

Fig C 4-26
Usual interstitial pneumonia. Diffuse, coarse reticulonodular pattern.

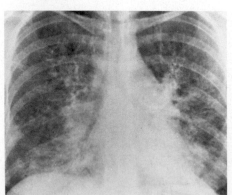

Fig C 4-27
Desquamative interstitial pneumonia.
Diffuse reticulonodular pattern indicating interstitial disease, combined with bibasilar air-space consolidation that obscures the borders of the heart.

Condition	Comments
Amyloidosis (Fig C 4-28)	More prominent in the lower lung zones. Hilar and mediastinal lymph nodes may be markedly enlarged (occasionally densely calcified).
Waldenström's macroglobulinemia	Rare lymphoproliferative disorder in which there is usually hepatosplenomegaly and palpable peripheral adenopathy.
Tuberous sclerosis	Diffuse interstitial fibrosis pattern with honeycombing that is more prominent in the lower lung zones. Chylous pleural effusion and pneumothorax are common. Sclerotic (occasionally lytic) bone lesions may occur.
Pulmonary lymphangiomyomatosis (Fig C 4-29)	Rare condition that produces a radiographic appearance identical to that of tuberous sclerosis. Part of a generalized syndrome characterized by an excessive accumulation of muscle in relation to extrapulmonary lymphatics.
Neurofibromatosis	Additional manifestations include skin nodules, multiple bullae, scoliosis, and mediastinal neurofibromas.
Niemann-Pick disease	Shows characteristic bone changes and splenomegaly.
Embolism from oily contrast material	Complication of lymphography. The fine reticular pattern usually clears within 72 hours.
Interstitial fibrosis secondary to pulmonary disease (see Fig C 1-26)	Common cause of localized or generalized interstitial thickening, though the offending agent is not always recognized. May be the sequela of recurrent infection, chronic aspiration, lung trauma, radiation, or thromboembolic disease.

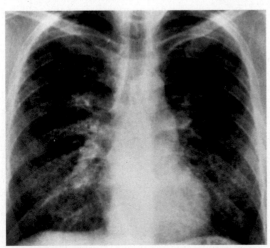

Fig C 4-28
Amyloidosis. Diffuse interstitial fibrosis pattern.

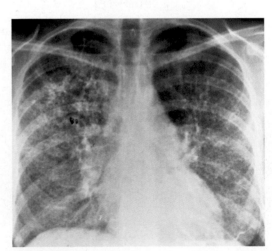

Fig C 4-29
Pulmonary lymphangiomyomatosis. Diffuse reticulonodular interstitial pattern throughout both lungs.

Honeycombing

Condition	Comments
Pneumoconiosis (Fig C 5-1)	Silicosis, asbestosis, berylliosis, coal-miner's lung, etc. Often associated with other radiographic manifestations (nodules, eggshell calcification, and progressive massive fibrosis in silicosis; pleural plaquing and calcification in asbestosis).
Sarcoidosis (Fig C 5-2)	Frequently associated with hilar and mediastinal lymph node enlargement, which often regresses spontaneously as the parenchymal disease develops.
Bronchiectasis (Fig C 5-3)	Irreversible dilatation of the bronchi related to a variety of causes, especially centrally obstructing lesions, infection or inflammation, congenital disorders, and pulmonary fibrosis.

A

B

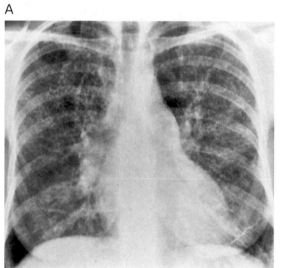

Fig C 5-1
Classic honeycomb pattern in pneumoconiosis. (A) Frontal and (B) lateral views.

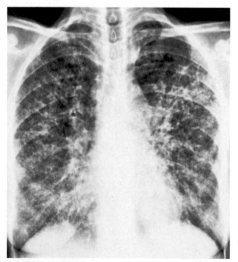

Fig C 5-2
Sarcoidosis. Coarse honeycomb pattern.

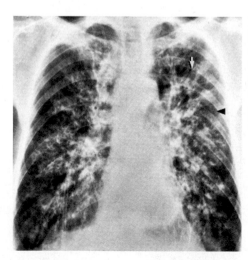

Fig C 5-3
Bronchiectasis (cystic fibrosis). Diffuse increase in interstitial markings radiating in a bronchovascular distribution with tramlines (arrows) and peribronchial cuffing (arrowhead).[16]

Condition	Comments
Idiopathic interstitial fibrosis (Hamman-Rich syndrome) (Fig C 5-4)	Usually most prominent at the bases and associated with progressive loss of lung volume. A similar diffuse interstitial fibrosis pattern may represent the end stage of a variety of pulmonary conditions, including chronic or recurrent pulmonary edema, the inhalation of noxious gases and organic dust, and drug therapy.
Pulmonary Langerhans cell histiocytosis (Fig C 5-5)	More prominent in the upper lung zones (sparing the bases). Spontaneous pneumothorax is a frequent complication.
Tuberculosis	Bronchiectasis and fibrosis may produce a localized honeycomb pattern in the upper lobes.
Connective tissue disorders (Fig C 5-6)	More prominent at the bases and usually associated with progressive loss of lung volume. Causes include scleroderma, rheumatoid lung, and dermatomyositis.
Ankylosing spondylitis	Rare manifestation that exclusively involves the upper lobes and resembles the fibrosis and bronchiectasis that may develop secondary to tuberculosis.
Desquamative interstitial pneumonia (DIP)	More prominent in the lower lung zones and associated with progressive loss of lung volume.

A   B

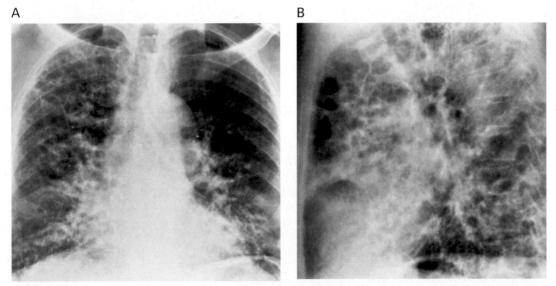

Fig C 5-4
Diffuse interstitial fibrosis. (A) Frontal and (B) lateral views of the chest demonstrate a coarse reticular pattern indicating pronounced fibrosis. Intervening small areas of lucency produce the appearance of a honeycomb lung, especially in the right upper lobe.

Condition	Comments
Amyloidosis (Fig C 5-7)	More prominent in the lower lung zones and often associated with hilar and mediastinal lymphadenopathy.
Neurofibromatosis (Fig C 5-8)	Additional manifestations include skin nodules, multiple bullae, scoliosis, and mediastinal neurofibromas.
Tuberous sclerosis	More prominent in the lower lung zones. Chylous pleural effusion and pneumothorax are common, and sclerotic (occasionally lytic) bone lesions may occur.
Niemann-Pick disease	Also characteristic bone changes and splenomegaly.
Lipoid pneumonia	Rare manifestation that usually involves a lower lobe.

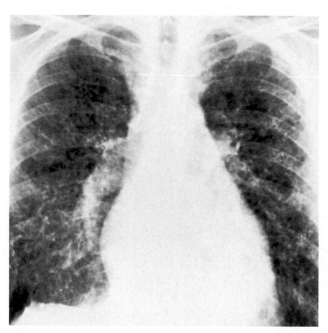

Fig C 5-5
Pulmonary Langerhans cell histiocytosis. Diffuse honeycomb pattern that is slightly more prominent in the upper lung zones.

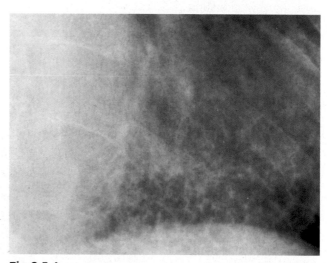

Fig C 5-6
Scleroderma. Coned view of the left lower lung demonstrates a honeycomb pattern, with small emphysematous areas combined with fibrosis and fine nodularity.

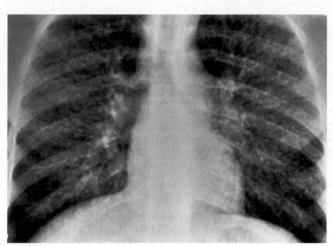

Fig C 5-7
Amyloidosis.

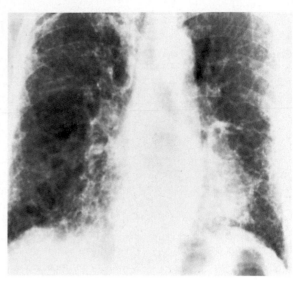

Fig C 5-8
Neurofibromatosis.

Solitary Pulmonary Nodule

Condition	Imaging Findings	Comments
Tuberculoma (Figs C 6-1 and C 6-2)	Round or oval, sharply circumscribed nodule that is seldom more than 4 cm in diameter. Central calcification and "satellite" lesions are common, as is calcification of hilar lymph nodes.	Primarily involves the upper lobes (especially the right). The draining bronchus may show irregular thickening or even frank stenosis.
Histoplasmoma (Figs C 6-3 and C 6-4)	Round or oval, sharply circumscribed nodule that is seldom more than 3 cm in diameter. Central calcification is common, and satellite lesions may occur.	Most frequently in the lower lobes. May be multiple and vary considerably in size. Often associated calcification of hilar lymph nodes.
Other fungal diseases (Fig C 6-5)	Usually a single, well-circumscribed nodule (may be multiple in coccidioidomycosis).	Actinomycosis, blastomycosis, coccidioidomycosis, cryptococcosis, and nocardiosis. Cavitation is common in actinomycosis, coccidioidomycosis, and nocardiosis. Empyema may complicate actinomycosis or nocardiosis.

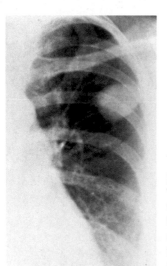

Fig C 6-1
Tuberculoma. Single smooth, well-defined pulmonary nodule in the left upper lobe. In the absence of a central nidus of calcification, this appearance is indistinguishable from that of a malignancy.

A
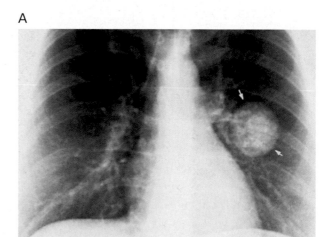

B
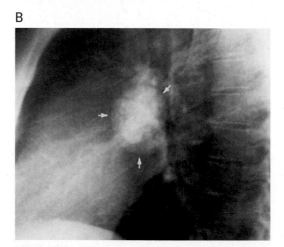

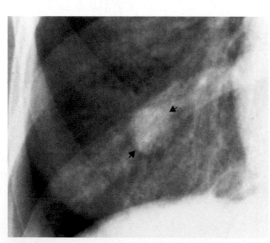

Fig C 6-3
Histoplasmoma. Solitary, sharply circumscribed granulomatous nodule (arrows) in the right lower lobe.

Fig C 6-2
Calcified tuberculoma. (A) Frontal and (B) lateral views of the chest show a large left lung soft-tissue mass (arrows) containing dense central calcification.

Condition	Imaging Findings	Comments
Echinococcal (hydatid) cyst (Fig C 6-6)	Solitary, sharply circumscribed, round or oval mass that tends to have a bizarre, irregular shape. Calcification is very rare.	Predilection for the lower lobes (especially the right). Communication with the bronchial tree causes an air-fluid level in the cyst (endocyst floats on the surface to produce the "water lily" sign [see Fig C 9-8] or "sign of the camalote") or the "crescent" sign (see Fig C 20-4) around its periphery.
Acute lung abscess (Fig C 6-7)	Round, often ill-defined mass that predominantly involves the posterior portions of the upper or lower lobes.	Bilateral in more than 60% of cases. Cavitation is very common (irregular, shaggy inner wall).

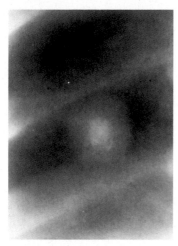

Fig C 6-4
Histoplasmoma. Characteristic central calcification in a solitary pulmonary nodule.

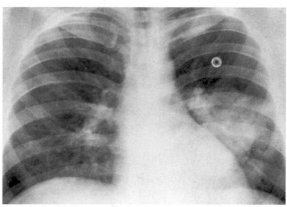

Fig C 6-5
Cryptococcosis. Single fairly well-circumscribed, mass-like consolidation in the superior segment of the left lower lobe.

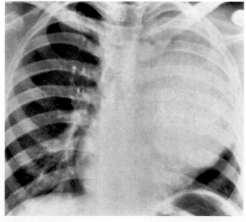

Fig C 6-6
Echinococcal cyst. Huge mass filling most of the left hemithorax.

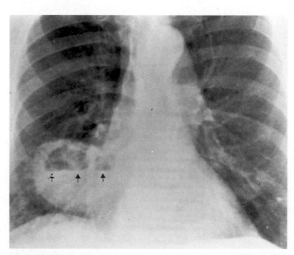

Fig C 6-7
Acute lung abscess. Large right middle lobe abscess containing an air-fluid level (arrows) in an intravenous drug abuser.

Condition	Imaging Findings	Comments
Bronchial adenoma (Fig C 6-8)	Solitary, round or oval, sharply circumscribed mass. Calcification and cavitation are very rare.	Approximately 25% appear as peripheral solitary nodules. The remaining 75% arise centrally in the bronchial lumen and cause segmental atelectasis or obstructive pneumonia. Hemoptysis occurs in more than half the patients.
Hamartoma (Figs C 6-9 and C 6-10)	Solitary, well-circumscribed, often lobulated mass. Popcorn calcification (multiple punctate calcifications in the lesion) is virtually diagnostic, but occurs in less than 10% of cases.	Serial examinations may show interval growth. An endobronchial lesion (10%) may cause segmental atelectasis or obstructive pneumonia.

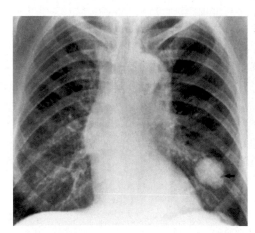

Fig C 6-8
Bronchial adenoma. Nonspecific solitary pulmonary nodule at the left base. Note the notched indentation of the lateral wall (arrow) of the mass. Although this "Rigler notch" sign was initially described as being pathognomonic of malignancy, an identical appearance is commonly seen in benign processes.

A   B

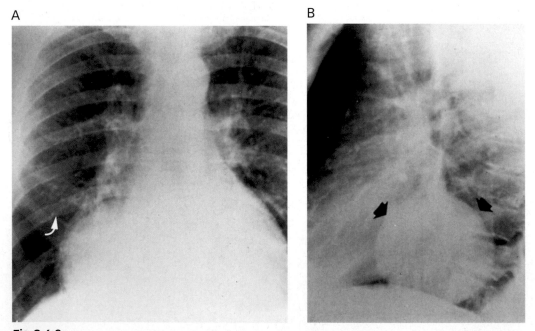

Fig C 6-9
Hamartoma. (A) Frontal view of the chest shows a large mass (arrow) in the right cardiophrenic angle; the mass mimics a pericardial cyst or herniation through the foramen of Morgagni, both of which tend to occur at this site. (B) Lateral view shows the mass to be posterior (arrows), effectively excluding the other diagnostic possibilities. The mass is indistinguishable from other benign or malignant processes in the lung.

Condition	Imaging Findings	Comments
Bronchogenic carcinoma (Fig C 6-11)	Ill-defined, lobulated, or umbilicated mass that usually exceeds 2 cm. Hilar and mediastinal lymph node enlargement is common, especially in oat-cell carcinoma.	Approximately 40% of solitary nodules are malignant. Bronchogenic carcinoma primarily involves the upper lobes with rare calcification and infrequent (2–10%) cavitation. Central or popcorn calcification virtually excludes a malignant lesion. The tumor almost invariably shows interval growth on serial films.
Hematogenous metastases (Fig C 6-12)	Single (25%) or multiple (75%) lesions that are generally well circumscribed with smooth or slightly lobulated margins and lower lobe predominance.	Represents approximately 5% of asymptomatic solitary pulmonary nodules. Calcification is rare (only in osteogenic sarcoma or chondrosarcoma). A malignant solitary pulmonary nodule is most likely a primary bronchogenic carcinoma in patients with carcinomas of the head and neck, bladder, breast, cervix, bile ducts, esophagus, ovary, prostate, or stomach. Conversely, patients with melanoma, sarcoma, or testicular carcinoma are more likely to have a solitary metastasis than a bronchogenic carcinoma.

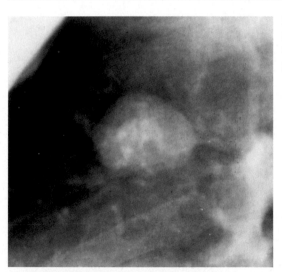

Fig C 6-10
Hamartoma. Well-circumscribed solitary nodule containing characteristic irregular scattered calcifications (popcorn pattern).

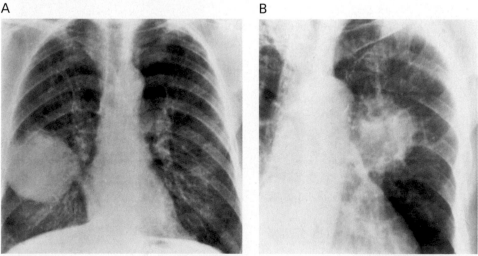

Fig C 6-11
Bronchogenic carcinoma. (A) Relatively well-defined mass. (B) Ill-defined solitary nodule.

Condition	Imaging Findings	Comments
Bronchioloalveolar (alveolar cell) carcinoma (Fig C 6-13)	Various patterns (smooth or lobulated, sharply circumscribed or ill defined).	Characteristic findings include an air bronchogram or bronchiologram in the mass and the "pleural tail" sign (linear strands extending from the lesion toward the pleura). The tumor tends to grow very slowly.
Non-Hodgkin's lymphoma	Single or, more commonly, multiple nodules that often have fuzzy outlines and strands of increased density extending into the adjacent lung.	May be a manifestation of primary or secondary disease. Hilar or mediastinal adenopathy is usually associated. Because the tumor rarely obstructs the bronchial tree (unlike carcinoma), air bronchograms often occur in the mass.
Multiple myeloma (plasmacytoma) (see Fig C 34-4)	Sharply circumscribed, extrapleural mass producing an obtuse angle with the chest wall.	Usually represents spread into the thorax of a primary rib lesion (therefore almost always a destructive process in one or more ribs).

A

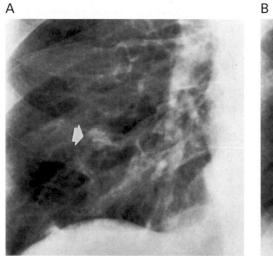

B

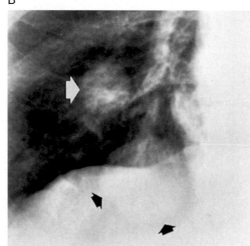

Fig C 6-12
Metastases. (A) Solitary metastasis (arrow). (B) Repeat examination 5 months later shows rapid growth of the previous solitary nodule (white arrow). There is a second huge nodule (black arrows) that was not appreciated on the previous examination because it projected below the right hemidiaphragm.

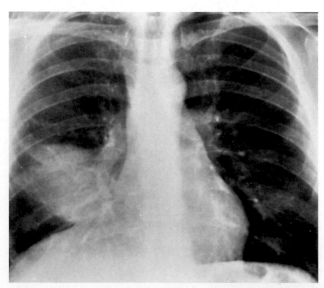

Fig C 6-13
Alveolar cell carcinoma. Large, well-circumscribed tumor mass.

Condition	Imaging Findings	Comments
Mesenchymal tumor	Usually solitary and well defined.	Rare tumor arising in the bronchial wall. May cause bronchial obstruction with peripheral atelectasis or obstructive pneumonia.
Carcinoid (Fig C 6-14)	Well-defined, round or ovoid mass that may have a lobulated margin.	Carcinoid tumors are sometimes located distal to segmental bronchi (peripheral carcinoids).
Pulmonary hematoma (Fig C 6-15)	Single or multiple, unilocular or multilocular, round or oval mass that may occasionally be huge. Usually in a peripheral subpleural location deep to the area of maximum trauma.	Results from hemorrhage into a pulmonary parenchymal laceration or a traumatic lung cyst. May communicate with the bronchial tree (air-fluid level). Generally shows a slow, progressive decrease in size (may persist for several months).
Lipoid pneumonia (Fig C 6-16)	Sharply circumscribed, smooth or lobulated mass that primarily occurs in the dependent portion of the lung. The lesion may have a shaggy border and simulate carcinoma.	Inflammatory reaction to aspirated oils (especially mineral oil). Characteristic streaky linear opacities may radiate outward from the periphery of the mass (interlobular septal thickening).

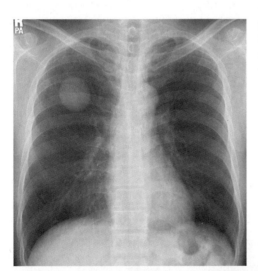

Fig C 6-14
Carcinoid. Well-defined round mass in the right upper lung.[17]

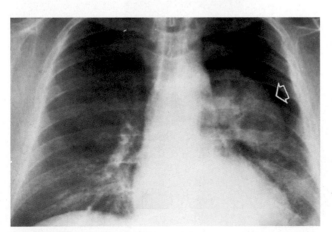

Fig C 6-15
Pulmonary hematoma. After a stab wound, a homogeneous kidney-shaped opacity (arrow) developed in the superior segment of the left lower lobe. There is blunting of the left costophrenic angle.

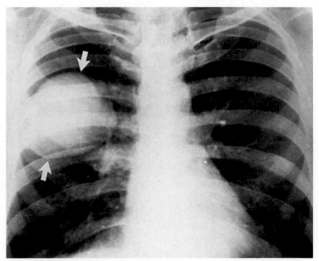

Fig C 6-16
Lipoid pneumonia. Sharply demarcated granulomatous-lipoid mass (arrows) simulating a neoplastic process.

Condition	Imaging Findings	Comments
Wegener's granulomatosis (see Fig C 9-14)	Round, solitary, or more commonly, multiple fairly well-circumscribed nodules that may simulate metastases.	Cavitation (thick walled with irregular shaggy inner margins) develops in about half the patients.
Rheumatoid necrobiotic nodule	Single or, more commonly, multiple smooth, well-circumscribed nodules that predominantly occur in a peripheral subpleural location.	Rare manifestation of rheumatoid lung disease that tends to wax and wane in relation to subcutaneous nodules. Cavitation is common (thick walled with smooth inner margins).
Bronchogenic cyst (see Figs C 23-3 and C 23-4)	Solitary round or oval, smooth, sharply circumscribed mass with a lower lobe predominance.	Approximately two-thirds of bronchogenic cysts are pulmonary (the rest are mediastinal). The cyst is homogeneous until a communication is established with contiguous lung (usually the result of infection).
Intralobar bronchopulmonary sequestration	Round, oval, or triangular mass that typically is well circumscribed and contiguous with the diaphragm (two-thirds of the cases are on the left).	Enclosed in visceral pleura of the affected lung. Although cystic, the mass appears homogeneous until a communication is established with contiguous lung (usually the result of infection). An intralobar sequestration is supplied by a systemic artery and drains via the pulmonary veins.
Extralobar bronchopulmonary sequestration (Fig C 6-17)	Well-defined, homogeneous mass that is related to the left hemidiaphragm (above or below it) in approximately 90% of cases.	Enclosed in its own visceral pleural layer (therefore seldom infected or air containing). An extralobar sequestration is supplied by a systemic artery (usually from the abdominal aorta) and drains via systemic veins (inferior vena cava or azygos system).

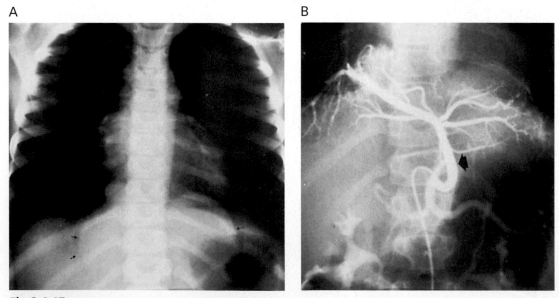

A B

Fig C 6-17
Bilateral pulmonary sequestration. (A) Frontal view of the chest shows bilateral oval, slightly lobulated paravertebral masses (arrows) in the juxtadiaphragmatic region. (B) Selective angiogram of a large anomalous artery (arrow) arising from the celiac trunk shows several branches supplying the bilateral paravertebral masses. The venous drainage was via the pulmonary veins.[18]

Condition	Imaging Findings	Comments
Pulmonary arteriovenous fistula (Fig C 6-18)	Sharply defined, round or oval, often slightly lobulated lesion that predominantly involves the lower lobes.	Diagnosis requires identification of the feeding artery and the draining vein. Approximately one-third of the fistulas are multiple (arteriography of both lungs required if surgical resection is contemplated). About 50% of the patients have hereditary hemorrhagic telangiectasia (Rendu-Osler-Weber disease).
Mucoid impaction (Fig C 6-19)	Generally a finger-like mass, although it may have a Y- or V-shaped configuration when a bronchial bifurcation is plugged.	Affects patients with bronchospasm (plugs present in dilated proximal segmental bronchi) and a sensitivity to *Aspergillus fumigatus*. Almost always associated with asthma or pre-existing chronic bronchial disease. Usually transient, but may persist for months and even enlarge. Cavitation (lung necrosis) is rare.

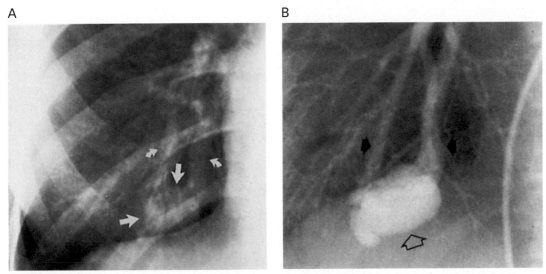

Fig C 6-18
Pulmonary arteriovenous fistula. (A) View of the right lung shows a round soft-tissue 8mass (straight arrows) at the left base. Feeding and draining vessels (curved arrows) extend to the lesion. (B) An arteriogram clearly shows the feeding artery and draining veins (closed arrows) associated with the arteriovenous malformation (open arrow).

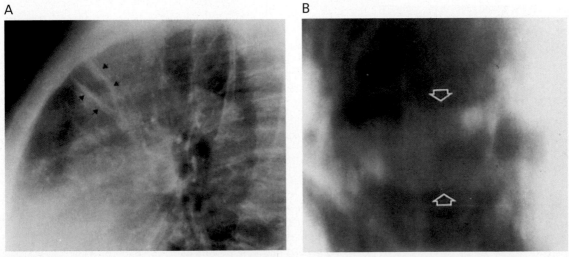

Fig C 6-19
Mucoid impaction. (A) V-shaped and (B) Y-shaped masses (arrows).

Condition	Imaging Findings	Comments
Congenital bronchial atresia	Smooth, sharply defined oval mass that has a strong predilection for the apicoposterior bronchus of the left upper lobe.	The mass consists of inspissated mucus that accumulates in the bronchus immediately distal to the point of obstruction. The lung parenchyma distal to the occlusion is overinflated because of collateral air drift. This very rare anomaly is usually asymptomatic and is discovered on a screening chest radiograph.
Pulmonary vein varix (Fig C 6-20)	Round or oval, lobulated, well-defined mass (may be multiple) involving the medial third of the lung.	Very rare congenital or acquired tortuosity and dilatation of a pulmonary vein just before its entrance into the left atrium. Typically, close association with adjacent pulmonary veins and often seen on only one of the orthogonal posterior and lateral views. Change in size and shape with Valsalva and Mueller maneuvers (as with arteriovenous fistulas).
Round pneumonia (Fig C 6-21)	Ranges from small dense mass to large ill-defined rounded opacity. The margins may be smooth, lobulated, or irregular or spiculated. Primarily involves the lower lobe.	Generally considered a disease of children, but may occur in adults. Often difficult to distinguish from bronchogenic carcinoma. Fewer than 20% demonstrate air bronchograms. Some patients present with no clinical symptoms, though they may give a history of cough and chills 1 week or longer previously.
Inflammatory pseudotumor	Solitary pulmonary nodule (or homogeneous consolidation) that may mimic a primary or metastatic neoplasm.	Probably represents a reparative process secondary to an unresolved pneumonia (though there is often no history of an acute respiratory illness).
Progressive massive fibrosis (PMF) (see Figs C 7-9 and C 7-10)	Large, often bilateral (but usually asymmetric), spindle-shaped mass in the upper half of the lungs. Typically arises near the periphery of the lung, with its lateral border (paralleling the rib cage) usually better defined than the medial edge. Tends to migrate toward the hila with time.	A manifestation of pneumoconiosis (especially silicosis or coal-miner's disease). Usually of homogeneous density unless there is cavitation (caused by ischemic necrosis or superimposed tuberculosis). May occasionally contain small calcifications (unlike bronchogenic carcinoma).

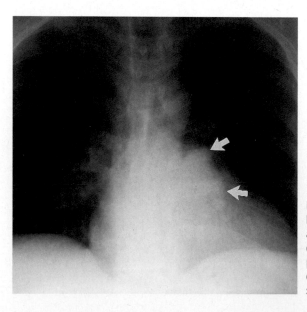

Fig C 6-20
Pulmonary vein varix. Frontal chest radiograph shows a round mass (arrows) inferior to the left hilum. The well-defined superior border and close association with the pulmonary veins inferiorly, as well as poor visualization on a lateral projection (not shown), are important features suggesting the diagnosis.[19]

A

B

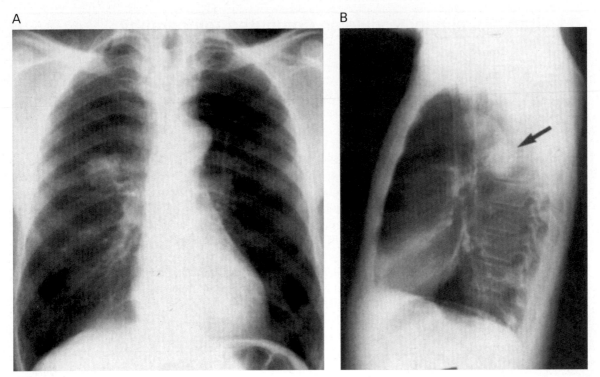

Fig C 6-21
Round pneumonia. Well-defined round mass (arrow) in the right mid-lung in posteroanterior (A) and lateral (B) chest radiographs that resolved completely after antibiotic therapy.[20]

Solitary Pulmonary Nodule on Computed Tomography

Condition	Comments
Benign versus malignant (Figs C 7-1 to C 7-3)	In general, the smaller the nodule, the more likely it is to be benign. About 80% of benign nodules are less than 2 cm in diameter. However, this does not exclude lung cancer, because about 15% malignant nodules are less than 1 cm in diameter and 40% are less than 2 cm. Although most nodules with smooth, well-defined margins are benign, approximately 20% of malignant nodules also have this appearance. A lobular contour implies uneven growth, which is associated with malignancy. However, this appearance can be seen in up to 25% of benign nodules. However, a nodule with an irregular, speculated margin with distortion of adjacent vessels (sunburst or corona radiate appearance) is likely to be malignant. When a benign lesion cavitates, the wall is typically smooth and thin (<4 mm), whereas those thick, irregular walls tend to be malignant. Although a substantial proportion of benign nodules are not calcified, the demonstration of central, diffuse solid, laminated, or popcorn calcification are reliable indicators of a benign cause.

Malignant calcification is usually diffuse and amorphous. Punctate calcification may also occur in lung cancer due to engulfment of a preexistent calcified granulomatous lesion or a metastasis (osteosarcoma or chondrosarcoma). Stability of a pulmonary nodule (>1 cm) for 2 years or more is a good sign of a benign process. The doubling time for most malignant nodules is between 30 and 400 days. Those that double either more rapidly or more slowly are typically benign. |

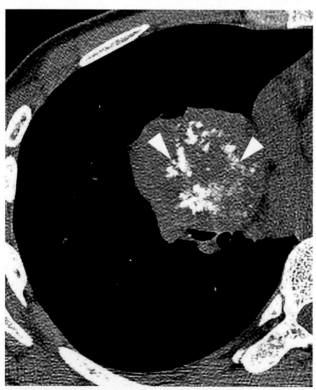

Fig C 7-1
Benign calcifications. Diffuse punctate calcifications in a large (6 cm), lobulated carcinoid.[17]

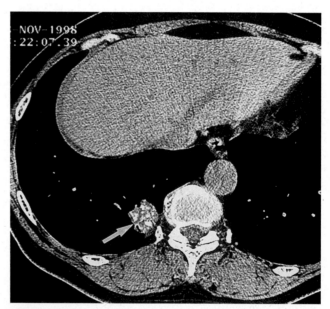

Fig C 7-2
Calcified metastasis mimicking hamartoma. Multiple punctuate calcifications in a mass (arrow) in the right lower lobe. A biopsy obtained because of prior resection of the rectum for a malignancy revealed a metastatic adenocarcinoma.[21]

Condition	Comments
Benign granuloma (Fig C 7-4)	Tuberculoma and histoplasmoma. Central calcification and "satellite" lesions are common, as is calcification of hilar lymph nodes. Tuberculomas primarily involve the upper lobes (especially the right); histoplasmomas are more common in the lower lobes.

A

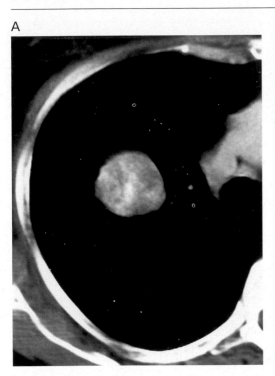

B

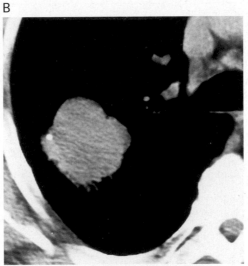

C

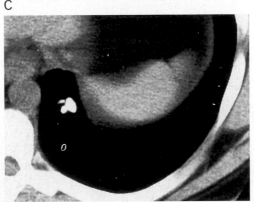

Fig C 7-3
Malignant calcification. (A) Amorphous calcification. (B) Peripheral punctuate calcification consistent with an "engulfed" granuloma. (C) Diffuse high-attenuation and lobulated contour in metastatic osteosarcoma.[22]

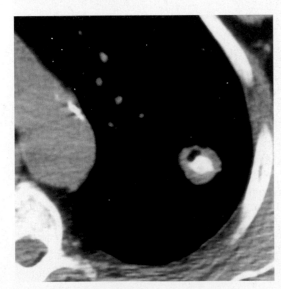

Fig C 7-4
Granuloma. Soft-tissue nodule with central calcification in an asymptomatic man. Note the eccentric calcification within the nodule.[22]

Condition	Comments
Other fungal diseases (Fig C 7-5 and C 7-6)	Actinomycosis, aspergillosis, blastomycosis, coccidiodomycosis, cryptococcosis, and nocardiosis. Cavitation is common in actinomycosis, coccidiodomycosis, and nocardiosis.
Echinococcal (hydatid cyst)	Frequently has a bizarre, irregular shape and rarely calcifies.
Acute lung abscess (Fig C 7-7)	Cavitation is very common (irregular, shaggy inner wall). Usually involves the posterior portions of the upper and lower lobes and is bilateral in more than 60% of cases.
Bronchial adenoma	About 25% appear as peripheral solitary nodules (the rest arise centrally in the bronchial lumen and cause segmental atelectasis or obstructive pneumonia)
Hamartoma (Figs C 7-8 and 7-9)	Popcorn calcification (multiple punctuate calcifications in the lesion) is virtually diagnostic, but occurs in less than 10% of cases. The presence of fat within a solitary pulmonary nodule is strongly suggestive of hamartoma (seen in about 50% of lesions and best seen on thin-section studies).
Hematoma	Results from hemorrhage into a pulmonary parenchymal laceration or a traumatic lung cyst. Usually in a peripheral subpleural location deep to the area of maximum trauma.

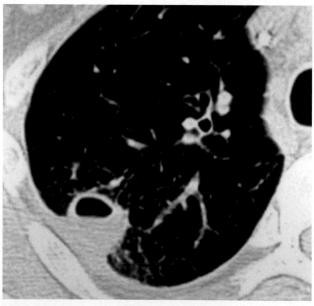

Fig C 7-5
Aspergillosis. Thin-walled cavitary nodule in the right lung of a patient with leukemia.[3]

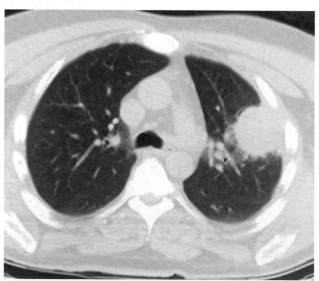

Fig C 7-6
Blastomycosis. Round, well-circumscribed left upper lobe mass with irregular borders in a heavy smoker. After a CT-guided biopsy was inconclusive, the patient underwent left upper lobectomy and mediastinal lymph node dissection for suspected lung carcinoma.[23]

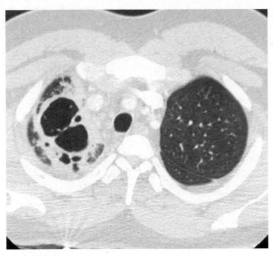

Fig C 7-7
Lung abscese (blastomycosis). Large apical thick-walled cavitary lesion in an acutely ill patient.[23]

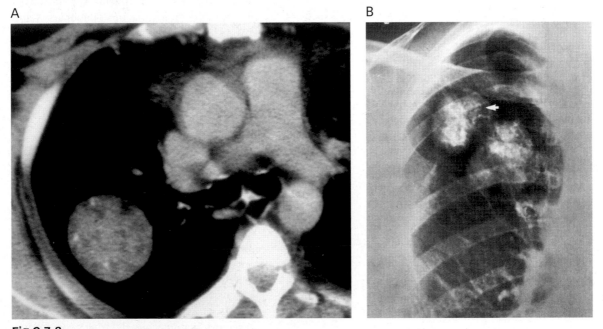

A

B

Fig C 7-8
Hamartoma. (A) Sharply marginated lesion with small focal areas of calcification and fat.[22] (B) Characteristic calcification of a hamartomatous nodule in another patient.[16]

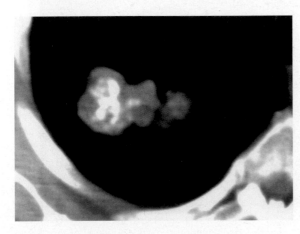

Fig C 7-9
Chondrohamartoma. Lobulated nodule with central popcorn-like in the right upper lobe (Reprinted from Bennett LL, Lesar MSL, Tellis. Multiple calcified chondrohamartomas of the lung: CT appearance. J Comput Assist Tomgr 9:180-182, 1985, cited in 24).

Condition	Comments
Lipoid pneumonia (Fig C 7-10)	Inflammatory reaction to aspirated oils (especially mineral oil) that primarily occurs in the dependent portion of the lung. The lesion may have a shaggy border and simulate malignancy.
Wegener's granulomatosis	Although more commonly multiple, there may be only a single nodule. The cavitation (thick walled with irregular shaggy inner margins) that develops in about half the patients may simulate malignancy.
Rheumatoid necrobiotic nodule	A single (more commonly multiple), often-cavitating nodule is a rare manifestation of rheumatoid lung disease.
Bronchopulmonary sequestration (Fig C 7-11)	Mass contiguous with the diaphragm. Intralobar sequestration drains via the pulmonary veins, while the extralobar type drains via systemic veins (inferior vena cava or azygos system).
Pulmonary arteriovenous fistula (Fig C 7-12)	Diagnosis requires identification of the feeding artery and the draining vein. About a third are multiple, and half are associated with hereditary hemorrhagic telangiectasia (Rendu-Osler-Weber disease).
Mucoid impaction (Fig C 7-13)	Usually a finger-like mass, although it may have a Y- or V-shaped configuration when a bronchial bifurcation is plugged. Affects patients with bronchospasm (plugs present in dilated proximal segmental bronchi) and a sensitivity to *Aspergillus fumigatus*.
Congenital bronchial atresia (Fig C 7-14)	Consisting of inspissated mucus that accumulates in the bronchus immediately distal to the point of obstruction, it has a strong predilection for the apical-posterior bronchus of the left upper lobe.

A
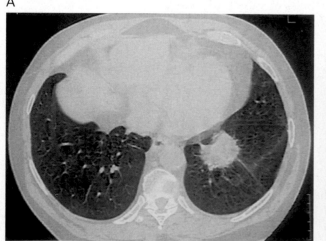

B
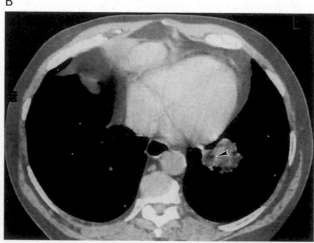

Fig C 7-10
Lipoid pneumonia. (A) Lung windowing shows a speculated mass in the left lower lobe. (B) Mediastinal windowing demonstrates that the mass contains fat attenuation, consistent with lipid deposits in the legion.

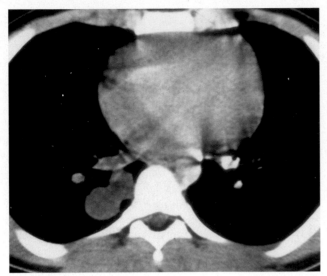

Fig C 7-11
Intralobar sequestration. Lobular, well-marginated nodule with homogeneous attenuation in the right lower lobe.[22]

A

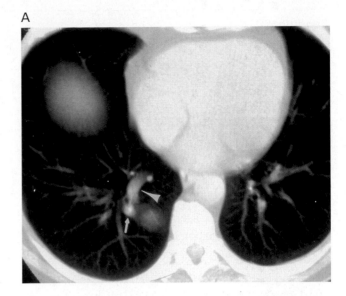

B

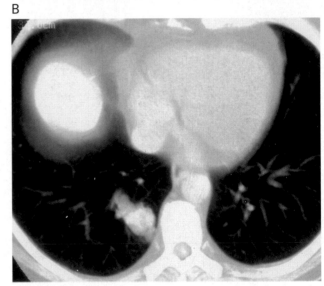

Fig C 7-12
Arteriovenous malformation. (A) Feeding artery (arrow) and an enlarged draining vein (arrowhead) associated with a right lower lung nodule. (B) Scan at a lower level shows the nidus of the malformation (Reprinted from Swensen SJ, Brown LR, Colby, et al. Lung nodule enhancement at CT: prospective findings. Radiology 201:447-455, 1996, cited in 24).

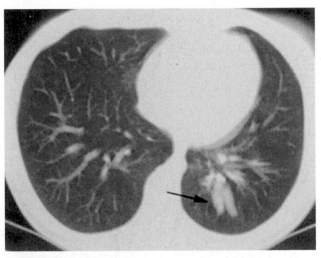

Fig C 7-13
Mucoid impaction. Characteristic V-shaped structure.[24]

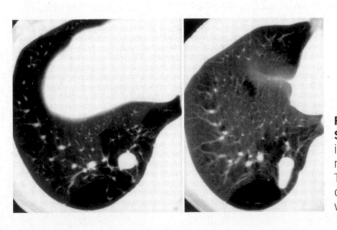

Fig C 7-14
Segmental bronchial atresia. Branching tubular area of increased attenuation in the right lower lobe as well as pulmonary parenchyma with lower-than-expected attenuation. This constellation of findings in teenager was considered so characteristic of segmental bronchial atresia that no further work-up was performed.[22]

Condition	Comments
Pulmonary vein varix	Very rare congenital or acquired tortuosity and dilatation of a pulmonary vein just before its entrance in the left atrium. Changes size and shape with Valsalva and Mueller maneuvers (as with arteriovenous fistulas).
Round pneumonia	Ranging from a small dense mass to a large, ill-defined rounded opacity, primarily in the lower lobe, it may be difficult to distinguish from malignancy. Some patients present with a history of cough and chills for 1 week or longer.
Inflammatory pseudotumor	Probably represents a reparative process secondary to an unresolved pneumonia (though there often is no history of an acute respiratory illness).
Amyloidoma (Fig C 7-15)	Limited form of amyloidosis that is usually misinterpreted as a neoplasm. Resection of the nodule is both diagnostic and curative.
Malignant Bronchogenic carcinoma (Fig C 7-16)	Primarily involves the upper lobes and almost invariably shows interval growth on serial studies. Usually an ill-defined, lobulated, or umbilicated mass that is generally more than 2 cm in diameter.
Hematogenous metastasis (Figs C 7-17 and C 7-18)	Single in about 25% of cases, metastases represent approximately 5% of asymptomatic pulmonary nodules. Calcification is rare (only in osteosarcoma or chondrosarcoma). A malignant solitary pulmonary nodule is most likely a primary bronchogenic carcinoma in patients with carcinomas of the head and neck, bladder, breast, cervix, bile ducts, esophagus, ovary, prostate, or stomach. Conversely, patients with melanoma, sarcoma, or testicular carcinoma are more likely to have a solitary metastasis than a primary lung cancer.

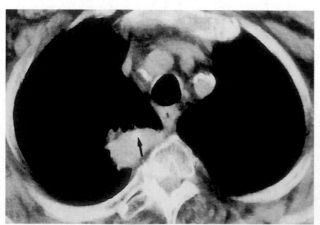

Fig C 7-15
Amyloidoma. Solid mass adjacent to the spine that contains amorphous calcification.[25]

A

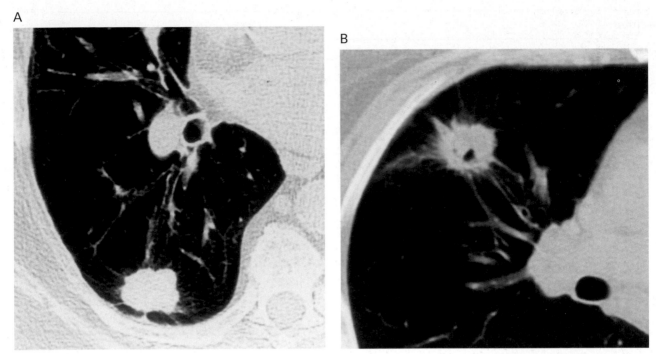

Fig C 7-16
Non–small cell cancer. (A) Lobulated and speculated nodule in the right lower lobe. (B) In another patient, there is eccentric cavitation within a speculated upper lobe nodule.[22]

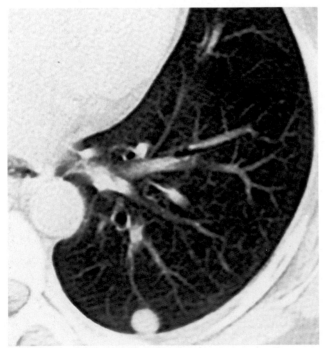

Fig C 7-17
Solitary metastasis. Smoothly marginated 1 cm peripheral nodule in a patient with bladder cancer.[22]

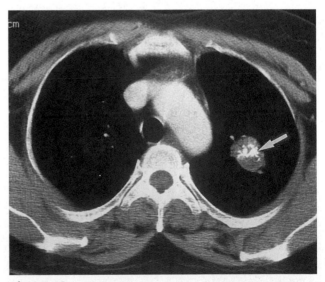

Fig C 7-18
Ossified metastasis. This left upper lobe nodule containing what appears to be dense calcification (arrow) proved to be a metastatic osteosarcoma.[21]

Condition	Comments
Bronchioloalveolar carcinoma (Fig C 7-19)	Smooth or lobulated, sharply circumscribed or ill-defined mass that tends to grow very slowly. Characteristic findings include an air bronchogram or bronchiologram in the mass and the "pleural tail" sign (linear strands extending from the lesion toward the pleura).
Non-Hodgkin's lymphoma	More commonly multiple and a manifestation of primary or secondary disease. There is usually associated hilar or mediastianal adenopathy. Because the tumor rarely obstructs the bronchial tree (unlike carcinoma), air bronchograms can often be detected within the mass.
Neuroendocrine tumor (Figs C 7-20 and C 7-21)	Up to 40% of carcinoids occur in the peripheral lung and present as solitary pulmonary nodules. They appear as round or ovoid, well-defined masses that may have slightly lobulated borders and usually show intense contrast enhancement. A punctuate or diffuse pattern of calcification or ossification can be seen in up to one-third of lesions on CT. Malignant neuroendocrine tumors usually show heterogeneous contrast enhancement due to intratumoral necrosis.
Plasmacytoma	Extrapleural mass that usually represents spread into the thorax of a primary rib lesion (therefore almost always a destructive process in one or more ribs).

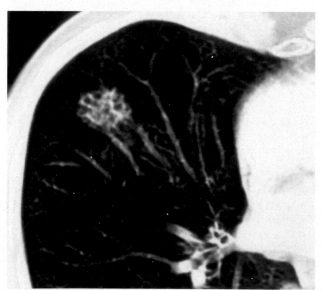

Fig C 7-19
Bronchioloalveolar carcinoma. Poorly marginated nodule in the right mid lung containing small focal areas of low attenuation, an appearance highly suggestive of bronchoalveolar cell carcinoma.[22]

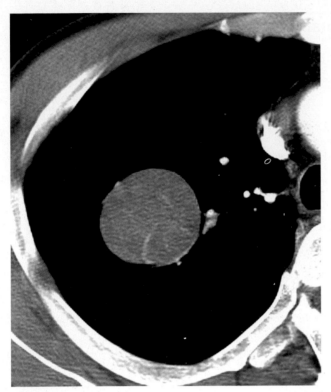

Fig C 7-20
Carcinoid. Well-defined, homogeneous mass in the right upper lobe.[17]

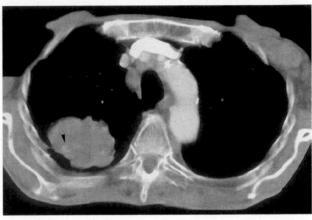

Fig C 7-21
Neuroendocrine carcinoma. Large mass containing punctuate calcifications (arrowhead) and low attenuation areas related to necrosis. Note the right paratracheal lymphadenopathy.[25]

Multiple Pulmonary Nodules

Condition	Imaging Findings	Comments
Pyogenic abscesses (Fig C 8-1)	Round, well-circumscribed masses (may have poor definition in the acute stage).	Cavitation (irregular, thick-walled) is very common. May reflect septic emboli in an intravenous drug addict.
Granulomatous infections (Figs C 8-2 and C 8-3)	Generally round or oval, well-circumscribed nodules. Irregular and poorly defined masses in *Pseudomonas*.	Histoplasmosis, tuberculosis, coccidioidomycosis, *Pseudomonas*. Calcification is common in histoplasmosis, tuberculosis, and coccidioidomycosis; cavitation is common in coccidioidomycosis and *Pseudomonas*.

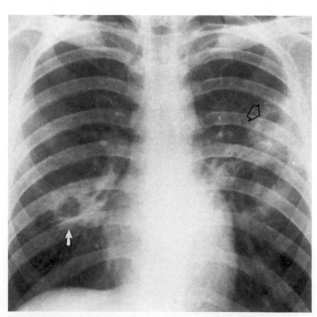

Fig C 8-1
Septic pulmonary emboli. Several round lesions, many with cavitation, are seen throughout the lungs in this intravenous drug abuser with staphylococcal tricuspid endocarditis.

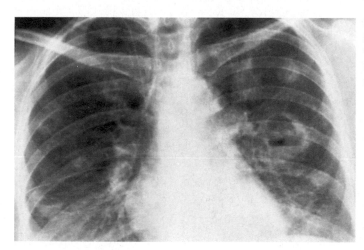

Fig C 8-2
Secondary tuberculosis. Bilateral cavitary lesions (arrows) with relatively thick walls.

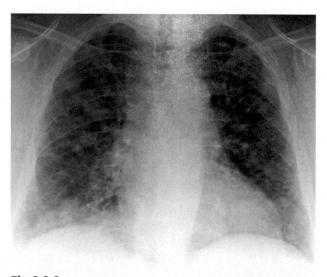

Fig C 8-3
Blastomycosis. Bilateral diffuse intermediate-sized nodules along with patchy consolidation at the lung bases.[24]

Condition	Imaging Findings	Comments
Viral infections (Figs C 8-4 and C 8-5)	Diffuse small, often ill-defined nodules throughout both lungs.	Varicella-zoster, cytomegalovirus (CMV), herpes simplex virus (HSV). Varicella (chickenpox) nodules often calcify 1 year or more after the initial infection (see Fig C 17-5).
Paragonimus westermani (Fig C 8-6)	Well-circumscribed cystic masses that have a predilection for the periphery of the lower lobes.	Characteristic appearance of multiple ring opacities or thin-walled cysts (may mimic cystic bronchiectasis).

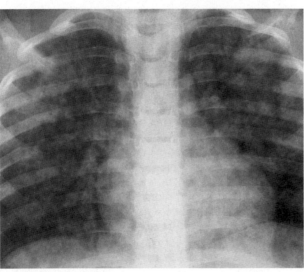

Fig C 8-4
Chickenpox pneumonia. Multiple ill-defined and occasionally confluent nodules throughout the lungs in a young child with severe combined immunodeficiency disease.[26]

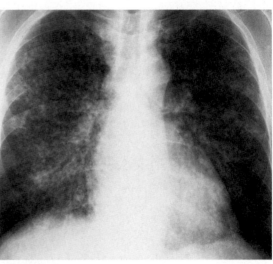

Fig C 8-5
CMV pneumonia. Multiple small, ill-defined nodules throughout the lungs that developed in a patient who had undergone a renal transplant 3 months earlier and was receiving immunosuppression therapy.[26]

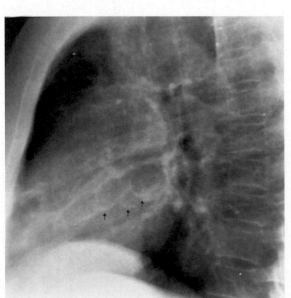

Fig C 8-6
Paragonimus westermani. Arrows point to a few of the multiple cysts in the right middle lobe. The cysts are thin walled, and most have a prominent crescent-shaped opacity along one side of their borders, the characteristic ring shadow of paragonimiasis.

Condition	Imaging Findings	Comments
Hematogenous metastases (Figs C 8-7 and C 8-8)	Various patterns (from diffuse micronodular shadows resembling miliary disease to multiple large, well-defined "cannonballs"). Tend to be more numerous in the lower lobes.	Nodules typically vary in size in the same patient. Calcification is rare but is virtually diagnostic of osteogenic sarcoma or chondrosarcoma. Cavitation occurs in approximately 4% and most commonly involves squamous cell neoplasms (also adenocarcinomas of the large bowel and sarcomas).
Bronchioloalveolar (alveolar cell) carcinoma (Fig C 8-9)	Poorly defined nodules scattered throughout both lungs.	Other presentations include a single well-circumscribed peripheral solitary nodule (see Fig C 6-13), focal "pneumonia" (see Fig C 1-25), and a miliary pattern (see Fig C 8-15).

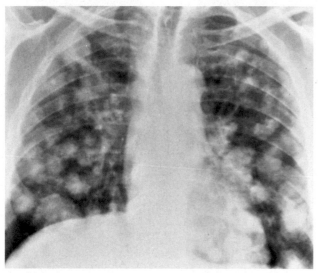

Fig C 8-7
Hematogenous metastases. Multiple well-circumscribed nodules scattered diffusely throughout both lungs.

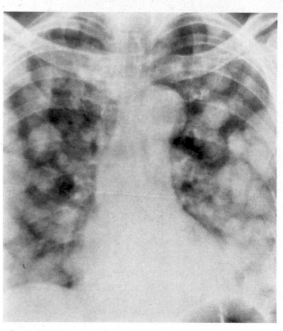

Fig C 8-8
Cannonball metastases in a patient with choriocarcinoma.

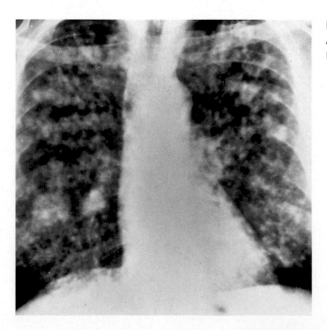

Fig C 8-9
Alveolar cell carcinoma. Multiple poorly defined nodules scattered throughout both lungs.

Condition	Imaging Findings	Comments
Papillomatosis of lung (see Fig C 11-18)	Round, sharply circumscribed nodules that frequently cavitate (often resembling advanced cystic bronchiectasis).	Usually associated with laryngeal or tracheal papillomas. Typically obstruct the airways, resulting in peripheral atelectasis and obstructive pneumonia.
Lymphoma	Multiple nodules that often have fuzzy outlines and are most numerous in the lower lobes.	Manifestation of secondary disease. Usually associated with mediastinal and hilar lymph node enlargement. Cyst-like lesions may simulate central cavitation.
Pulmonary arteriovenous fistulas (see Fig C 6-17)	Sharply defined, round or oval, often slightly lobulated nodules that predominantly involve the lower lobes. The lesions may change in size between the Valsalva and the Mueller maneuvers.	Diagnosis requires identification of the feeding artery and the draining vein. Approximately one-third of the fistulas are multiple (arteriography of both lungs required if surgical resection is contemplated). About 50% have hereditary hemorrhagic telangiectasia (Rendu-Osler-Weber disease).
Wegener's granulomatosis (see Fig C 11-14)	Round, fairly well-circumscribed nodules that may simulate metastases.	Cavitation (thick walled with irregular, shaggy inner margins) develops in approximately half the patients.
Rheumatoid necrobiotic nodules (Fig C 8-10)	Smooth, well-circumscribed nodules that predominantly occur in peripheral subpleural locations. Cavitation is common (thick walled with smooth inner margins).	Rare manifestation of rheumatoid lung disease that tends to wax and wane in relation to the activity of the rheumatoid arthritis and the presence of subcutaneous nodules. May be associated with pneumoconiosis (Caplan's syndrome).
Amyloidosis	Multiple nodules that may cavitate and show calcification or ossification.	Discrete masses of amyloid may develop in the rare parenchymal form of the disease. The nodular parenchymal form of the disease has a better prognosis than the tracheobronchial (obstructive) or diffuse interstitial types (see Fig C 4-27).
Pulmonary hematomas (see Fig C 6-14)	Unilocular or multilocular, round or oval nodules that are occasionally huge. Usually in peripheral subpleural locations deep to areas of maximum trauma.	Result from hemorrhage into pulmonary parenchymal lacerations or traumatic lung cysts. May communicate with the bronchial tree (air-fluid level). Generally a slow, progressive decrease in size (may persist for several months).

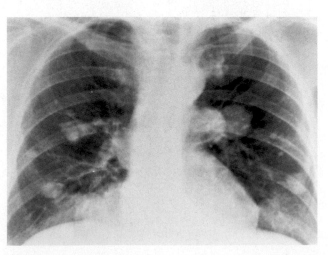

Fig C 8-10
Caplan's syndrome. Multiple well-circumscribed, rounded nodules of varying size in a patient with subcutaneous rheumatoid nodules.

Condition	Imaging Findings	Comments
Hamartomas (Fig C 8-11)	Characteristic popcorn calcification.	This most common benign tumor of the lung is usually solitary.
Sarcoidosis (Fig C 8-12)	Sharply circumscribed and widely distributed nodules that may simulate metastatic disease.	Rare manifestation. Usually associated with a reticulonodular pattern and often concomitant hilar and mediastinal adenopathy.
Pulmonary ossification	Small, densely calcified or ossified nodules throughout the lungs.	Primarily a manifestation of mitral stenosis (or other causes of elevated left atrial pressure).
Pneumoconiosis (progressive massive fibrosis) (Figs C 8-13 and C 8-14)	Conglomerate masses that predominantly involve the upper lobes and are usually irregular and ill defined with peripheral stranding.	Masses represent confluence of individual silicotic nodules, sometimes associated with superimposed tuberculous infection. They typically develop in the mid-zone or periphery of the lung and tend to migrate toward the hilum.
Polyarteritis	Poorly defined nodules that are often associated with patchy consolidations.	The pulmonary manifestations typically show progression and regression of lesions on serial films, reflecting the appearance of new lesions and the healing of old ones. The angiographic demonstration of multiple arterial aneurysms in one or more abdominal organs is considered virtually diagnostic of this disease.

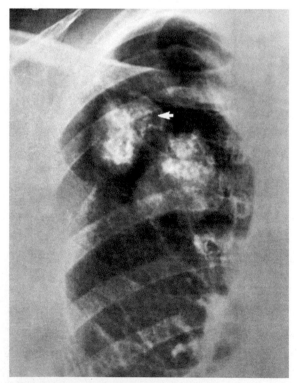

Fig C 8-11
Hamartomas. Characteristic calcification of the cartilaginous matrix (arrow).[16]

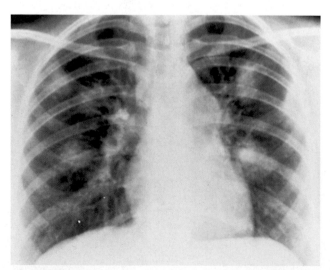

Fig C 8-12
Sarcoidosis. Patchy, ill-defined areas of air-space consolidation scattered throughout both lungs.

Condition	Imaging Findings	Comments
Pulmonary varices	Multiple, round, well-defined opacities that most commonly appear on lateral radiographs projecting posterior and inferior to the hilar structures.	Congenital or acquired tortuosity and dilatation of pulmonary veins just before their entrance into the left atrium. The varicosities change shape and size with the Valsalva and Mueller maneuvers (similar to arteriovenous fistulas).
Mucoid impactions (see Fig C 6-18)	Multiple (more commonly single), round, oval, or elliptical opacities caused by plugs in dilated bronchi.	Usually associated with hypersensitivity bronchopulmonary aspergillosis in patients with asthma or pre-existing chronic bronchial disease.

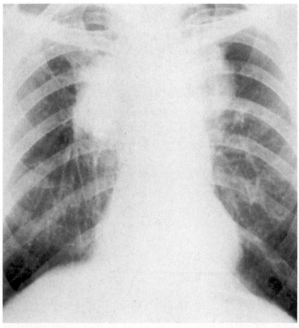

Fig C 8-13
Progressive massive fibrosis in silicosis. Non-segmental areas of homogeneous density in both upper lobes.

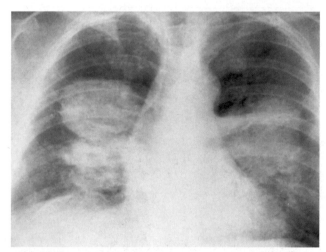

Fig C 8-14
Progressive massive fibrosis in silicosis. Large, irregular nodules in both perihilar regions.

Multiple Pulmonary Nodules on Computed Tomography

Condition	Imaging Findings	Comments
Pyogenic abscesses (Fig C 9-1)	Round, well-circumscribed masses (may have poor definition in the acute stage).	Cavitation (irregular, thick walled) is very common. May reflect septic emboli in an intravenous drug addict.
Granulomatous infections (Fig C 9-2)	Generally round or oval, well-circumscribed nodules.	Histoplasmosis, tuberculosis, coccidioidomycosis, and blastomycosis. Calcification is common in histoplasmosis, tuberculosis, and coccidioidomycosis; cavitation is common in coccidioidomycosis.
Hematogenous metastases (Figs C 9-3 and C 9-4)	Various patterns (from diffuse micronodular shadows resembling miliary disease to multiple large, well-defined "cannonballs"). Tend to be more numerous in the lower lobes.	Nodules typically vary in size in the same patient. Calcification is rare but is virtually diagnostic of osteogenic sarcoma or chondrosarcoma. Cavitation occurs in approximately 4% and most commonly involves squamous cell neoplasms (also adenocarcinomas of the large bowel and sarcomas).
Bronchioloalveolar (alveolar cell) carcinoma (Fig C 9-5)	Poorly defined nodules scattered throughout both lungs. Ground-glass opacification, with areas of increased density representing elements of adenocarcinoma.	BAC may also appear as a single well-circumscribed peripheral solitary nodule, Focal "pneumonia," a miliary pattern, or thin-walled cystic lesions.

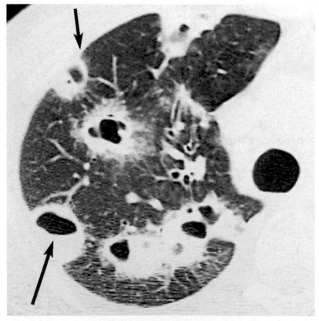

Fig C 9-1
Septic pulmonary emboli. Multiple cavitating nodules (*Nocardia*) in a young immunocompromised man. Note the feeding vessel sign (vessel leading directly to the nodule) in several nodules (arrows).[30]

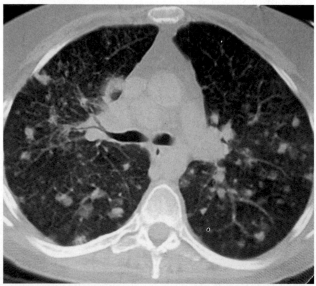

Fig C 9-2
Blastomycosis. Multiple intermediate-sized nodules in a patient with persistent and worsening symptoms of cough, chest pain, and fevers.[23]

Condition	Imaging Findings	Comments
Papillomatosis of lung (Fig C 9-6)	Round, sharply circumscribed nodules that frequently cavitate (often resembling advanced cystic bronchiectasis).	Usually associated with laryngeal or tracheal papillomas. Typically obstruct the airways, resulting in peripheral atelectasis and obstructive pneumonia.

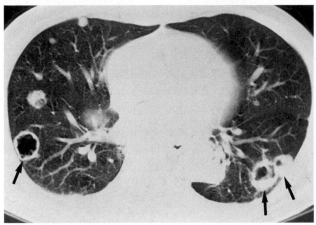

Fig C 9-3
Hematogenous metastases. Several cavitating nodules (arrows) in both lower lobes with irregular thickening of the walls in a patient with metastatic squamous cell cancer of the lungs.[22]

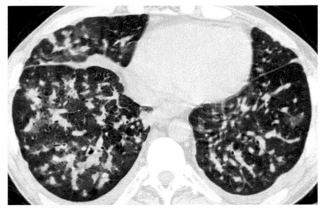

Fig C 9-4
Kaposi's sarcoma. Innumerable, bilateral, poorly defined peribronchovascular micronodules, some of which exhibit coalescence.[6]

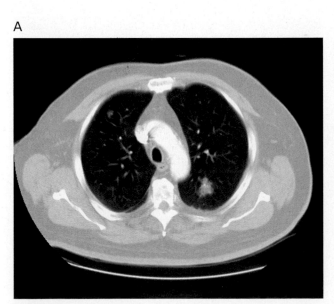

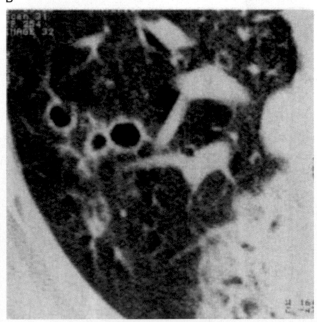

Fig C 9-5
Bronchioloalveolar carcinoma. (A) Ground-glass lesions bilaterally. The mass in the left lower lobe also contains solid elements, consistent with the diagnosis of bronchoialveolar carcinoma with adenocarcinoma features. (Courtesy of Diana Litmanovich, M.D., Boston) (B) Multiple thin-walled cystic lesions in the right lower lobe.[122]

Condition	Imaging Findings	Comments
Lymphoma (Fig C 9-7)	Multiple nodules that often have fuzzy outlines and are most numerous in the lower lobes.	Manifestation of secondary disease. Usually associated with mediastinal and hilar lymph node enlargement. Cyst-like lesions may simulate central cavitation.
Pulmonary arteriovenous fistulas	Sharply defined, round or oval, often slightly lobulated nodules that predominantly involve the lower lobes.	Diagnosis requires identification of the feeding artery and the draining vein. Approximately one-third of the fistulas are multiple (arteriography of both lungs required if surgical resection is contemplated). About 50% have hereditary hemorrhagic telangiectasia (Rendu-Osler-Weber disease).
Wegener's granulomatosis (Fig C 9-8)	Round, fairly well-circumscribed nodules that may simulate metastases.	Cavitation (thick walled with irregular, shaggy inner margins) develops in approximately half the patients.

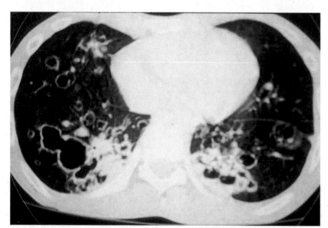

Fig C 9-6
Pulmonary papillomatosis. Multiple cavitating lung nodules, some of which contain air-fluid levels.[25]

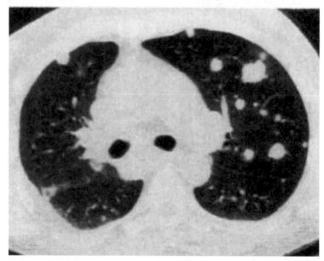

Fig C 9-7
Lymphoma. Multiple pulmonary nodules on a study obtained 10 months after cardiac transplantation.[123]

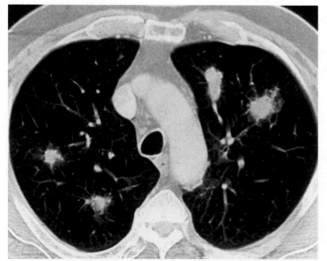

Fig C 9-8
Wegener's granulomatosis. Multiple irregular nodules in a peribronchovascular distribution.[109]

Condition	Imaging Findings	Comments
Rheumatoid necrobiotic nodules (Fig C 9-9)	Smooth, well-circumscribed nodules that predominantly occur in peripheral subpleural locations. Cavitation is common (thick walled with smooth inner margins).	Rare manifestation of rheumatoid lung disease that tends to wax and wane in relation to the activity of the rheumatoid arthritis and the presence of subcutaneous nodules. May be associated with pneumoconiosis (Caplan's syndrome).
Amyloidosis	Multiple nodules that may cavitate and show calcification or ossification.	Discrete masses of amyloid may develop in the rare parenchymal form of the disease.
Pulmonary hematomas	Unilocular or multilocular, round or oval nodules that are occasionally huge. Usually in peripheral subpleural locations deep to areas of maximum trauma	Result from hemorrhage into pulmonary parenchymal lacerations or traumatic lung cysts. May communicate with the bronchial tree (air-fluid level). Generally a slow, progressive decrease in size (may persist for several months).
Sarcoidosis (Fig C 9-10)	Sharply circumscribed and widely distributed nodules that may simulate metastatic disease.	Rare manifestation. Usually associated with a reticulonodular pattern and often concomitant hilar and mediastinal adenopathy.
Pneumoconiosis (progressive massive fibrosis) (Fig C 9-11)	Conglomerate masses that predominantly involve the upper lobes and are usually irregular and ill defined with peripheral stranding.	Masses represent confluence of individual silicotic nodules, sometimes associated with superimposed tuberculous infection. They typically develop in the mid-zone or periphery of the lung and tend to migrate toward the hilum.

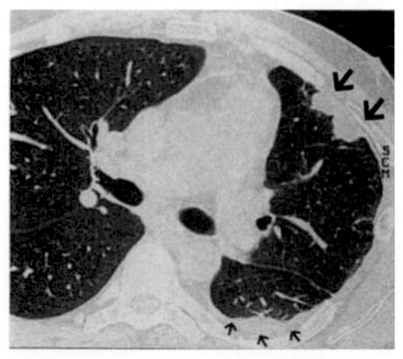

Fig C 9-9
Rheumatoid necrobiotic nodules. Two large, pleural-based nodules (large arrows) are seen at the level of the left upper lobe. The nodules are associated with marked posterior left-sided pleural thickening (small arrows).[147]

Condition	Imaging Findings	Comments
Talc injection (Fig C 9-12)	Irregular nodular in the middle and upper areas of the lungs that may coalesce to form conglomerate masses that resemble progressive massive fibrosis. Diffuse small nodules may be the first manifestation of talc-induced lung disease.	Talc (magnesium silicate) is an insoluble filler used in several oral medications to bind the active medicinal agent within the individual tablets. When oral medications are crushed, dissolved, and injected intravenously, talc particles embolize small pulmonary vessels and may then migrate into the pulmonary interstitium, where they induce a foreign-body reaction and fibrosis.
Polyarteritis	Poorly defined nodules that are often associated with patchy consolidations.	The pulmonary manifestations typically show progression and regression of lesions on serial films, reflecting the appearance of new lesions and the healing of old ones.
Mucoid impactions	Multiple (more commonly single), round, oval, or elliptical opacities caused by plugs in dilated bronchi.	Usually associated with hypersensitivity broncho-pulmonary aspergillosis in patients with asthma or pre-existing chronic bronchial disease.

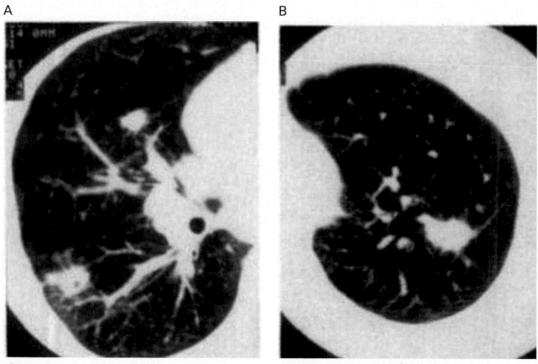

A B

Fig C 9-10
Sarcoidosis. Two images show parenchymal nodules of high attenuation involving both lungs.[148]

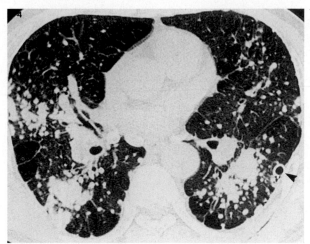

Fig C 9-11
Progressive massive fibrosis. Conglomerate masses and adjacent small nodules in coal workers' pneumoconiosis. The arrowhead points to a thoracostomy tube that was placed in the left hemithorax for a pneumothorax.[149]

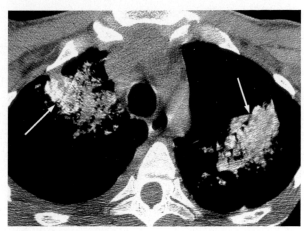

Fig C 9-12
Talc-induced lung disease. Bilateral irregular nodular areas of high attenuation in the upper lobes.[10]

Miliary Nodules*

Condition	Comments
Tuberculosis (Fig C 10-1)	Hematogenous dissemination that almost invariably leads to a dramatic febrile response with night sweats and chills. There may be minimal symptoms in severely debilitated patients, especially elderly persons and those receiving steroids.
Fungal diseases (Figs C 10-2 and C 10-3)	Hematogenous dissemination, most commonly of histoplasmosis but also coccidioidomycosis, blastomycosis, and candidiasis. May represent the healing phase of the acute epidemic form of histoplasmosis.
Disseminated hematogenous metastases (Fig C 10-4)	Most commonly thyroid carcinoma ("snowstorm"), which may remain unchanged for a long time because of the very low grade of malignancy. Other causes include trophoblastic disease, bone sarcomas, renal cell carcinoma, and, infrequently, melanoma and carcinomas of the breast and gastrointestinal tract.
Bronchioloalveolar (alveolar cell) carcinoma (Fig C 10-5)	Other presentations include a well-circumscribed, peripheral solitary nodule (see Fig C 6-13), focal "pneumonia" (see Fig C 1-25), and multiple poorly defined nodules (see Fig C 7-6).

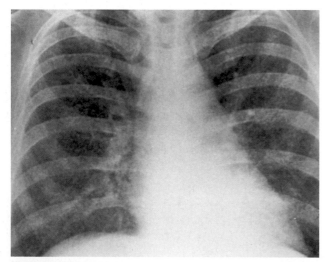

Fig C 10-1
Tuberculosis.

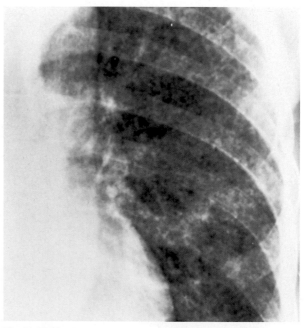

Fig C 10-2
Coccidioidomycosis. Coned view of the left lung shows a diffuse pattern of fine nodules simulating miliary tuberculosis.

*Diffuse fine nodules less than 5 mm in diameter

A

B

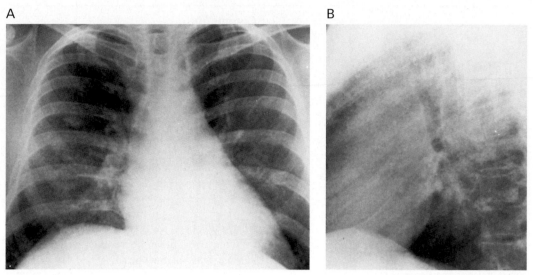

Fig C 10-3
Histoplasmosis. (A) Frontal and (B) lateral views.

B

A

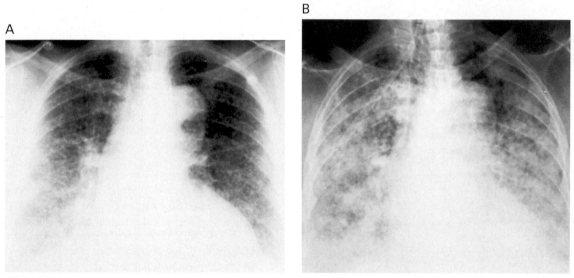

Fig C 10-4
Metastatic thyroid carcinoma. (A) Multiple fine miliary nodules scattered throughout both lungs. (B) At a later stage, there is a coarser miliary pattern.

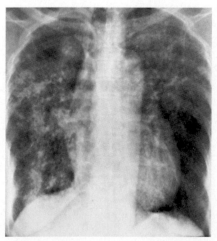

Fig C 10-5
Alveolar cell carcinoma. Miliary pattern diffusely involving both lungs represents bronchogenic spread.

Condition	Comments
Pneumoconiosis (Figs C 10-6 and C 10-7)	Silicosis, coal-workers' pneumoconiosis, and berylliosis. The nodules represent localized areas of fibrosis (or the summation of linear shadows).
Pulmonary Langerhans histiocytosis	Early active stage of the disease. The nodules represent individual granulomatous foci.
Sarcoidosis (see Fig C 14-8)	Associated bilateral and symmetric hilar adenopathy is virtually pathognomonic (though the adenopathy classically regresses as the parenchymal disease progresses).
Allergic alveolitis (farmer's lung)	Allergy involving the alveolar wall due to a variety of noninvasive fungi. Represents the subacute or chronic phase of the illness.
Viral pneumonia (Fig C 10-8)	Primarily chickenpox pneumonia (adults more than children). May heal with the development of multiple calcified nodules (as in histoplasmosis).
Alveolar microlithiasis (see Fig C 2-15)	Diffuse, very fine micronodules of calcific density that are usually asymptomatic. Characteristic black pleura sign (due to contrast between the extreme density of the lung parenchyma on one side of the pleura and the ribs on the other side).
Pulmonary hemosiderosis (Fig C 10-9)	Develops in patients with long-standing severe mitral stenosis who have had multiple episodes of hemoptysis.
Amyloidosis	Rare manifestation in which amyloid infiltrates almost every alveolar septum and is deposited around capillaries and within interstitial tissue.
Bronchiolitis obliterans	End result of lower respiratory tract damage in which the bronchioles become obstructed by organizing exudate and polypoid masses of granulation tissue.
Oil embolism	Complication of lymphography (lipid material in the extravascular interstitial tissue).
Interstitial fibrosis	Early stage before the development of the more classic reticulonodular and reticular patterns.
Niemann-Pick disease	Rare lipid storage disease. The miliary nodule pattern (and early age of onset) is a differential point from Gaucher's disease.
Parasitic disease (Fig C 10-10)	Schistosomiasis, filariasis.
Listeriosis (Fig C 10-11)	Rare bacterial disease that primarily occurs as an intrauterine infection with a high mortality rate, or as a disease of the newborn.

Condition	Comments
Rheumatoid disease	Miliary pattern occurs in the early "subacute" stage of the disease before the development of the more characteristic diffuse interstitial pulmonary fibrosis.
Wegener's granulomatosis	Rare manifestation representing a diffuse granulomatous reaction occurring around vessels. The small fine nodules usually develop in combination with larger, more ill-defined densities that often cavitate.

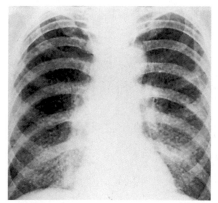

Fig C 10-6
Silicosis.

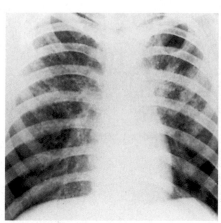

Fig C 10-7
Coal-workers' pneumoconiosis.

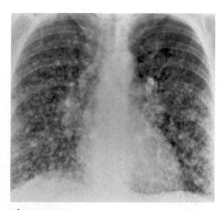

Fig C 10-8
Chickenpox pneumonia. Bilateral, coarse miliary infiltrates distributed diffusely throughout both lungs.

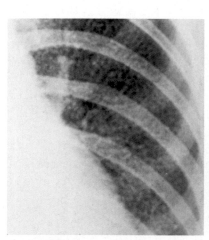

Fig C 10-9
Pulmonary hemosiderosis.[27]

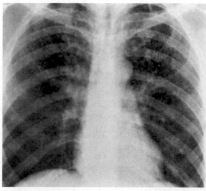

Fig C 10-10
Schistosomiasis. Perivascular granulomas produce small nodular and linear densities that are distributed diffusely throughout the lungs in a miliary pattern simulating tuberculosis.

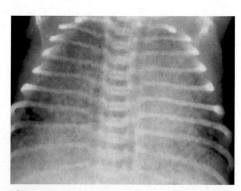

Fig C 10-11
Listeriosis. Diffuse miliary pattern of coarse, irregular granular densities is distributed throughout both lungs.

Cavitary Lesions of the Lungs

Condition	Imaging Findings	Comments
Bacterial lung abscess (Fig C 11-1)	Generally a thick-walled cavity with a shaggy inner lining.	Most frequently *Staphylococcus, Klebsiella, Pseudomonas,* and *Proteus*. An empyema is commonly associated. Multiple cavities often occur with anaerobic organisms.
Pneumatocele (Fig C 11-2)	Thin-walled cystic space (may be multiple).	Develops in approximately 50% of children with staphylococcal pneumonia. Results from a check-valve obstruction of the communication between a peribronchial abscess and the bronchial lumen.

A   B

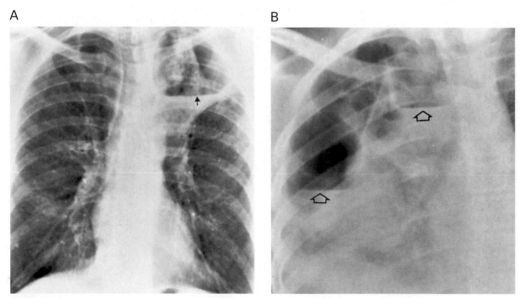

Fig C 11-1
Bacterial lung abscess. (A) *Proteus* pneumonia. Large, thick-walled left upper lobe abscess with an air-fluid level (arrow) and an associated infiltrate. (B) *Staphylococcal pneumonia*. Multiple lung abscesses with air-fluid levels (arrows) associated with diffuse air-space consolidation and a large pleural effusion.

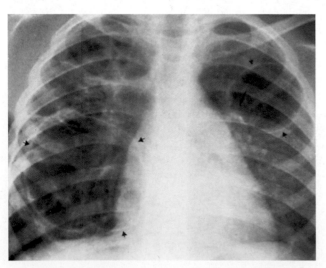

Fig C 11-2
Pneumatocele. Residual thin-walled cystic spaces (arrows) in the pulmonary parenchyma many years after a childhood staphylococcal pneumonia.

Condition	Imaging Findings	Comments
Mycobacteria (Figs C 11-3 and C 11-4)	Wall of the cavity is usually of moderate thickness and has a generally smooth inner lining.	Cavitation (often multiple) tends to be a more prominent feature of atypical mycobacterial disease than of *Mycobacterium tuberculosis*. Tuberculous cavities predominantly involve the apical and posterior regions of the upper lobes and the posterior segments of the lower lobes. Thin-walled cavities may persist after chemotherapy in the absence of acute disease.

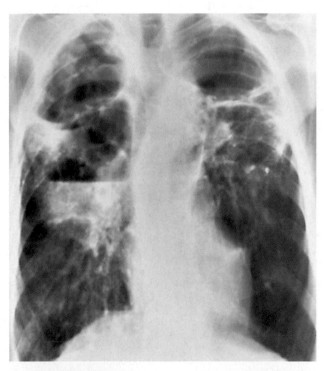

Fig C 11-3
Tuberculosis. Multiple large cavities with air-fluid levels in both upper lobes. Note the chronic fibrotic changes and upward retraction of the hila.

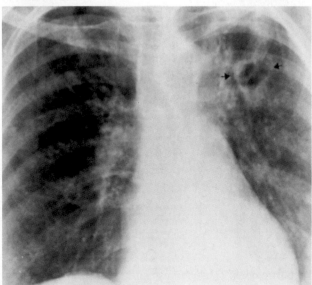

Fig C 11-4
Atypical mycobacteria. Cavitary lesion (arrows) in the left upper lobe. The wall of the cavity is mildly irregular, and there is minimal parenchymal disease

Condition	Imaging Findings	Comments
Fungal lung abscess (Figs C 11-5 to C 11-7)	Single or multiple cavities, most of which are thick walled (coccidioidomycosis tends to produce a very thin-walled lesion).	Pleural effusion and extension into the chest wall are common in actinomycosis and nocardiosis. Histoplasmosis typically involves the apical and posterior segments of the upper lobes (indistinguishable from tuberculosis), whereas coccidioidomycosis is characteristically located in the anterior segment. Candidiasis, aspergillosis, sporotrichosis, and mucormycosis are essentially limited to debilitated patients and those with underlying diseases (diabetes mellitus, lymphoma, leukemia).

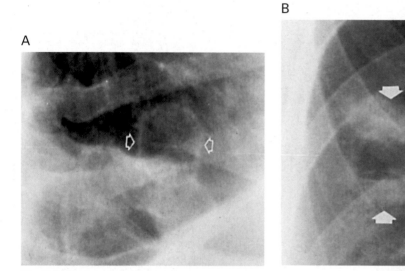

Fig C 11-5
Coccidioidomycosis. (A) Thin-walled cavity (arrows). (B) Irregular, thick-walled cavity with surrounding infiltrate (arrows).

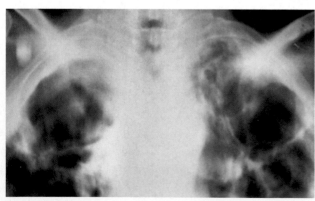

Fig C 11-6
Sporotrichosis. Frontal tomogram shows extensive bilateral upper lobe cavities.[15]

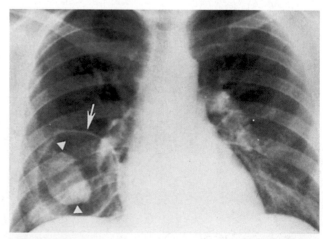

Fig C 11-7
Mucormycosis. Large thin-walled cavity (arrow) containing a smooth, elliptical, homogeneous mass (arrowheads) representing a fungus ball.

Condition	Imaging Findings	Comments
Amebic lung abscess	Thick-walled cavity with a ragged inner lining.	Almost always in the right lower lobe and associated with a right pleural effusion (organisms from a liver abscess enter the thorax by direct extension via the right hemidiaphragm).
Hydatid cyst (*Echinococcus granulosus*) (Fig C 11-8)	Thin-walled cavity, typically with a lower lobe predominance.	Rupture of the cyst into a bronchus results in part or all of its liquid contents being expelled into the bronchial system, producing the characteristic "meniscus sign" and "water lily sign" (irregularity of the air-fluid layer caused by collapsed cyst membranes). A hydropneumothorax may also occur.
Paragonimus westermani (Fig C 11-9)	Thin-walled cysts (ring shadows) that are generally multiple and have a predilection for the periphery of the lower lobes.	Typically a crescent-shaped opacity along one aspect of the inner lining. May mimic cystic bronchiectasis.

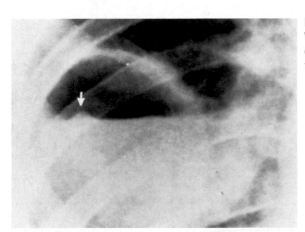

Fig C 11-8
Water lily sign in pulmonary echinococcal cyst. The endocyst membranes (arrow) are floating on the surface of fluid in a ruptured hydatid cyst.[28]

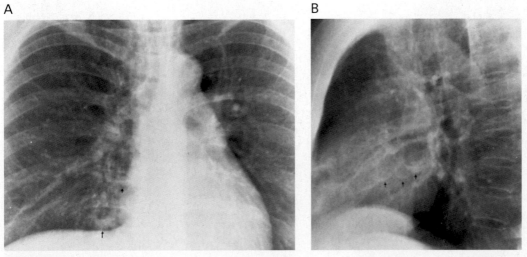

Fig C 11-9
Paragonimiasis. (A) Frontal and (B) lateral chest radiographs demonstrate multiple cysts (arrows) in the right middle lobe. The cysts are thin walled, and most have a prominent crescent-shaped opacity along one side of their borders, the characteristic ring shadow of paragonimiasis.

Condition	Imaging Findings	Comments
Pneumocystis carinii (Fig C 11-10)	Single or multiple thin-walled cavities.	Primarily seen in patients with AIDS.
Bronchogenic carcinoma (Fig C 11-11)	Generally a thick-walled cavity with an irregular, nodular inner lining (occasionally a thin-walled cavity simulating a bronchogenic cyst).	Cavitation in 2% to 10% of cases, most commonly in peripheral squamous cell tumors of the upper lobes. Multiple primaries are very rare.
Hematogenous metastases (Fig C 11-12)	Thin- or thick-walled cavities may develop in a few or multiple metastatic nodules. Most commonly involves upper lobe lesions.	Cavitation in approximately 4% of cases. Most commonly involves squamous cell neoplasms (also adenocarcinomas of the large bowel and sarcomas).
Hodgkin's disease	Single or multiple thick-walled cavities with irregular inner linings.	Cavitation typically develops in peripheral parenchymal consolidations (most often in the lower lobes). Usually, enlargement of mediastinal and hilar lymph nodes is also seen.
Septic embolism (Figs C 11-13 and C 11-14)	Generally thin-walled cavities (less commonly thick walled with shaggy inner linings).	Almost always multiple with lower lobe predominance. A wide variation in size may reflect recurrent showers of emboli.
Silicosis	Thick-walled cavity with an irregular inner lining. Often multiple with strong upper lobe predominance.	Generally a background of nodular or reticulonodular disease and associated hilar lymph node enlargement. Cavitation in conglomerate lesions is more often the result of superimposed tuberculosis than ischemic necrosis. Cavitation also occurs in coal-workers' pneumoconiosis.
Wegener's granulomatosis (Fig C 11-15)	Usually multiple thick-walled cavities with irregular inner linings (may eventually become thin-walled cystic spaces).	Cavitation eventually occurs in approximately half of patients. With treatment, the cavitary lesions may disappear or heal with scar formation.

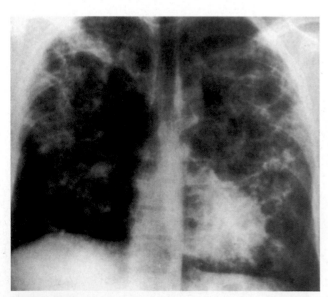

Fig C 11-10
Pneumocystis carinii. Innumerable thin-walled cavities.[29]

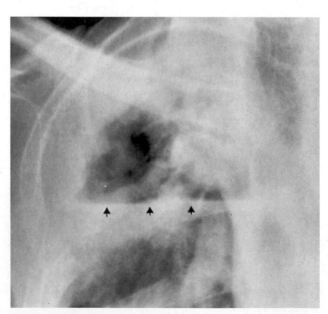

Fig C 11-11
Bronchogenic carcinoma. Large cavitary right upper lobe mass with an air-fluid level (arrows) and associated rib destruction.

Condition	Imaging Findings	Comments
Rheumatoid necrobiotic nodule	Thick-walled cavity with a smooth inner lining (may become thin-walled and even disappear with remission of the arthritis).	Often multiple and generally in a peripheral subpleural location (most often the lower lobe). May be associated with pleural effusion or spontaneous pneumothorax.

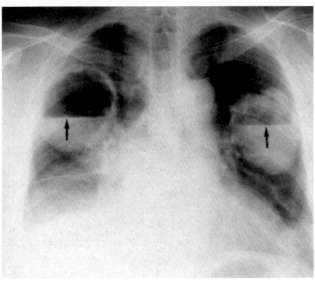

Fig C 11-12
Hematogenous metastases. Extensive cavitation with air-fluid levels (arrows) of squamous cell carcinoma on a film obtained after two cycles of chemotherapy.[22]

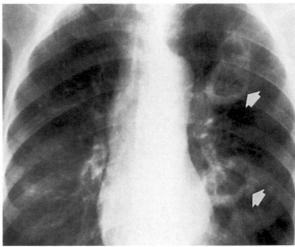

Fig C 11-13
Septic pulmonary emboli. Large cavity lesions (arrows) in the left lung of an intravenous drug abuser with septic thrombophlebitis.

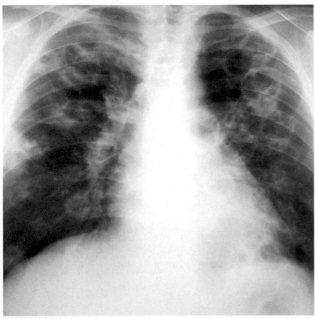

Fig C 11-14
Septic pulmonary emboli. Multiple cavitary nodules throughout both lungs representing *Nocardia* septic emboli in an intravenous drug abuser with AIDS.[30]

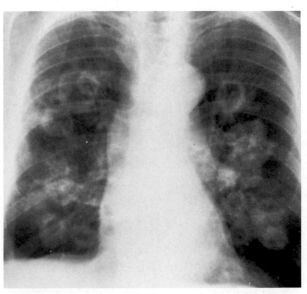

Fig C 11-15
Wegener's granulomatosis. Multiple thick-walled cavities with irregular, shaggy inner linings.

Condition	Imaging Findings	Comments
Cystic bronchiectasis (Fig C 11-16)	Multiple thin-walled cavities with lower lobe predominance. Often a tiny air-fluid level at the bottom of the ring shadow.	Cavities represent severely dilated segmental bronchi. Generally a considerable loss of volume in the affected region.
Bleb/bulla (Fig C 11-17)	Very thin-walled cystic space. Usually multiple with upper lobe predominance.	Air-fluid levels develop with infection. Often radiographic evidence of diffuse pulmonary emphysema.
Traumatic lung cyst	Single or several thin-walled cavities that may contain air-fluid levels.	Typically occurs in a peripheral subpleural location immediately underlying the point of maximum injury.
Sarcoidosis	Cystic lesions developing on a background of diffuse reticulonodular pulmonary disease.	Very uncommon manifestation (should suggest superimposed tuberculosis or fungal disease). A mycetoma may occur in a cavitary lesion.
Intralobar bronchopulmonary sequestration	Thin- or thick-walled cystic mass that is often multilocular or multiple.	Almost invariably arises contiguous to the diaphragm (two-thirds are on the left). May be obscured by pneumonia in the surrounding parenchyma.
Bronchogenic cyst	Solitary thin-walled cystic mass that may contain an air-fluid level.	Approximately 75% of bronchogenic cysts that are originally opaque and fluid filled eventually become air containing because of an infectious communication with the contiguous lung.
Congenital cystic adenomatoid malformation (see Fig C 15-7)	Multiple air-containing cysts scattered irregularly throughout a mass of soft-tissue density.	Expands the ipsilateral hemithorax (depresses the hemidiaphragm and shifts the mediastinum to the contralateral side). May occasionally be confused with a diaphragmatic hernia containing bowel loops. The malformation can often be detected by fetal ultrasound.

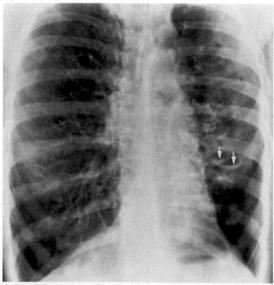

Fig C 11-16
Cystic bronchiectasis. Multiple cystic spaces, some with air-fluid levels (arrows), predominantly involve the left lung.

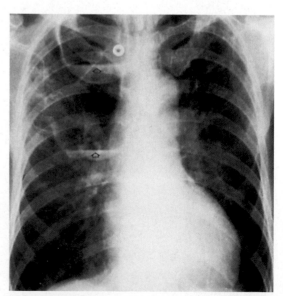

Fig C 11-17
Pulmonary emphysema. Large bullae in the right upper lung. The presence of air-fluid levels (arrows) in the cystic spaces indicates superimposed infection.

Condition	Imaging Findings	Comments
Cystic fibrosis (mucoviscidosis) (Fig C 11-18)	Thin-walled cystic lesions with or without air-fluid levels associated with diffuse, coarse, reticular changes, hyperinflation, and pulmonary arterial hypertension.	Ring shadows in this condition can be caused by cystic bronchiectasis, bullae, microabscesses, or honeycombing.
Papillomatosis (Fig C 11-19)	Multiple thin-walled cysts.	Laryngeal papillomatosis is a common disease in children that infrequently seeds distally in the tracheobronchial tree to produce excavating lesions in the lung.
Plombage (Fig C 11-20)	Plastic (lucite) spheres appear radiographically as multiple perfectly round, cavity-like lucencies.	Former therapy for pulmonary tuberculosis that consisted of filling of the extrapleural space with a sufficient volume of inert material to collapse the adjacent lung. The spheres are often not entirely watertight, so that a small amount of fluid may collect in each. On upright views, the resulting air-fluid levels can simulate cavitation and suggest the incorrect diagnosis of acute infection.

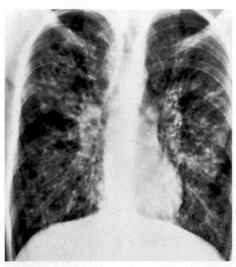

Fig C 11-18
Cystic fibrosis. Multiple small cysts superimposed on a diffuse, coarse, reticular pattern.

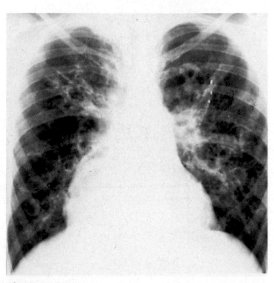

Fig C 11-19
Papillomatosis. Multiple thin-walled cystic lesions.

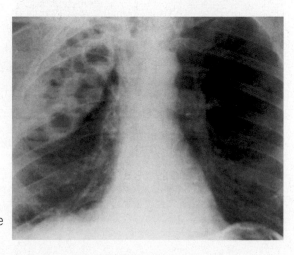

Fig C 11-20
Plombage. Air-fluid levels in the plastic spheres simulate cavitation.

Unilateral Hilar Enlargement

Condition	Comments
Inflammatory lymphadenopathy (Figs C 12-1 and C 12-2)	Histoplasmosis, tuberculosis, coccidioidomycosis. The hilar nodes often calcify and are usually associated with ipsilateral parenchymal disease.
Intrabronchial neoplasm	Hilar mass generally represents local nodal metastases (the endobronchial lesion itself usually produces only a minimal mass effect).
Metastatic neoplasm (Fig C 12-3)	Often bilateral, with involvement of mediastinal lymph nodes. In lymphangitic spread, there is generally a diffuse reticular or reticulonodular pattern.
Lymphoma	Primarily Hodgkin's disease, which often produces asymmetric bilateral hilar adenopathy. There may be pulmonary involvement or pleural effusion. The nodes may calcify after mediastinal irradiation.

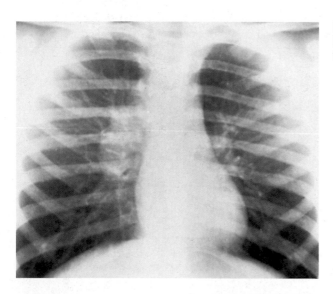

Fig C 12-1
Primary tuberculosis. Enlargement of right hilar nodes without a discrete parenchymal infiltrate.

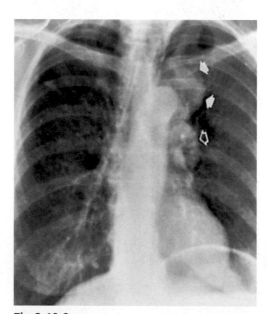

Fig C 12-3
Lymphadenopathy due to oat cell carcinoma of the lung. In addition to left hilar adenopathy (open arrow), there is enlargement of anterior mediastinal lymph nodes (closed arrows).

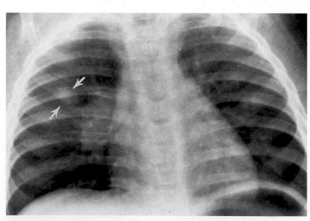

Fig C 12-2
Primary tuberculosis. The combination of a focal parenchymal lesion (arrows) and enlarged right hilar lymph nodes produces the classic primary complex.

Condition	Comments
Valvular pulmonic stenosis (see Fig CA 15-6)	Poststenotic dilatation of the left pulmonary artery. There is usually enlargement of the right ventricle. Central dilatation of the right pulmonary artery also occurs, but the dilated segment is hidden in the mediastinum (left-sided enlargement is not due to the direction of the jet emanating from the constricted valve).
Pulmonary embolism (Fig C 12-4)	Result of vascular distention by bulk thrombus (not increased vascular resistance in the affected lung). The occluded vessel is often more sharply delineated than normal and may terminate suddenly ("knuckle" sign).
Pulmonary artery aneurysm	Congenital or posttraumatic.
Pulmonary artery coarctation	Poststenotic dilatation of the affected pulmonary artery.
Pulmonary arteriovenous fistula	Enlargement of hilar vessels is due to increased blood flow on the affected side. There is often evidence of single or multiple parenchymal nodules with characteristic feeding arteries and draining veins.
Normal variant (see Fig CA 15-1)	Prominence of the left pulmonary artery occurs in adults younger than 30 (especially women).
Narrowed or occluded pulmonary artery	Unilateral enlargement of the opposite hilum may develop in patients with carcinoma, Swyer-James syndrome, or congenital absence of the pulmonary artery.

A

B

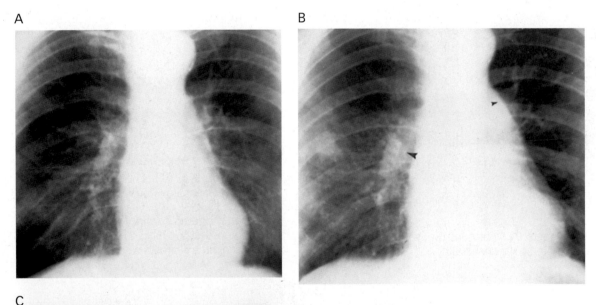

C

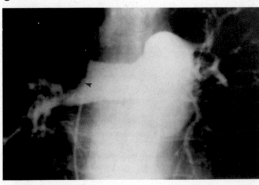

Fig C 12-4
Pulmonary embolism. (A) Baseline chest radiograph demonstrates normal-sized pulmonary arteries. (B) Enlargement of the main pulmonary artery (small arrow) and right pulmonary artery (large arrow) coincides with the onset of the patient's symptoms. (C) Arteriogram demonstrates multiple bilateral pulmonary emboli and a large right saddle embolus (arrow).

Bilateral Hilar Enlargement

Condition	Imaging Findings	Comments
Lymphadenopathy (Figs C 13-1 through C 13-6)	Bilateral enlargement of hilar nodes that may be associated with reticular or reticulonodular parenchymal disease.	Causes include infectious agents (especially tuberculosis, histoplasmosis, mycoplasma, and viral pneumonias), malignancy (carcinoma, lymphoma), silicosis, and sarcoidosis.
Congenital heart disease (see Fig CA 13-4)	Bilateral enlargement of pulmonary vessels that is usually associated with cardiomegaly.	Severe left-to-right shunts (atrial septal defect, ventricular septal defect, patent ductus arteriosus). Also cyanotic admixture lesions (transposition of great vessels, persistent truncus arteriosus).
Pulmonary arterial hypertension (Fig C 13-7)	Bilateral enlargement of central pulmonary arteries with rapid tapering and small peripheral vessels. Also cardiac enlargement (especially the right ventricle).	Primary or secondary to such conditions as widespread peripheral pulmonary emboli, Eisenmenger's syndrome (reversed left-to-right shunt), and chronic obstructive emphysema. Rare causes include metastases from trophoblastic neoplasms, immunologic disorders (Raynaud's phenomenon, rheumatoid disease), schistosomiasis, multiple pulmonary artery stenoses or coarctations, and vasoconstrictive diseases.

A

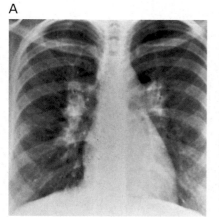

B

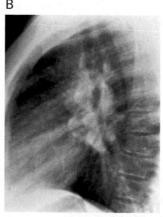

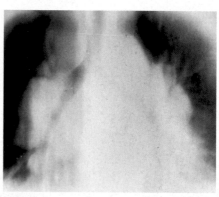

Fig C 13-1
Infectious mononucleosis. (A) Frontal and (B) lateral views of the chest demonstrate marked bilateral hilar adenopathy.

Fig C 13-2
Bronchogenic carcinoma. Tomography demonstrates bilateral bulky hilar adenopathy typical of oat cell carcinoma.

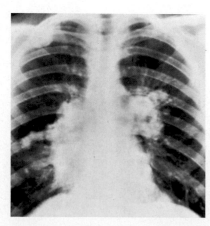

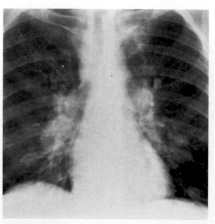

Fig C 13-3
Ossified metastases to hilar lymph nodes bilaterally from osteogenic sarcoma. There are also multiple parenchymal metastases.

Fig C 13-4
Lymphoma. Frontal view shows bilateral hilar adenopathy.

Condition	Imaging Findings	Comments
Pulmonary embolism	Bilateral enlargement of central pulmonary arteries. Usually obliteration of peripheral vessels and right-sided cardiac enlargement.	May reflect massive bilateral central emboli or widespread peripheral emboli.
Pulmonary venous hypertension	Bilateral enlargement of central pulmonary veins associated with cardiomegaly and cephalization of pulmonary blood flow.	Causes include left-sided heart failure and mitral stenosis.
Primary polycythemia	Generalized bilateral increase in central and peripheral pulmonary vascularity.	Increased blood volume produces prominence of the pulmonary vascular shadows, usually without the cardiomegaly associated with the increased pulmonary vascularity in patients with congenital heart disease. Intravascular thrombosis may cause pulmonary infarctions that appear as focal consolidations or bands of fibrosis.

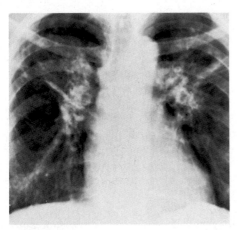

Fig C 13-5
Silicosis. Characteristic eggshell lymph node calcification associated with bilateral perihilar masses.

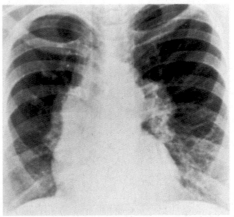

Fig C 13-6
Sarcoidosis. Prominent bilateral hilar adenopathy with a suggestion of enlarged nodes in the right and left paratracheal regions.

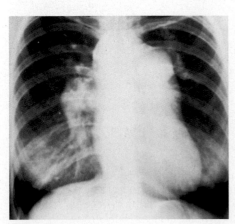

Fig C 13-7
Pulmonary arterial hypertension. Frontal chest film in a patient with atrial septal defect and Eisenmenger's physiology demonstrates a huge pulmonary outflow tract and central pulmonary arteries with abrupt tapering and sparse peripheral vasculature.[31]

Hilar and Mediastinal Lymph Node Enlargement

Condition	Imaging Findings	Comments
Primary tuberculosis (see Figs C 12-1 and C 12-2)	Enlarged hilar and paratracheal nodes that often calcify. Bilateral involvement in approximately 20% of cases.	Almost always associated with ipsilateral parenchymal disease (may even obscure the lymphadenopathy).
Histoplasmosis	Unilateral or bilateral enlargement of hilar, mediastinal, and, occasionally, intrapulmonary nodes.	Usually associated with parenchymal disease (often absent in children). The enlarged nodes may extrinsically obstruct the airways and cause distal infection or atelectasis. Calcification of nodes is common and may even lead to erosion into the bronchial lumen.
Coccidioidomycosis	Unilateral or bilateral enlargement of hilar or paratracheal nodes.	There may be associated parenchymal disease. Enlargement of paratracheal lymph nodes may indicate imminent dissemination.
Mycoplasma pneumoniae	Unilateral or bilateral enlargement of hilar nodes.	Common in children, rare in adults. Always associated with ipsilateral parenchymal disease.
Viral diseases (Fig C 14-1; see Fig C 13-1)	Hilar node enlargement that is often bilateral.	Psittacosis, infectious mononucleosis (also splenomegaly), rubeola, echovirus, varicella. Usually parenchymal involvement or increased bronchovascular markings.
Bacterial infections (Figs C 14-2 and C 14-3)	Various patterns of nodal enlargement.	Unilateral in pertussis (whooping cough) and tularemia (ipsilateral hilar enlargement in 25% to 50% of tularemic pneumonias); bilateral involvement in anthrax and plague.

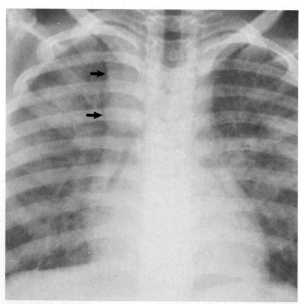

Fig C 14-1
Measles pneumonia. Diffuse, reticular interstitial infiltrate with a focal area of consolidation in the right upper lobe. Note the striking right hilar and mediastinal adenopathy (arrows).

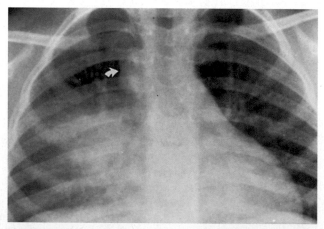

Fig C 14-2
Tularemia pneumonia. Air-space consolidation involving the right middle lobe and a portion of the right upper lobe. Note the right paratracheal nodal enlargement (arrow).

Condition	Imaging Findings	Comments
Bronchogenic carcinoma (Fig C 14-4)	Usually unilateral enlargement of hilar nodes.	Presenting sign in up to one-third of patients (primary carcinoma arising in a major hilar bronchus or metastasis from a small primary tumor in adjacent or peripheral parenchyma). Bulky, even bilateral, nodal enlargement suggests oat cell carcinoma.

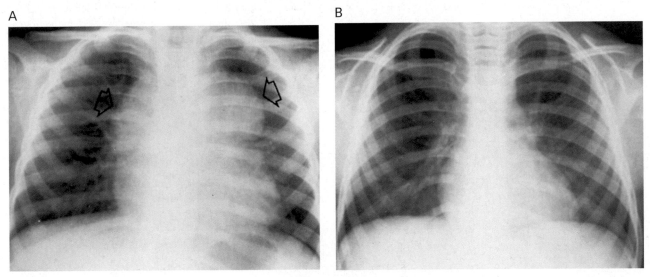

A   B

Fig C 14-3
Bubonic plague. (A) Initial film demonstrates massive enlargement of the mediastinal lymph nodes (arrows). (B) After chloramphenicol therapy, a repeat chest film demonstrates complete clearing of the lymphadenopathy.[32]

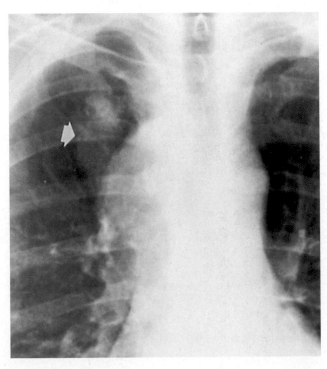

Fig C 14-4
Oat cell carcinoma. Prominent right mediastinal lymphadenopathy associated with an ill-defined primary malignant lesion (arrow).

Condition	Imaging Findings	Comments
Lymphoma (Figs C 14-5 and C 14-6)	Enlargement of all hilar and mediastinal nodes (the anterior mediastinal and retrosternal nodes are frequently affected). Typically bilateral but asymmetric (unilateral node enlargement is very rare).	Most common radiographic finding in Hodgkin's disease (visible on the initial chest films of ~50% of patients). Pulmonary involvement or pleural effusion occurs in about 30%. Calcification may develop in intrathoracic lymph nodes after mediastinal irradiation.
Leukemia (Fig C 14-7)	Symmetric enlargement of hilar and mediastinal nodes in approximately 25% of patients.	Lymphadenopathy occurs more commonly in lymphocytic than in myelocytic leukemia. There may also be pleural effusion and parenchymal involvement.
Metastases (lymphangitic spread)	Unilateral or bilateral enlargement of hilar or mediastinal nodes.	Usually associated with a diffuse reticular or reticulonodular pattern that predominantly involves the lung bases (see Fig C 4-1).

A B

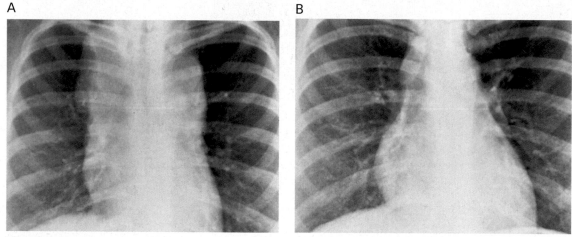

Fig C 14-5
Lymphoma. (A) Initial chest film demonstrates marked widening of the upper half of the mediastinum due to pronounced lymphadenopathy. (B) After chemotherapy, there is a marked decrease in the width of the upper mediastinum.

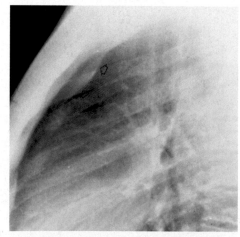

Fig C 14-6
Lymphoma. Lateral view of the chest shows subtle enlargement of a retrosternal (internal mammary) lymph node (arrows).

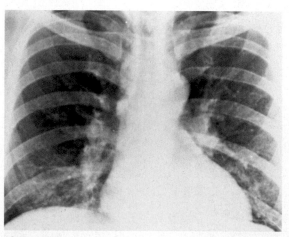

Fig C 14-7
Leukemia. Bilateral hilar and right paratracheal lymphadenopathy.

Condition	Imaging Findings	Comments
Silicosis (see Fig C 13-5)	Bilateral hilar node enlargement. Typical eggshell calcification (in approximately 10% of patients) is almost pathognomonic (occasionally occurs in sarcoidosis or radiated Hodgkin's disease) and can involve mediastinal, peritoneal, and retroperitoneal nodes.	Usually associated with a diffuse nodular or reticulonodular pattern throughout both lungs. A similar appearance may occur in chronic berylliosis.
Sarcoidosis (Fig C 14-8)	Bilaterally symmetric enlargement of hilar and paratracheal nodes develops in up to 90% of patients. The outer borders of the enlarged hila are usually lobulated.	Approximately half of patients have diffuse parenchymal disease. Nodal enlargement often resolves as the parenchymal disease develops, unlike lymphoma or tuberculosis. The bilateral symmetry is unlike tuberculosis, whereas the lack of retrosternal involvement is unlike lymphoma.
Pulmonary Langerhans cell histiocytosis	Symmetric enlargement of hilar and mediastinal nodes is a rare manifestation.	Early diffuse micronodular pattern that may become coarse in later stages. Lack of lymph node enlargement in a patient with diffuse interstitial pulmonary disease favors a diagnosis of histiocytosis X rather than sarcoidosis.
Idiopathic pulmonary hemosiderosis/ Goodpasture's syndrome	Symmetric enlargement of hilar nodes primarily occurs in the acute stage.	Episodes of pulmonary hemorrhage produce diffuse alveolar and interstitial disease.
Cystic fibrosis	Unilateral or bilateral hilar node enlargement is an uncommon finding.	Diffuse increase in pulmonary markings with hyperinflation and areas of atelectasis and bronchiectasis.
Bronchopulmonary amyloidosis	Symmetric enlargement of hilar and mediastinal nodes (may be densely calcified).	Rare manifestation of this plasma cell dyscrasia. Sometimes associated with diffuse pulmonary involvement.
Heavy-chain disease	Symmetric enlargement of mediastinal nodes.	Unusual manifestation of this rare plasma cell dyscrasia. Hepatosplenomegaly is common, whereas lung involvement is rare.
Drug-induced changes	Bilateral hilar or mediastinal lymph node enlargement.	May develop during diphenylhydantoin or trimethadione therapy.

B

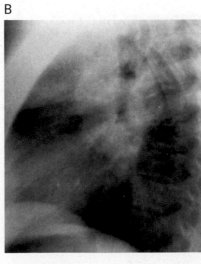

A

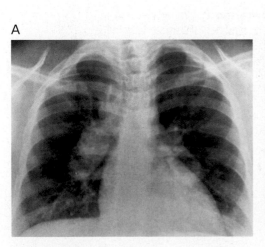

Fig C 14-8
Sarcoidosis. (A) Frontal and (B) lateral views of the chest demonstrate enlargement of the right hilar, left hilar, and right paratracheal lymph nodes, producing the classic 1-2-3 pattern of adenopathy.

Unilateral Lobar or Localized Hyperlucency of the Lung

Condition	Imaging Findings	Comments
Local obstructive emphysema	Localized hyperlucency of the lung associated with thin, attenuated vessels (predominantly involves the lower zones).	Approximately 50% of cases of emphysema have local rather than diffuse involvement radiographically. Affected zones show air trapping on expiration and overinflation at full lung capacity.
Bulla/bleb (Figs C 15-1 and C 15-2)	Sharply defined, air-containing spaces that are bounded by curvilinear, hairline shadows and vary in size from 1 cm to an entire hemithorax.	Predominantly unilateral. Unlike local obstructive emphysema, the vascular markings are absent rather than attenuated. Overinflation and air trapping usually occur.
Foreign body aspiration (see Fig C 31-3)	Segmental distribution with lower lobe predominance (especially on the right). Characteristic air trapping on expiratory films and often local oligemia.	Most common manifestation of foreign body aspiration. An opaque foreign body may be demonstrated.
Compensatory overaeration (Fig C 15-3)	Overinflation and oligemia of the remaining lobe(s).	Lobar collapse or agenesis causes overdistention of the normal portions of the lung.

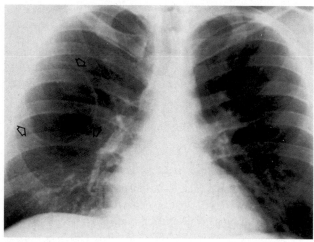

Fig C 15-1
Congenital emphysematous bulla. Large thin-walled air cyst (arrows) in the mid-portion of the right lung.

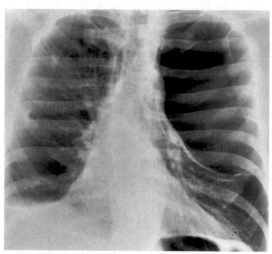

Fig C 15-2
Giant emphysematous bulla. The air-containing mass fills most of the left hemithorax.

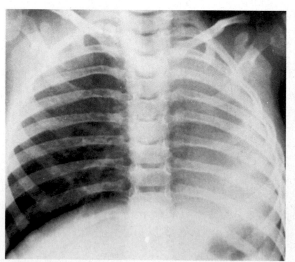

Fig C 15-3
Compensatory overaeration in agenesis of the left lung. There is virtually total absence of aerated lung in the left hemithorax. The right lung is markedly overinflated and has herniated across the midline. The entire mediastinum lies within the left hemithorax. The chest wall is asymmetric, and the ribs are somewhat close together on the left.

Condition	Imaging Findings	Comments
Pulmonary neoplasm	Segmental, lobar, or entire lung involvement. Air trapping on expiratory films.	Benign or malignant endobronchial neoplasms are a rare cause of unilateral or segmental hyperlucent lung (more commonly bronchial obstruction is complete and results in atelectasis or postobstructive pneumonia). Metastases to hilar lymph nodes occasionally compress a bronchus and cause oligemia.
Thromboembolic disease (Fig C 15-4)	Affected segment often shows moderate loss of volume but may still appear hyperlucent due to local oligemia (Westermark's sign).	Almost invariably associated with obstruction of a major lobar or segmental pulmonary artery. The affected artery is typically widened and is sharper than normal.

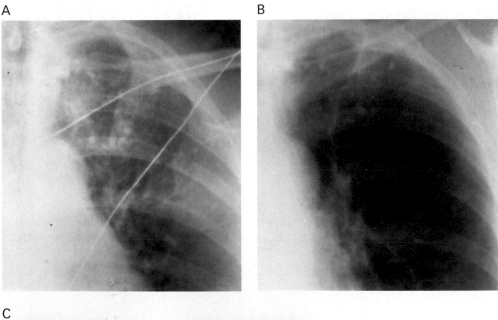

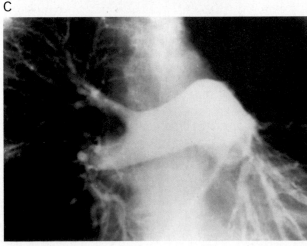

Fig C 15-4
Westermark's sign of pulmonary embolism. (A) Baseline chest radiograph demonstrates normal vascularity in the left upper lobe. (B) Striking hyperlucency of the left upper lobe coincided with the onset of the patient's symptoms. (C) Arteriogram performed on the same day the film in (B) was made shows an occluding clot in the left upper lobe and multiple emboli in the right lung.

Condition	Imaging Findings	Comments
Unilateral or lobar emphysema (Swyer–James syndrome) (Fig C 15-5)	Usually involvement of an entire lung (unilateral radiolucency), though a single lobe is occasionally affected. Air trapping during expiration (mediastinal shift toward the normal lung).	Probably results from acute pneumonia during infancy or childhood that causes bronchiolitis obliterans and an emphysema-like picture. The hilar and peripheral vessels are small.
Congenital lobar emphysema (Fig C 15-6)	Severe overinflation of a pulmonary lobe (especially the right upper or the right middle lobe).	Approximately one-third of cases apparent at birth (others noted several weeks later). Severe air trapping causes marked lobar enlargement, contralateral displacement of the mediastinum, and ipsilateral depression of the diaphragm.

A   B   C

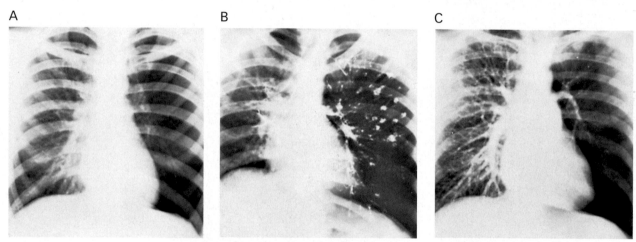

Fig C 15-5
Unilateral hyperlucent lung. (A) Frontal radiograph exposed at total lung capacity reveals a marked discrepancy in the radiolucency of the two lungs, with the left showing severe oligemia but normal lung volume. (B) Frontal radiograph at residual volume after bronchography demonstrates severe air trapping in the left lung and little change in volume from total lung capacity. Because the deflation of the right lung is normal, the mediastinum has swung sharply to the right. (C) A pulmonary arteriogram shows the discrepancy in blood flow to the two lungs. The left pulmonary artery is present, although diminutive, differentiating this appearance from congenital absence of the left pulmonary artery.[7]

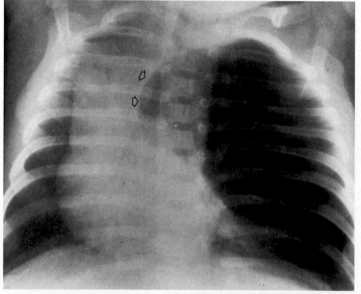

Fig C 15-6
Congenital lobar emphysema. Severe overdistension of the left upper lobe causes marked radiolucency of the left hemithorax along with depression of the ipsilateral hemidiaphragm and displacement of the mediastinum into the right hemithorax. The hyperinflated left upper lobe has herniated into the right side of the chest (arrows). Note the small and widely separated bronchovascular markings in the lucent left lung.

Condition	Imaging Findings	Comments
Cystic adenomatoid malformation (Fig C 15-7)	Usually appears as a mass composed of numerous air-containing cysts scattered irregularly throughout a soft-tissue density in a single lobe. Occasionally, a single air-filled cyst predominates, simulating infantile lobar emphysema.	Rare congenital anomaly consisting of an intralobar mass of disorganized pulmonary tissue that is classified as a hamartoma, though it is not neoplastic. If the malformation does not communicate with the bronchial tree, it contains only fluid and appears radiographically as a large pulmonary mass. The lesion expands the ipsilateral hemithorax by depressing the hemidiaphragm and shifting the mediastinum toward the contralateral side.
Hypogenetic lung syndrome (see Fig CA 8-8)	Small, often hyperlucent right lung associated with a small or absent pulmonary artery. May be associated with an anomalous draining vein that forms a broad, gently curved shadow descending to the diaphragm just to the right of the heart (scimitar sign).	Very rare anomaly in which the right lung is supplied partly or completely by systemic arteries (left-to-right shunt). Other cardiopulmonary anomalies are common.
Pulmonary branch stenosis	Ipsilateral lung is hypoplastic and has reduced volume, and there is an absent or diminutive hilum. No air trapping on forced expiration (unlike Swyer–James syndrome).	Very rare anomaly in which the involved lung is supplied by a hypertrophied bronchial circulation. The anomalous artery is usually on the side opposite the aortic arch (when on the left, there is a high incidence of associated cardiovascular anomalies).
Anomalous origin of left pulmonary artery from right pulmonary artery	Hyperlucent right lung due to air trapping and overinflation (anomalous vessel compresses the right main bronchus).	Very rare anomaly in which severe compression may collapse the lung. Compression of the trachea causes bilateral overinflation and air trapping on expiration. An esophagram shows pathognomonic posterior displacement of the esophagus and anterior displacement of the trachea by the interposed anomalous artery.

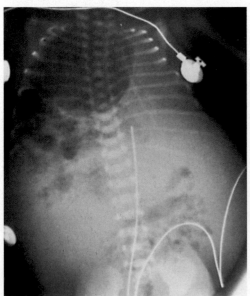

Fig C 15-7
Cystic adenomatoid malformation. Frontal radiograph of an infant's chest and abdomen at 1 hour of age demonstrates a large lucent mass in the right hemithorax with shift of the mediastinal structures to the left. In the lower right chest, the mass appears multicystic and resembles air-filled loops of bowel. Ascites is also present.[33]

Condition	Imaging Findings	Comments
Congenital bronchial atresia	Characteristic elliptical mass in the hilar region representing inspissated mucus distal to the point of atresia. May have a linear or branched pattern.	Very rare anomaly that most commonly involves the apicoposterior segment of the left upper lobe (can affect various segments). The bronchial tree peripheral to the point of obliteration is patent and air enters the affected segment by collateral air drift.
Tuberculosis	Overinflation and oligemia due to partial bronchial obstruction from ipsilateral hilar lymph node enlargement.	Primarily involves the anterior segment of an upper lobe or the medial segment of the middle lobe. May be the result of bronchostenosis from a tuberculous granuloma. Complete obstruction causes atelectasis.
Staphylococcal infection (pneumatocele) (see Fig C 11-2)	Characteristic thin-walled cystic spaces develop in approximately 50% of affected children. May be large and even fill an entire hemithorax. Often contain air-fluid levels.	Cystic spaces usually appear during the first week of a pneumonia and tend to disappear spontaneously within 6 weeks. Rare in adults. Probably results from check-valve obstruction of a communication between a peribronchial abscess and the bronchial lumen.
Hydrocarbon poisoning (Fig C 15-8)	Inhalation in children can lead to the formation of pneumatoceles simulating those in staphylococcal pneumonia.	Ingestion or inhalation of hydrocarbons is the leading cause of poisoning in children. Inhaled hydrocarbon initially produces perihilar infiltrates and pulmonary edema; ingested hydrocarbon is absorbed through the gastrointestinal tract and is carried by the bloodstream to the lungs, where it adds to the pulmonary injury.
Broncholith	Overinflation and oligemia due to partial bronchial obstruction from an endobronchial calcified mass.	Erosion of a calcified lymph node (usually from histoplasmosis) into the bronchial lumen.
Sarcoidosis	Hyperlucency of the lung due to air trapping and overinflation.	Rare cause. May be due to bronchial compression from enlarged nodes but more commonly results from endobronchial sarcoid deposits.

A   B

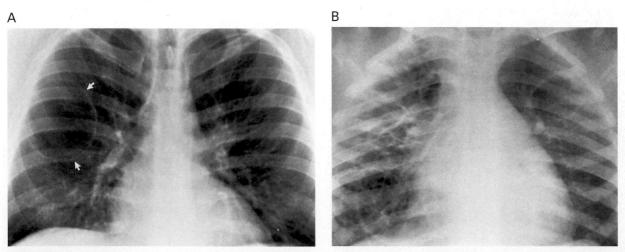

Fig C 15-8
Hydrocarbon poisoning. (A) Large thin-walled pneumatocele (arrows). (B) Multiple thin-walled pneumatoceles bilaterally but more marked on the right.

Condition	Imaging Findings	Comments
Nonpulmonary causes (normal vessels)		
Mastectomy	Unilateral hyperlucent lung. Absent breast shadow.	May be bilateral.
Absent pectoralis muscles (Fig C 15-9)	Unilateral hyperlucent lung.	Disparity in thickness of the supraclavicular soft tissues and axillary folds.
Faulty radiographic technique	Unilateral hyperlucent lung.	Most commonly due to patient rotation, which projects the soft tissues and the spine over one side of the chest while rotating them off the opposite, more lucent side (especially prominent in women with large pendulous breasts). Another cause is improper centering of the x-ray beam.

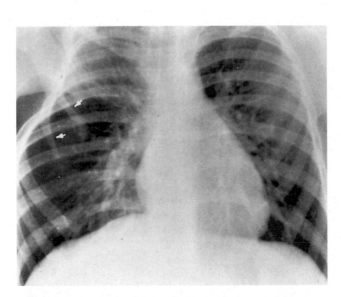

Fig C 15-9
Absence of the right pectoralis muscles. Asymmetry of the thoracic cage with hypoplasia of the anterior ribs (arrows). The lower portion of the right lung appears hyperlucent, whereas the apex seems comparatively opaque.

Bilateral Hyperlucent Lungs

Condition	Imaging Findings	Comments
Chronic obstructive emphysema (Fig C 16-1)	Severe hyperinflation (low, flat, or concave diaphragm; increased posteroanterior diameter of the chest; increased retrosternal space).	Marked attenuation and stretching (even virtual absence) of pulmonary vessels. Often evidence of pulmonary hypertension (enlargement of central pulmonary arteries with rapid peripheral tapering). The heart tends to be small and relatively vertical, and there are often single or multiple bullae. In α_1-antitrypsin deficiency, the emphysema predominantly involves the lower lobes.
Acute asthmatic attack (Fig C 16-2)	Severe overinflation of the lungs with air trapping. Characteristic tubular shadows ("tramlines") represent edema or thickening of bronchial walls.	Unlike emphysema, in this condition the vascular markings throughout the lungs are of normal caliber. Usually there is no radiographic abnormality between acute attacks.

A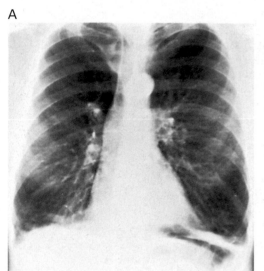
B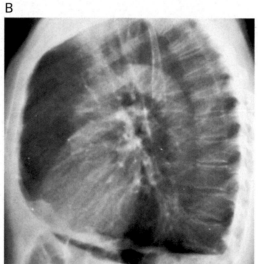

Fig C 16-1
Pulmonary emphysema. (A) Frontal and (B) lateral views of the chest demonstrate severe overinflation of the lungs along with flattening and even a superiorly concave configuration of the hemidiaphragms. There is also increased size and lucency of the retrosternal air space, an increase in the anteroposterior diameter of the chest, and a reduction in the number and caliber of peripheral pulmonary arteries.

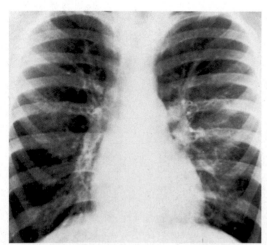

Fig C 16-2
Asthma. Frontal view of the chest demonstrating hyperexpansion of the lungs with depression of the hemidiaphragms, increased anteroposterior diameter of the chest and retrosternal air space, and prominence of the interstitial structures. The heart and pulmonary vascularity are normal.

Condition	Imaging Findings	Comments
Acute bronchiolitis	Severe overinflation of the lungs that is often associated with a reticulonodular pattern that predominantly involves the lower lobes.	Usually a viral infection of small airways that primarily affects children younger than the age of 3 years and is generally self-limited. May affect adults with pre-existing respiratory disease.
Bullous disease of the lung (Figs C 16-3 and C 16-4)	Multiple thin-walled, sharply demarcated, air-filled avascular spaces in the lung that most commonly occur in the upper lobes and may grow. Although there is overinflation as in chronic obstruction emphysema, there is no diffuse oligemia of the remaining pulmonary parenchyma.	Generally affects males, who remain asymptomatic until there is severe compression of the uninvolved lung parenchyma. Spontaneous pneumothorax from a ruptured bulla is a common complication.
Cystic fibrosis (mucoviscidosis) (Fig C 16-5)	Overinflation of the lungs associated with accentuation of interstitial markings and episodes of atelectasis and recurrent local pneumonia.	Obstruction of air passages by the tenacious mucus that is characteristic of this condition.
Diffuse infantile bronchopneumonia	Diffuse or patchy overinflation of the lungs that is usually associated with areas of consolidation and enlargement of peribronchial lymph nodes.	This pattern of bilateral pneumonia commonly complicates influenza, measles, or whooping cough. It may rarely occur with bacterial organisms.
Tracheal or laryngeal obstruction or compression	Overinflation of the lungs that may be associated with various tracheal abnormalities. Often recurrent pneumonias or evidence of parenchymal scarring from previous inflammatory disease.	Causes include vascular ring, tumor (squamous cell carcinoma, adenoid cystic carcinoma, osteochondroma, papilloma), tracheobronchomegaly (dilatation of deficient cartilage rings), relapsing polychondritis, localized tracheomalacia or stenosis (late complication of endotracheal intubation or tracheostomy), and saber-sheath trachea (narrowed coronal diameter due to chronic obstructive pulmonary disease).
Faulty radiographic technique	Bilateral "hyperlucent" lungs.	Overpenetrated film (especially portable radiographs and films on patients with very thin body habitus).

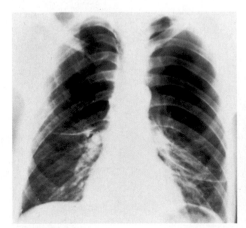

Fig C 16-3
Massive bilateral bullae. There is striking hyperlucency of both lungs.

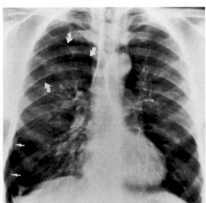

Fig C 16-4
Bullous emphysema. A small right pneumothorax (straight arrows) resulting from the rupture of a bulla. The curved arrows point to the walls of three of the multiple bullae in the upper portion of the right lung.

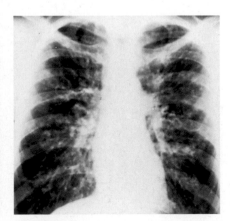

Fig C 16-5
Cystic fibrosis. Bilateral overinflation of the lungs associated with coarse interstitial markings.

Lobar Enlargement

Condition	Comments
Klebsiella pneumonia (Fig C 17-1)	Tends to form a voluminous inflammatory exudate that produces a homogeneous parenchymal consolidation (containing an air bronchogram) and bulging of an interlobar fissure. High frequency of abscess and cavity formation (rare in pneumococcal pneumonia).
Pneumococcal pneumonia	Appearance similar to *Klebsiella* pneumonia although cavitation is rare.
Haemophilus influenzae pneumonia (Fig C 17-2)	Most often develops in compromised hosts (chronic pulmonary disease, immune deficiency, alcoholism, diabetes).
Plague pneumonia	Hilar and paratracheal lymph node enlargement is common.
Tuberculous pneumonia	Manifestation of primary parenchymal involvement.
Lung abscess (Fig C 17-3)	Lobar expansion in an acute lung abscess (large mass, usually with cavitation) is probably related to air trapping by a check-valve mechanism in the communicating airway.
Bronchogenic carcinoma (Fig C 17-4)	Any large space-occupying mass that occupies a significant volume or is contiguous with a fissure.

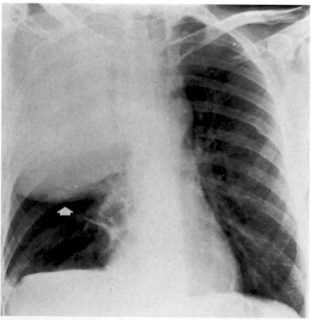

Fig C 17-1
***Klebsiella* pneumonia.** Downward bulging of the minor fissure (arrow) due to massive enlargement of the right upper lobe with inflammatory exudate.

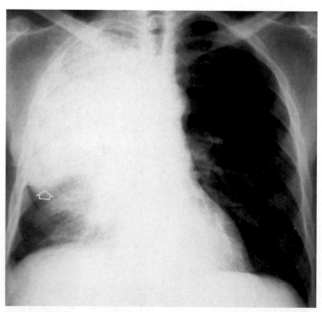

Fig C 17-2
***Haemophilus influenzae* pneumonia.** Acute lobar consolidation with downward bulging of the minor fissure (arrow) due to enlargement of the right upper lobe.[34]

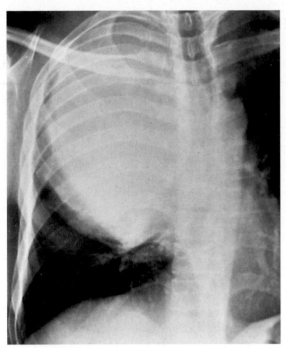

Fig C 17-3
Streptococcal pneumonia and empyema. A large
mottled opacity over the right upper lung represents
an extensive empyema that obscures the underlying
parenchymal pneumonia and produces an appearance
indistinguishable from that of lobar enlargement. The
patchy air densities in the empyema indicate commu-
nication with the bronchial tree.

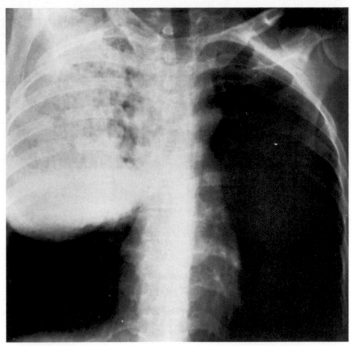

Fig C 17-4
Bronchogenic carcinoma. Appearance of massive lobar enlargement in a 30-year-old asymptomatic man.

Lobar or Segmental Collapse*

Condition	Imaging Findings	Comments
Bronchogenic carcinoma (Fig C 18-1)	Lobar collapse associated with a hilar mass (representing metastases to regional lymph nodes).	Because bronchial obstruction is a slowly progressive process, there is usually a distal infection with inflammatory exudate that prevents collapse once the bronchus is totally occluded. Characteristic Golden's S sign in right upper lobe collapse (upper laterally concave segment of the S is formed by the elevated minor fissure; lower medial convexity is caused by the tumor mass responsible for the collapse).
Bronchial adenoma (Fig C 18-2)	Lobar collapse.	Most common radiographic finding of a central adenoma. Collateral air drift may present complete collapse.
Foreign body	Lobar or segmental collapse. An opaque foreign body may be detectable.	In adults, collapse is usually associated with aspiration of food (eg, a large piece of meat). Bizarre variety of causes in children (who more commonly present with overaeration of the lung distal to the site of obstruction due to collateral air drift).

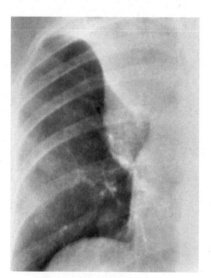

Fig C 18-1
Bronchogenic carcinoma. Typical reverse S-shaped curve (Golden's sign) representing collapse of the right upper lobe associated with malignant bronchial obstruction.

A

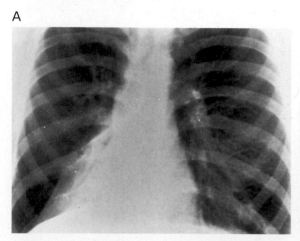

B

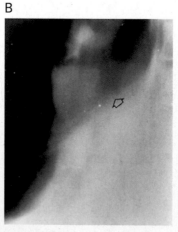

Fig C 18-2
Central bronchial adenoma. (A) Frontal chest radiograph demonstrates a right lower lobe density with obscuration of the right hemidiaphragm and relative preservation of the right border of the heart, consistent with right lower lobe collapse. (B) Tomography shows an ill-defined mass causing a high-grade obstruction of the right lower lobe bronchus (arrow).

*See Figs C 18-6 through 18-11.

Condition	Imaging Findings	Comments
Malpositioned endotracheal tube (Figs C 18-3 and C 18-4)	Usually collapse of the left lung.	Advancing the tube too far (into the bronchus intermedius) occludes the left main-stem bronchus.
Mucous plug (Fig C 18-5)	Primarily segmental collapse.	Most common cause of small airway obstruction. Frequent complication of abdominal and thoracic surgery, anesthesia and respiratory depressant drugs, and infectious diseases (eg, tetanus) that produce respiratory depression and impaired clearance of tracheobronchial secretions.

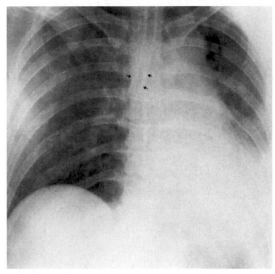

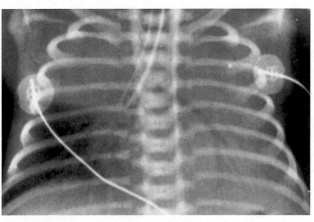

Fig C 18-4
Malpositioned endotracheal tube. Inordinately low position of the endotracheal tube in the bronchus intermedius causes collapse of the right upper lobe and the entire left lung.

Fig C 18-3
Malpositioned endotracheal tube. Collapse of the left lung, especially the left lower lobe, due to an endotracheal tube (arrows) in the right main-stem bronchus that effectively blocks the passage of air into the left bronchial tree.

A

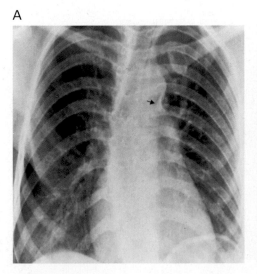

B

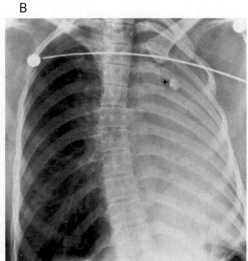

Fig C 18-5
Mucous plug in a paraplegic. (A) Baseline radiograph is within normal limits. Note the calcified granuloma in the left perihilar region (arrow). (B) Complete collapse of the left lung after the lodging of a mucous plug in the left main-stem bronchus. Note the change in position of the calcified granuloma when the left lung collapses (arrow).

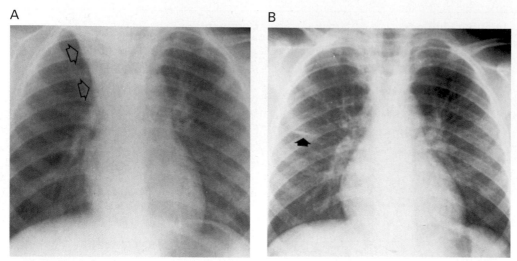

Fig C 18-6
Right upper lobe collapse. (A) Initial chest radiograph demonstrates the collapsed right upper lobe, which appears as a homogeneous soft-tissue mass (arrows) in the right apex along the upper mediastinum. (B) As the collapsed lobe expands, the soft-tissue has disappeared and the minor fissure (arrow) has reappeared.

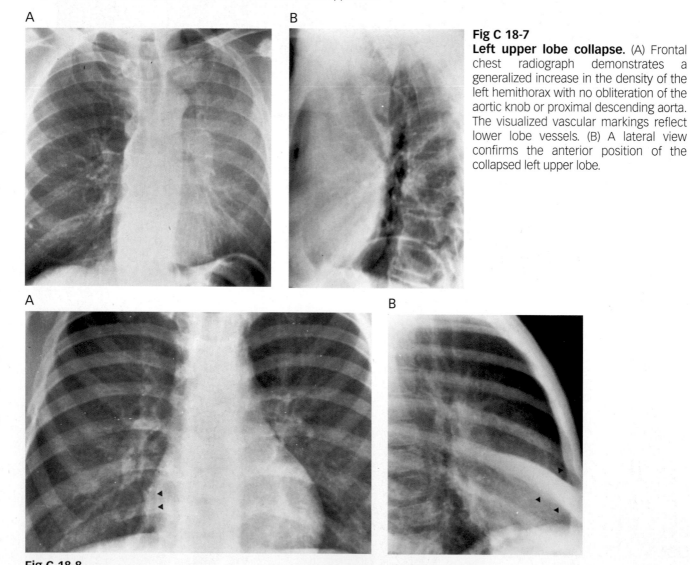

Fig C 18-7
Left upper lobe collapse. (A) Frontal chest radiograph demonstrates a generalized increase in the density of the left hemithorax with no obliteration of the aortic knob or proximal descending aorta. The visualized vascular markings reflect lower lobe vessels. (B) A lateral view confirms the anterior position of the collapsed left upper lobe.

Fig C 18-8
Right middle lobe collapse. (A) Frontal chest radiograph demonstrates minimal obliteration of the lower part of the right border of the heart (arrows). (B) Lateral view demonstrates collapse of the right middle lobe (arrows).

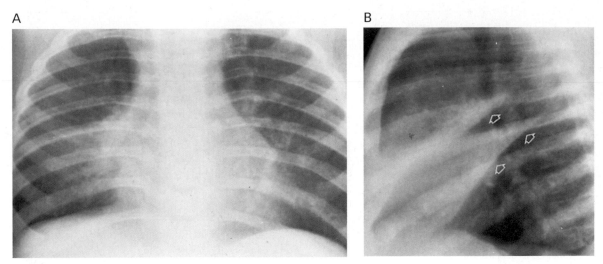

Fig C 18-9
Right middle lobe and lingular collapse. (A) Frontal chest radiograph demonstrates obliteration of the right and left borders of the heart. (B) Lateral view demonstrates collapse of both the right middle lobe and the lingula (arrows).

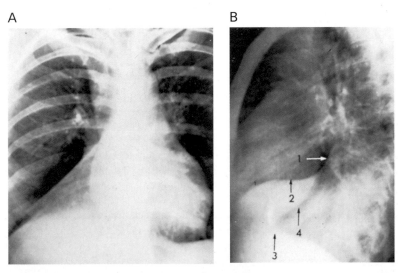

Fig C 18-10
Right lower lobe collapse. (A) Frontal chest radiograph demonstrates a right lower lung density with preservation of the right border of the heart. The right hemidiaphragm is obscured. (B) Lateral view confirms the presence of right lower lobe collapse (due to bronchogenic carcinoma) with posterior displacement of the major fissure (1). The elevated right hemidiaphragm (2) is obliterated posteriorly by the airless right lower lobe, and the anterior third of the left hemidiaphragm (3) is obscured by the bottom of the heart. The overlapping shadows of the back of the heart (4), which lies in the left hemithorax, and the right hemidiaphragm simulate interlobar effusion.[35]

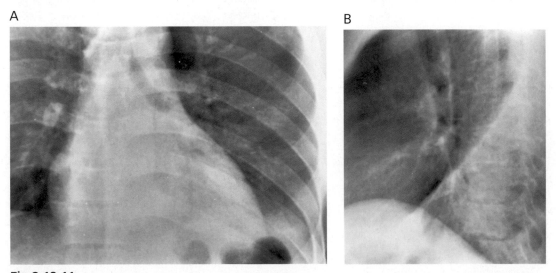

Fig C 18-11
Left lower lobe collapse. (A) Frontal chest radiograph demonstrates obliteration of the descending thoracic aorta and obscuration of much of the left hemidiaphragm. (B) Lateral view confirms the posterior portion of the collapsed left lower lobe.

Condition	Imaging Findings	Comments
Mucoid impaction	Segmental or subsegmental collapse.	Develops in patients with asthma and hypersensitivity (allergic) bronchopulmonary aspergillosis.
Bronchial metastases	Lobar or segmental collapse.	Most frequently renal cell carcinoma. Also breast carcinoma and melanoma.
Chronic obstructive pulmonary disease	Segmental or subsegmental collapse (also evidence of underlying disease).	Obstruction of small airways with the formation of small intraluminal mucous plugs (most commonly in acute exacerbations of asthma, chronic bronchitis, emphysema, and bronchiolitis obliterans).
Pneumonia	Segmental or subsegmental collapse.	Peribronchial inflammation may lead to small airway obstruction followed by collapse. Develops occasionally in bacterial, viral, and mycoplasma pneumonias.
Cystic fibrosis	Lobar, segmental, or subsegmental collapse superimposed on a coarse interstitial pattern.	Small airway obstruction due to excessively viscous mucus that is poorly cleared from the tracheobronchial tree.
Cardiac enlargement	Usually collapse of the left lower lobe.	Dilated left atrium (mitral stenosis, atrial septal defect).
Aortic aneurysm	Lobar or segmental collapse.	Extrinsic pressure on the bronchial tree.
Mediastinal neoplasm	Lobar or segmental collapse.	Extrinsic pressure on the bronchial tree.
Inflammatory bronchial stricture	Lobar, segmental, or subsegmental collapse. Usually evidence of an alveolar or interstitial infiltrate.	Most commonly because of tuberculosis (volume loss of the upper lobe). Also histoplasmosis and other granulomatous infections.
Fractured bronchus	Lobar or segmental collapse with characteristic rounded bronchial occlusion.	Result of severe thoracic trauma. Causes a pronounced collapse because it is sudden and complete.
Pulmonary embolism	Lobar or segmental collapse.	Unusual manifestation (precise mechanism unclear).
Bronchiectasis	Lobar or segmental collapse.	Caused by retained secretions in advanced disease. More commonly, there is only moderate volume loss.
Middle lobe syndrome	Collapse of the right middle lobe. The lymph node producing the compression may contain calcium.	Chronic process caused by quiescent granulomatous lymphadenitis (histoplasmosis, tuberculosis, occasionally silicosis). A similar process may involve other lobes or segments.

Condition	Imaging Findings	Comments
Lymphadenopathy	Lobar or segmental collapse.	Hilar adenopathy is often cited as the cause of collapse, although the volume loss probably reflects the underlying pathologic process (eg, primary bronchogenic carcinoma, tuberculosis). To support this view, sarcoidosis is associated with profound hilar adenopathy yet rarely causes any volume loss.
Radiation therapy	Lobar or segmental collapse (often a peculiar nonanatomic distribution of volume loss that coincides with the radiation port).	Late scarring may produce a substantial loss of volume superimposed on a characteristic interstitial pattern.
Broncholithiasis	Lobar or segmental collapse associated with intrabronchial calcification.	Results from erosion of a calcified lymph node into a bronchus.

Pulmonary Parenchymal Calcification

Condition	Imaging Findings	Comments
Histoplasmoma (Figs C 19-1 and C 19-2)	Central calcification that may be multiple or widespread.	Most common form of pulmonary calcification. Often associated with calcifications in regional lymph nodes and the spleen. Eccentric calcification in the mass may indicate a bronchogenic carcinoma growing around the histoplasmoma.
Other granulomatous infections (Fig C 19-3)	Central calcification that may be multiple or widespread.	Tuberculosis, coccidioidomycosis. There may be calcification of regional lymph nodes. Eccentric calcification in the mass may indicate a bronchogenic carcinoma growing around the granuloma.
Plasma cell granuloma (Fig C 19-4)	Fine or coarse calcification in a parenchymal nodule.	Common inflammatory pseudotumor of the lung that represents a benign proliferative response to pulmonary infection or injury. Occasionally the process is aggressive and encases bronchi or invades mediastinal structures, chest wall, or diaphragm.
Fungus ball	Various patterns of calcification of the mycelial mass may occur.	Scattered small nodules of calcification, a fine rim around the periphery of the mass, or an extensive process involving most of the mycelial ball.
Chickenpox (varicella) pneumonia (Fig C 19-5)	Tiny widespread calcifications.	Develops in adults 1 or more years after pulmonary chickenpox infection. The calcifications vary in size and number and predominate in the lower half of the lungs. No calcification of hilar lymph nodes (unlike histoplasmosis or tuberculosis).
Parasites	Multiple small pulmonary calcifications. May be solitary.	Paragonimiasis, schistosomiasis, cysticercosis, guinea worm, *Armillifer armillatus* (also in thoracic muscles or subcutaneous tissues).

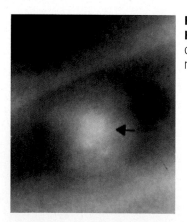

Fig C 19-1
Histoplasmoma. Central calcification (arrow) in a solitary pulmonary nodule.

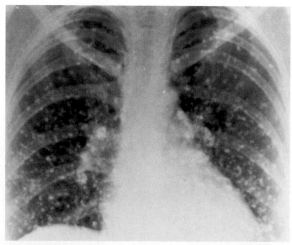

Fig C 19-2
Histoplasmosis. Diffuse calcifications in the lungs produce a snowball pattern.

Condition	Imaging Findings	Comments
Pulmonary arteriovenous fistula	Single or multiple calcifications.	Rare manifestation that is probably due to phleboliths. The feeding artery and draining vein can often be detected.
Bronchogenic cyst	Curvilinear calcification about the periphery of the mass.	Cyst wall calcification is rare.

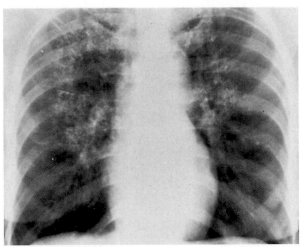

Fig C 19-12
Secondary hyperparathyroidism. Heterotopic calcification in a patient with chronic renal failure.

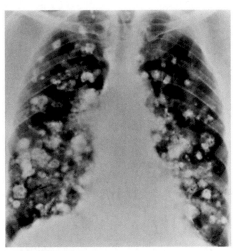

Fig C 19-13
Broncholithiasis. Innumerable calcified masses scattered throughout the lungs.

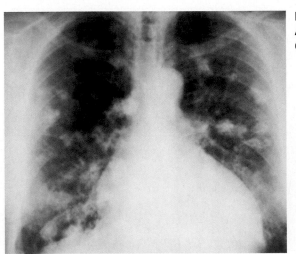

Fig C 19-14
Amyloidosis. Dystrophic calcification in nodular deposits in the lung.[36]

Pulmonary Disease with Eosinophilia

Condition	Imaging Findings	Comments
Acute idiopathic eosinophilic pneumonia (Löffler's syndrome) (Fig C 20-1)	Patchy parenchymal consolidation with blood eosinophilia.	Characteristic transitory and migratory pattern of ill-defined infiltrates that are nonsegmental in distribution and tend to involve the periphery of the lung. "Reversed pulmonary edema pattern" (involvement of the lung periphery in contrast to the perihilar or central distribution of pulmonary edema).
Chronic eosinophilic pneumonia	Patchy parenchymal consolidation with eosinophilic infiltration of the lung.	Pattern identical to that in Löffler's syndrome, except that the lesions tend to persist unchanged for weeks unless corticosteroid therapy is instituted. Blood eosinophilia occurs in most patients although it is not essential for the diagnosis.
Drug sensitivity (Figs C 20-2 and C 20-3)	Patchy nonsegmental, peripheral parenchymal consolidation with blood eosinophilia.	Sulfonamides, penicillin, isoniazid, and many other medications. Nitrofurantoin causes a diffuse reticular pattern. Withdrawal of the drug results in prompt disappearance of the clinical and radiographic manifestations.
Parasitic disease (Figs C 20-4 to C 20-8)	Patchy nonsegmental, peripheral parenchymal consolidation with blood eosinophilia.	Ascariasis, strongyloidiasis, tropical pulmonary eosinophilia (filariasis), ancylostomiasis (hookworm), visceral larva migrans (dog or cat roundworm), schistosomiasis. Amebiasis produces basilar consolidation (not peripheral) that may cavitate.
Hypersensitivity bronchopulmonary aspergillosis (Fig C 20-9)	Round, oval, or elliptical opacities (mucous plugs) that usually develop in segmental bronchi of the upper lobes. May have homogeneous consolidation. Blood eosinophilia.	Mucous plugs contain aspergilli and eosinophils. Usually a history of long-standing bronchial asthma. Involvement of several bronchi may produce a "cluster of grapes," or Y-shaped, shadow.

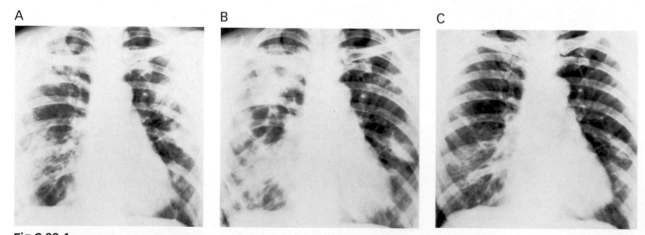

A   B   C

Fig C 20-1
Löffler's syndrome. (A) Initial frontal chest radiograph shows numerous bilateral areas of consolidation that have no precise segmental distribution. Note particularly the broad shadow of increased density along the lower axillary zone of the right lung. (B) One week later, the anatomic distribution of the consolidation has changed considerably, being more extensive in the right upper and lower lobes and less extensive in the left upper lobe. (C) One week later, after adrenocorticotropic hormone (ACTH) therapy, the radiographic abnormalities have completely resolved.[7]

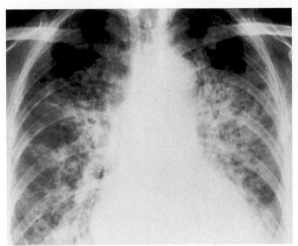

Fig C 20-2
Nitrofurantoin-induced lung disease. Mixed alveolar and interstitial pattern in an elderly woman who presented with progressive cough and dyspnea after the long-term use of nitrofurantoin for recurring urinary tract infections.[14]

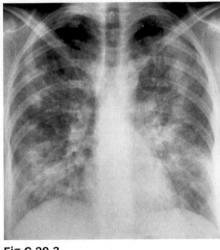

Fig C 20-3
Methotrexate-induced lung disease. The diffuse, bilateral, patchy densities were changeable and fleeting during the illness. The radiographic findings cleared completely after steroid therapy.[37]

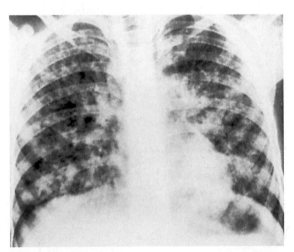

Fig C 20-4
Ascariasis. Extensive pulmonary infiltrates due to the presence of *Ascaris* larvae in the lungs.[38]

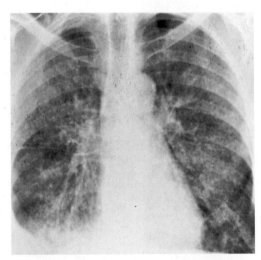

Fig C 20-5
Strongyloidiasis. Chest radiograph during the stage of larval migration shows a pattern of miliary nodules diffusely distributed throughout both lungs. There is also a large right pleural effusion.

Condition	Imaging Findings	Comments
Asthma (Fig C 20-10)	Hyperexpansion of the lungs with bronchial wall thickening (tubular shadows). Eosinophils in the sputum and slight blood eosinophilia.	Chest radiograph is often normal (especially in patients with mild disease and late age of onset). Increased incidence of pneumonia and atelectasis (mucous plugging or impaction).
Hypereosinophilic syndrome (eosinophilic leukemia)	Various patterns of eosinophilic infiltration of the pulmonary parenchyma.	Rare condition characterized by mature eosinophil infiltration of multiple organs. Occurs almost exclusively in males.
Wegener's granulomatosis (see Fig C 11-14)	Patchy parenchymal consolidation with minimal blood and tissue eosinophilia.	Almost invariably multiple and frequently cavitates.

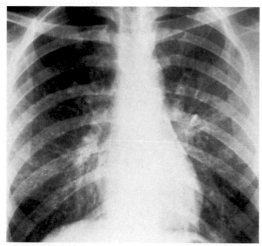

Fig C 20-6
Tropical pulmonary eosinophilia. Multiple small nodules with indistinct outlines produce a pattern of generalized increase in lung markings.[39]

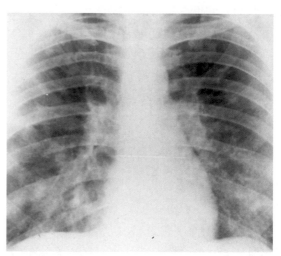

Fig C 20-7
Cutaneous larva migrans. Multiple small irregular areas of air-space consolidation widely scattered throughout both lungs.[40]

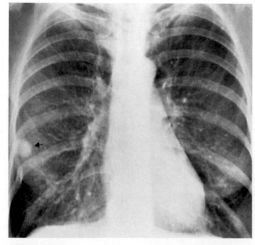

Fig C 20-8
Dirofilariasis. Well-circumscribed solitary pulmonary nodule (arrow) that is indistinguishable from a malignant coin lesion.

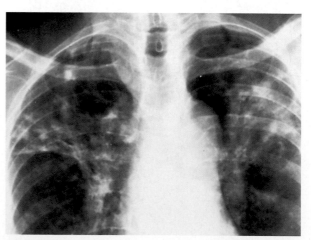

Fig C 20-9
Hypersensitivity bronchopulmonary aspergillosis. Patchy opacifications in segmental bronchi of the upper lobes in a patient with asthma and pronounced peripheral eosinophilia.

Condition	Imaging Findings	Comments
Allergic granulomatosis	Patchy parenchymal consolidation with considerable blood and tissue eosinophilia.	Granulomatous disease involving many organs and restricted to patients with a history of asthma. The consolidation is almost always multiple and frequently cavitates.
Polyarteritis nodosa	Fleeting nonsegmental patchy consolidation with tissue eosinophilia.	Hypersensitivity angiitis that typically involves the kidneys and may cause systemic hypertension. Other findings include pulmonary edema, accentuated interstitial markings, and miliary nodules.
Desquamative interstitial pneumonia (DIP) (Fig C 20-11)	Generalized reticular pattern with small numbers of eosinophils in the interstitium.	Progressive loss of lung volume on sequential studies. Spontaneous pneumothorax and pleural effusion may occur.
Coccidioidomycosis (Fig C 20-12)	Various patterns of pulmonary disease, often with significant blood eosinophilia.	May produce parenchymal consolidation, nodules (single, multiple, miliary) that may cavitate, and lymph node enlargement.

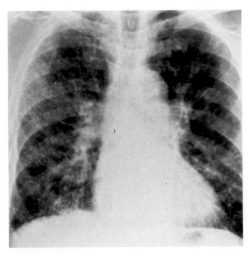

Fig C 20-10
Asthma. Recurrent pulmonary infections have led to the development of diffuse pulmonary fibrosis.

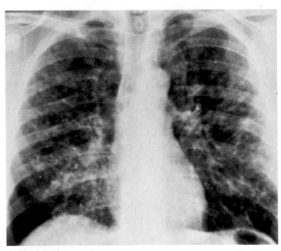

Fig C 20-11
Desquamative interstitial pneumonia. Generalized reticular pattern throughout both lungs.

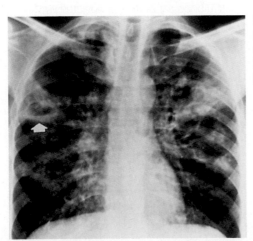

Fig C 20-12
Coccidioidomycosis. Patchy areas of air-space consolidation in both lungs. There is an air-fluid level (arrow) in a right upper lobe cavity abutting the minor fissure.

Skin Disorder Combined with Widespread Lung Disease

Condition	Imaging Findings	Comments
Systemic lupus erythematosus (see Figs C 36-4 and C 36-9)	Pericardial and pleural effusions. Nonspecific, poorly defined patchy areas of parenchymal consolidation that are usually in the lung bases and situated peripherally (probably reflect acute pneumonia). Fleeting basilar atelectasis may occur.	Cutaneous manifestations (in 80% of patients) include butterfly rash, discoid lupus, alopecia, and photosensitivity. Arthritis and arthralgia occur in approximately 95% of cases.
Sarcoidosis (Fig C 21-1)	Bilateral hilar and paratracheal adenopathy. Diffuse reticulonodular or fluffy alveolar pattern.	Cutaneous involvement (approximately 30% of cases) includes slightly raised, often purplish nodules (lupus pernio) that usually appear about the face, neck, shoulders, and digits. Large plaques resembling psoriasis may occur over the trunk or extremities.
Scleroderma (see Fig C 5-5)	Diffuse interstitial pattern that predominantly involves the lower lung zones.	Characteristic thickened and inelastic skin. Erosion of terminal phalangeal tufts with calcification in the fingertips.
Dermatomyositis	Diffuse interstitial pattern that predominantly involves the lung bases.	Cutaneous changes include puffiness of the face and an erythematous rash involving the neck, ears, chest, and shoulders. Bilateral and symmetric muscle weakness and diffuse subcutaneous and muscular calcification. Traditionally associated with an increased incidence of malignancy.
Rheumatoid arthritis (see Fig C 4-12)	Diffuse reticulonodular pattern, more prominent in the lung bases. Discrete nodular lesions (similar to subcutaneous nodules). Pleural effusion.	The hands are often cool and damp (reflecting autonomic nervous system dysfunction) and palmar erythema often occurs. In long-standing disease, the skin over the distal extremities often becomes atrophic and bruises easily. Nail-fold thrombi, small infarcts on the volar surface of the hands, digital gangrene, and ulcers of the lower part of the leg and ankle are manifestations of rheumatoid vasculitis.

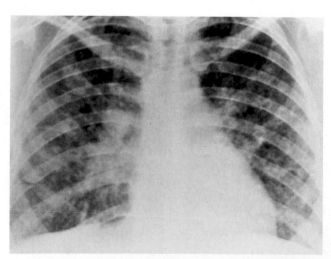

Fig C 21-1
Sarcoidosis. Diffuse reticulonodular pattern associated with hilar adenopathy.

Condition	Imaging Findings	Comments
Neurofibromatosis	Diffuse interstitial pulmonary fibrosis and bullae. Cutaneous nodules may project over the lungs.	Multiple fibromas and neuromas of the skin with café au lait spots. There may be posterior mediastinal masses and skeletal deformities (scoliosis and rib lesions).
Tuberous sclerosis (Fig C 21-2)	Diffuse interstitial fibrosis with honeycombing. Pneumothorax is common.	Cutaneous manifestations include adenoma sebaceum (acneform butterfly rash on the face) and subungual fibromas. Potato-like tumor masses also involve the brain, kidneys, and eyes.
Wegener's granulomatosis (see Fig C 11-14)	Multiple bilateral nodules. Thick-walled cavities in approximately half the cases.	Skin ulcerations and vesicular or hemorrhagic cutaneous lesions.
Hereditary hemorrhagic telangiectasis (Rendu–Osler–Weber disease)	Single or multiple pulmonary arteriovenous fistulas (prominent feeding artery and draining vein).	Cutaneous and mucous membrane telangiectasia.
Metastases from skin neoplasm	Multiple pulmonary nodules.	Melanoma (pigmented elevation), Kaposi's sarcoma (multiple bluish, hemorrhagic skin lesions). Often "bull's-eye" lesions in the gastrointestinal tract.
Mycosis fungoides	Various patterns (reticulonodular, multiple larger nodules, pleural effusion, enlargement of mediastinal lymph nodes).	Lymphomatous process that predominantly affects the skin (scaly cutaneous plaques or frank ulcerating tumors). Clinically resembles eczema or psoriasis and has a poor prognosis.
Lymphoma (see Figs C 13-4 and C 14-5)	Various patterns (reticulonodular, multiple larger nodules, enlargement of mediastinal lymph nodes).	Lymphomatous lesions in the skin are dermal or subcutaneous nodules that typically have a purple or red-brown color and are usually covered by relatively normal intact epidermis. Skin infiltrates may be the initial manifestation or may appear at any time during the course of the disease.
Erythema nodosum	Enlargement of hilar lymph nodes (usually bilateral). Occasional pulmonary infiltrates.	Acute skin eruption (especially of legs) consisting of symmetrically distributed, red, tender nodules. Associated with sarcoidosis. May represent an allergic reaction resulting from a variety of bacterial, chemical, and toxic agents.

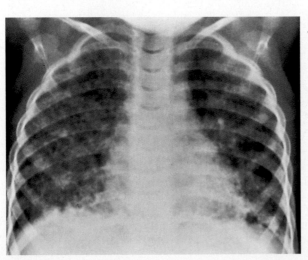

Fig C 21-2
Tuberous sclerosis. Diffuse interstitial fibrosis with honeycombing.

Condition	Imaging Findings	Comments
Fungal infections (Fig C 21-3)	Various patterns (parenchymal nodules, lymphadenopathy, pleural effusion).	Scaling macules and papules of the epidermis, hair, toenails, and fingernails. Certain fungi (especially *Candida* species) invade the epidermis when the skin is exposed to high humidity and becomes macerated (most commonly in the intertriginous areas under the breasts and in the umbilicus, groin, and axillae).
Pulmonary Langerhans cell histiocytosis (Fig C 21-4)	Diffuse coarse reticulonodular pattern (honeycomb lung). Pneumothorax is common.	Variety of skin lesions (may be the presenting sign), including scaly papules or vesicles, pruritic seborrheic or eczematous lesions in intertriginous areas, petechiae (due to perivascular infiltrates or thrombocytopenia), scaly or exudative eruptions of the scalp, and xanthomas.
Acquired immunodeficiency syndrome (AIDS)	Broad spectrum of pulmonary findings.	Variety of skin lesions of both infectious and noninfectious origins.
Chickenpox (Fig C 21-5)	Patchy, diffuse air-space pneumonia. In the healed phase, characteristic innumerable tiny widespread calcifications throughout both lungs.	Scarlatiniform rash with rapid development of typical vesicles and papules.
Measles (Fig C 21-6)	Reticular pattern in primary pneumonia. Segmental consolidation and atelectasis indicate bacterial superinfection.	Red maculopapular rash that breaks out first on the forehead; spreads downward over the face, neck, and trunk; and appears on the feet on the third day. Characteristic Koplik's spots (small, red, irregular lesions with blue-white centers) appear 1 to 2 days before the onset of the rash on the mucous membranes of the mouth and occasionally on the conjunctiva or intestinal mucosa.
Acanthosis nigricans	Increased incidence of bronchogenic carcinoma.	Bilateral, symmetric hyperkeratosis and hyperpigmentation of the skin (especially in the flexural and intertriginous areas). High incidence of abdominal malignancy (especially of the stomach).

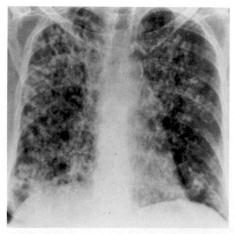

Fig C 21-3
Pulmonary candidiasis. Diffuse pattern of ill-defined nodules throughout both lungs.

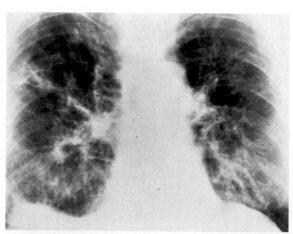

Fig C 21-4
Pulmonary Langerhans cell histiocytosis. Coarse reticular pattern diffusely involving both lungs.

Condition	Imaging Findings	Comments
Amyloidosis (Fig C 21-7)	Various patterns (intra-airway mass causing atelectasis or obstructive pneumonitis, parenchymal form with solitary or multiple masses, miliary form, lymphadenopathy, reticulonodular pattern).	Skin lesions are one of the most characteristic manifestations of amyloidosis and consist of slightly raised waxy papules or plaques that are usually clustered in the folds of the axillary, anal, or inguinal regions; the face and neck; or mucosal areas such as the ear or tongue. Gentle rubbing may induce bleeding into the skin, leading to purpura.
Hypersensitivity reaction (Fig C 21-8)	Various patterns depending on the stage of the condition.	Many forms of allergy, drug sensitivity, and parasitic infestation.
Burns	Various patterns (patchy pulmonary consolidation, atelectasis, pulmonary edema).	Cutaneous manifestations vary depending on the severity of the burn.
Bleeding disorders (see Fig C 2-11)	Alveolar infiltrates that may eventually produce interstitial fibrosis after repeated episodes of bleeding.	Spectrum of appearances—from extensive macules (ecchymoses) to tiny petechiae.

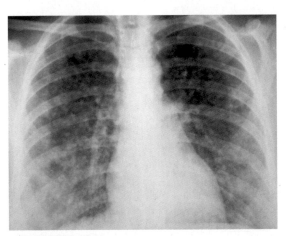

Fig C 21-5
Chickenpox pneumonia. Patchy, diffuse air-space consolidation.

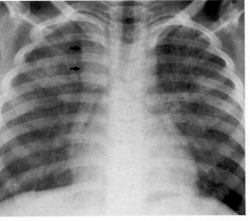

Fig C 21-6
Measles pneumonia. Diffuse, reticular interstitial infiltrate with a focal area of consolidation in the right upper lobe. Note the striking right hilar and mediastinal adenopathy (arrows).

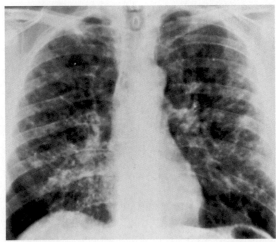

Fig C 21-7
Amyloidosis. Diffuse reticulonodular pattern.

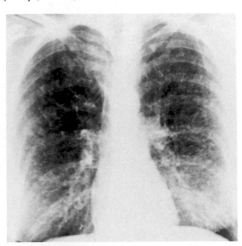

Fig C 21-8
Busulfan-induced lung disease. Diffuse coarse reticulonodular pattern.

Meniscus (Air-Crescent) Sign*

Condition	Comments
Aspergillus fungus ball (Figs C 22-1 through C 22-3)	Aspergillosis is the most common cause of this appearance. It generally develops in immuno-compromised patients (especially those with disseminated malignancy).
Fungus ball of other etiology	Candidiasis, coccidioidomycosis, nocardiosis, and cryptococcosis.
Hydatid (echinococcal) cyst (Fig C 22-4)	Rupture between the pericyst and the exocyst permits the entry of air between these layers.

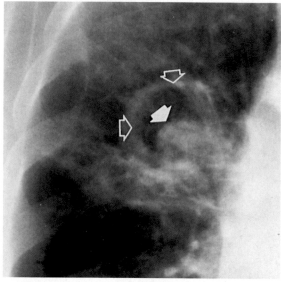

Fig C 22-1
Aspergillosis. A mycetoma (solid arrow) appears as a homogeneous rounded mass that is separated from the thick wall of the cavity by a crescent-shaped air space (open arrows).

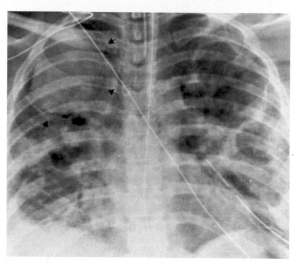

Fig C 22-2
Aspergillosis. Multiple cavities of various sizes are superimposed on a diffuse pulmonary infiltrate. A fungus ball almost fills the large cavity in the right upper lobe (arrows). A right pleural effusion is also seen in this patient with chronic lymphocytic leukemia.

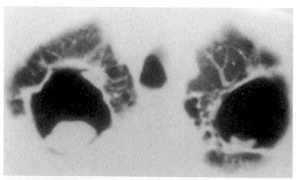

Fig C 22-3
Aspergillosis. Bilateral aspergillomas in an elderly man with residual tuberculosis. CT scan shows large cavities in the upper lobes containing fungus balls of different sizes.[41]

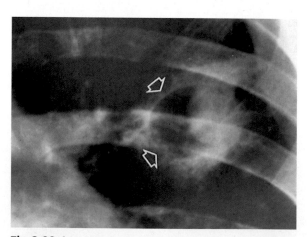

Fig C 22-4
Hydatid cyst. A crescent of air (arrows) is seen about the periphery of the echinococcal cyst.

*Lucent crescent along the inner border of a cavity or between a dense parenchymal lesion and surrounding lung structures.

Condition	Comments
Lung abscess with inspissated pus	Various infectious agents.
Neoplasm	Bronchogenic carcinoma, bronchial adenoma, sarcoma, and sclerosing hemangioma.
Granuloma	Tuberculous, fungal, or idiopathic.
Gangrene of lung	Large mass of necrotic lung in an abscess cavity. Most frequent in pneumococcal or *Klebsiella* pneumonia.
Intracavitary blood clot	Blood clot in a tuberculous cavity, infarct, or pulmonary laceration.

Anterior Mediastinal Lesions

Condition	Imaging Findings	Comments
Substernal thyroid (Fig C 23-1)	Sharply defined, smooth or lobulated mass that occurs in the superior portion of the mediastinum and may calcify.	Typically compresses the trachea or the esophagus or both. Occasionally occurs in the posterior mediastinum (almost exclusively on the right).
Thymoma (Figs C 23-2 and C 23-3)	Round or oval, smooth or lobulated mass that often calcifies and may protrude to one or both sides of the mediastinum. Usually arises near the junction of the heart and great vessels (displacing them posteriorly).	High fat content (relatively lucent on plain films and easily apparent on CT). As many as 25% to 50% of patients have myasthenia gravis (approximately 15% of patients with myasthenia gravis have thymic tumors). The normal thymus appears as an anterior mediastinal mass in neonates.

A   B

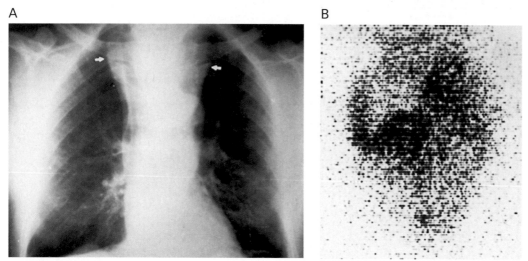

Fig C 23-1
Substernal thyroid. (A) Marked widening of the superior mediastinum to both sides (arrows) and severe deviation of the trachea to the right. (B) Iodine-131 scan shows increased uptake of the radionuclide in the area of the mass seen on the radiograph.[42]

A   B

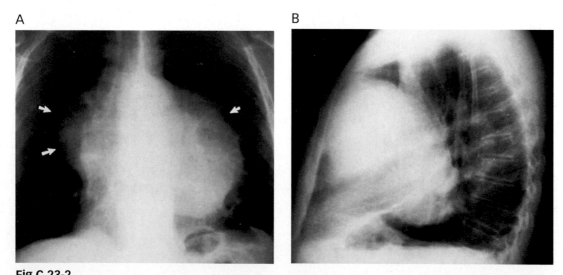

Fig C 23-2
Thymoma. (A) Frontal view shows a large bilateral lobulated mass (arrows) extending to both sides of the mediastinum. (B) Lateral view shows filling of the anterior precardiac space by a mass and posterior displacement of the left side of the heart.

Condition	Imaging Findings	Comments
Teratoma and other germinal cell neoplasms (Fig C 23-4)	Round or oval, smooth or lobulated mass that may protrude to one or both sides of the mediastinum.	Calcification (bone, teeth) or fat may occur in teratomas and dermoid cysts. Benign lesions tend to be smooth and cystic, whereas malignant lesions are often lobulated and solid.
Lymphoma (especially Hodgkin's)/leukemia (Fig C 23-5)	Enlargement of anterior mediastinal and retrosternal lymph nodes commonly occurs.	The presence of anterior mediastinal nodes in lymphoma is a differential point from sarcoidosis (which also affects hilar nodes but not nodes in the anterior compartment). There is often symmetric widening of the superior mediastinum on frontal views.

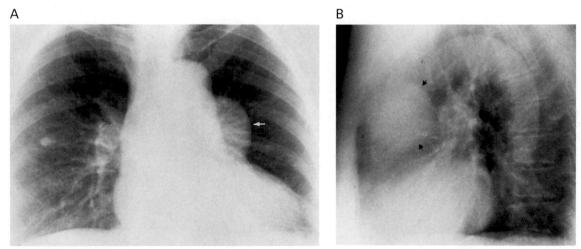

A   B

Fig C 23-3
Thymoma with myasthenia gravis. (A) Frontal and (B) lateral views of the chest demonstrate a large mass in the anterior mediastinum (arrows).

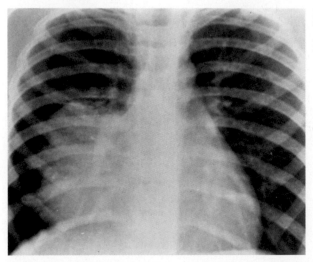

Fig C 23-4
Teratodermoid tumor. Large lobulated mass confluent with the right border of the heart.

Condition	Imaging Findings	Comments
Lymphangioma (hygroma)	Smooth or lobulated mass in the superior portion of the mediastinum.	Benign or invasive lesion that is often associated with a soft-tissue mass in the neck. Chylothorax may develop.
Mesenchymal tumor (Fig C 23-6)	Various patterns.	May be benign or malignant. A striking lucency suggests a lipoma or lipomatosis (steroid therapy). Phleboliths are diagnostic of a hemangioma.
Parathyroid tumor	Smooth or lobulated mass that may be too small to be detectable on plain films.	May displace the esophagus. There is often evidence of hyperparathyroidism in the thoracic spine.
Aneurysm of ascending aorta or sinus of Valsalva (Fig C 23-7)	Saccular or fusiform mass that tends to extend anteriorly and to the right.	May erode the sternum. Calcification is relatively uncommon.
Morgagni hernia (see Fig C 46-7)	Round or oval lower mediastinal mass that is almost invariably on the right.	Presence of gas-filled bowel (or contrast-filled colon from an enema) in the mass is diagnostic. The hernia appears as a homogeneous opacity if it is filled with liver or omentum (mimics a fat pad or a pericardial cyst).
Pericardial cyst (Fig C 23-8)	Round or lobulated, sharply demarcated lower mediastinal mass that is usually located in the right cardiophrenic angle.	Typically touches both the anterior chest wall and the anterior portion of the right hemidiaphragm. Usually asymptomatic.

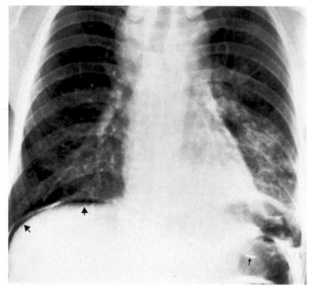

Fig C 23-5
Lymphoma. Diffuse widening of the upper portion of the mediastinum due to lymphadenopathy. There is an ill-defined lymphomatous parenchymal infiltrate at the left base. The metallic clip overlying the region of the spleen (small arrow) and the small amount of free intraperitoneal gas seen under the right hemidiaphragm (large arrows) are evidence of a recent exploratory laparotomy and splenectomy for staging of the lymphoma.

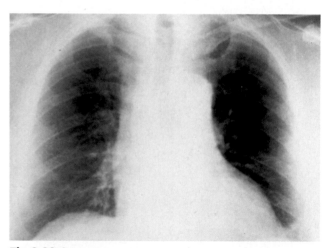

Fig C 23-6
Mediastinal lipomatosis. Generalized widening of the upper mediastinum.[43]

Condition	Imaging Findings	Comments
Mediastinal hemorrhage/hematoma	Uniform, symmetric widening of the mediastinum, especially the superior portion.	Generally a history of trauma, surgery, or dissecting aneurysm. A discrete hematoma may compress the superior vena cava and calcify. Any mediastinal compartment may be involved.
Mediastinitis (see Figs C 25-6 and C 25-7)	Generalized widening of the mediastinum, usually most evident superiorly. A lobulated paratracheal mass predominantly projecting to the right may develop in chronic disease.	Acute mediastinitis is most often because of esophageal rupture and may be associated with mediastinal air. Chronic mediastinitis (granulomatous or sclerosing) may calcify and compress vessels (especially the superior vena cava) or a major airway.
Benign lymphoid hyperplasia (Castleman's disease)	Solitary and sharply defined mass.	Although most common in the middle and posterior compartments, in the anterior mediastinum the lesion tends to be lobulated (suggesting a thymoma or teratoma).

A
B

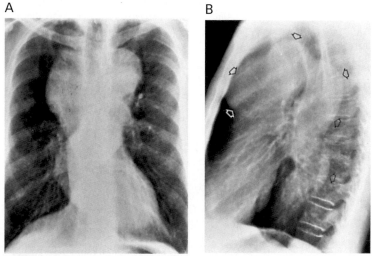

Fig C 23-7
Aneurysm of the thoracic aorta. (A) Frontal and (B) lateral views of the chest demonstrate marked dilatation of both the ascending and descending portions of the thoracic aorta (arrows, B), producing anterior and posterior mediastinal masses, respectively.

A

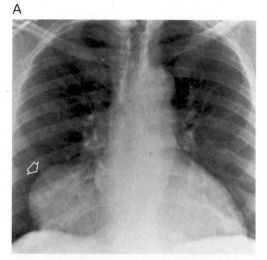

B

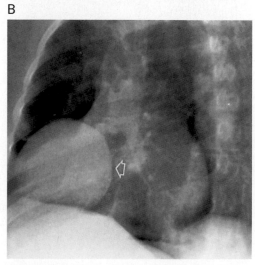

Fig C 23-8
Pericardial cyst. (A) Frontal and (B) oblique views demonstrate a smooth mass (arrows) in the right cardiophrenic angle.

Anterior Mediastinal Lesions on Computed Tomography

Condition	Comments
Fat density (–20 to –100 H) Lipomatosis	Frequent cause of generalized mediastinal widening. Excess fat deposition in the mediastinum may be associated with moderate obesity, steroid therapy, Cushing's syndrome, or diabetes or may be a normal variant in nonobese patients. Fat deposition localized to the superior portion of the anterior compartment may simulate a mass or aortic dissection.
Lipoma (Figs C 24-1 and C 24-2)	Benign collection of fatty tissue that is most common in the anterior mediastinum although it can also occur in the middle and posterior mediastina and adjacent to the diaphragm. Thymolipomas are anterior mediastinal masses that may be indistinguishable from lipomas. Liposarcomas are extremely rare, more commonly occur in the posterior mediastinum, generally have a higher density than benign fat, are inhomogeneous, and tend to show features of mediastinal invasion.

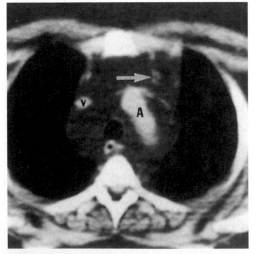

Fig C 24-1
Mediastinal lipomatosis. Abundant fat throughout the superior mediastinum that has a homogeneous attenuation similar to that of subcutaneous fat. (Arrow, residual thymic tissue or mediastinal lymph node; v, right innominate vein; A, aortic arch.)[44]

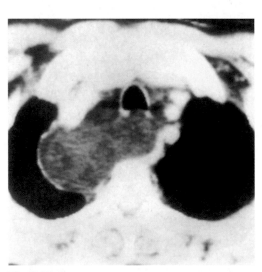

Fig C 24-2
Liposarcoma. Large, relatively inhomogeneous mass in the right side of the mediastinum. Note that the mass has a slightly higher attenuation than does the subcutaneous fat. The mass extended into the right side of the neck to involve the recurrent laryngeal nerve, paralyzing the right vocal cord.[44]

Condition	Comments
Fibrosing mediastinitis (Fig C 24-14)	Rare benign proliferation of acellular collagen and fibrous tissue within the mediastinum. Although often idiopathic, many cases are thought to be the result of an abnormal immunologic response *Histoplasma capsulatum* infection. Fibrosing mediastinitis primarily affects the middle mediastinum.
Vascular/enhancing	Aneurysms, ectatic vessels.
Intrinsic high density (more than 90 H)	Retrosternal thyroid.

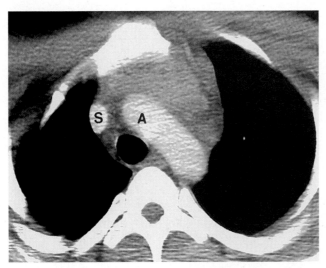

Fig C 24-14
Fibrosing mediastinitis. Soft-tissue attenuation mass in the anterior mediastinum. A, aorta; S, superior vena cava.)[50]

Middle Mediastinal Lesions

Condition	Imaging Findings	Comments
Lymph node enlargement (Fig C 25-1)	Unilateral or bilateral hilar and paratracheal masses.	Most commonly due to metastases, tuberculosis, histoplasmosis, lymphoma, pneumoconiosis, or sarcoidosis.
Aneurysm of aorta or major branch (Fig C 25-2)	Various patterns depending on the location of the aneurysm.	Transverse arch aneurysms typically obliterate the aorticopulmonary window and are symptomatic. Mural calcification is relatively common. Mediastinal masses may also be caused by pseudocoarctation of the aorta and by dilatation of the superior vena cava or azygos vein.

A   B

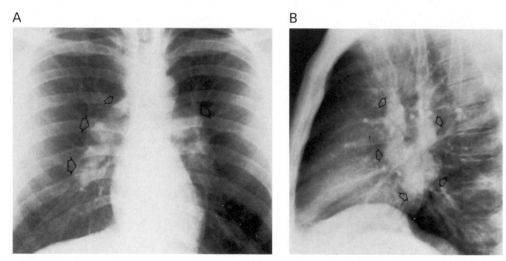

Fig C 25-1
Mediastinal lymphadenopathy in sarcoidosis. (A) Frontal and (B) lateral views of the chest demonstrate enlarged mediastinal lymph nodes (arrows).

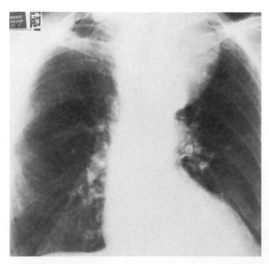

Fig C 25-2
Aneurysm of the left subclavian artery.
Left superior mediastinal widening in an elderly woman without chest symptoms.[43]

Condition	Imaging Findings	Comments
Bronchogenic cyst (Figs C 25-3 and C 25-4)	Round or oval, well-defined mass that is often lobulated and tends to mold itself to surrounding structures (because of its fluid contents).	Most commonly located just inferior to the carina. Often protrudes to the right and overlaps the right hilar shadow. Rarely communicates with the tracheobronchial tree.

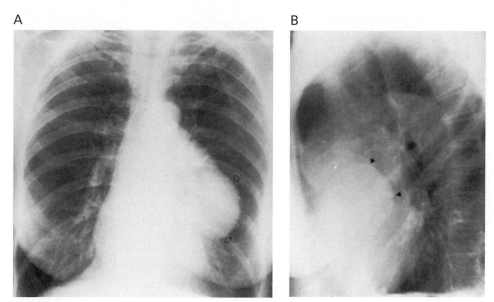

A   B

Fig C 25-3
Bronchogenic cyst. (A) Frontal and (B) lateral views of the chest demonstrate a smooth-walled, spherical mediastinal mass (arrows) projecting into the left lung and left hilum.

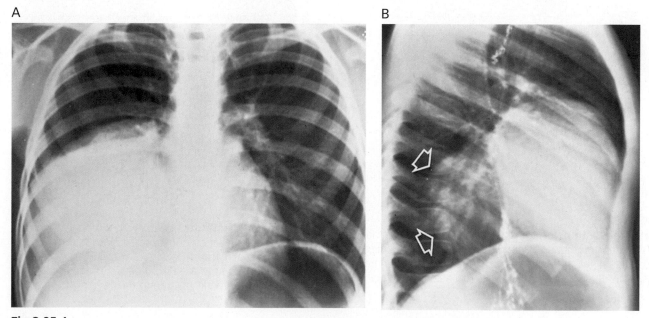

A   B

Fig C 25-4
Bronchogenic cyst. (A) Frontal and (B) lateral views of the chest demonstrate a huge middle mediastinal mass (arrows, B) protruding to the right and filling much of the lower half of the right hemithorax. The patient was asymptomatic.

Condition	Imaging Findings	Comments
Mediastinal hemorrhage/hematoma (Fig C 25-5)	Uniform, symmetric widening of the mediastinum (especially the superior portion).	Generally a history of trauma, surgery, or dissecting aneurysm. A discrete hematoma may compress the superior vena cava and calcify.
Mediastinitis (Figs C 25-6 and C 25-7)	Generalized widening of the mediastinum, usually most evident superiorly. A lobulated paratracheal mass predominantly projecting to the right may develop in chronic disease.	Acute mediastinitis is most often due to esophageal rupture and may be associated with mediastinal air. Chronic mediastinitis (granulomatous or sclerosing) may calcify and compress vessels (especially the superior vena cava) or a major airway.
Pleuropericardial (mesothelial) cyst	Round, oval, or teardrop mass with smooth margins.	Fluid-filled cyst that is almost always asymptomatic and may change shape with respiration or alteration in body position. May also involve the anterior mediastinum.
Intrapericardial hernia (Fig C 25-8)	Gas-filled loops of bowel that lie alongside the heart and remain in conformity with the heart border on multiple projections (including decubitus views).	Extremely rare congenital or posttraumatic lesion that can contain (in decreasing order of frequency) omentum, colon, small bowel, liver, or stomach. Although often asymptomatic for long periods, most patients eventually present with cardiorespiratory or gastrointestinal complaints.
Benign lymphoid hyperplasia (Castleman's disease)	Smooth or lobulated solitary mass.	Rare condition that most often involves the posterior mediastinum.

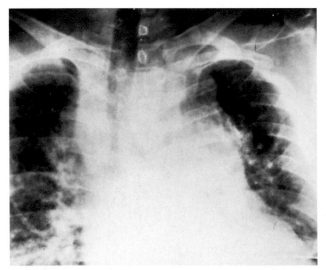

Fig C 25-5
Aortic transection. Frontal chest radiograph taken immediately after trauma demonstrates mediastinal widening, obscuration of the aorta, deviation of the trachea to the right, and downward displacement of the left main-stem bronchus.[51]

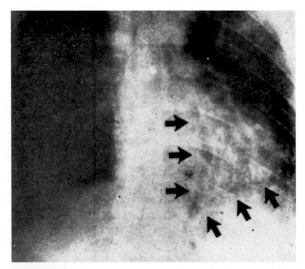

Fig C 25-6
Acute mediastinitis due to rupture of the esophagus. Plain radiograph demonstrates linear lucent shadows (arrows) that represent localized mediastinal emphysema and correspond to the fascial planes of the mediastinal and diaphragmatic pleurae in the region of the lower esophagus.[52]

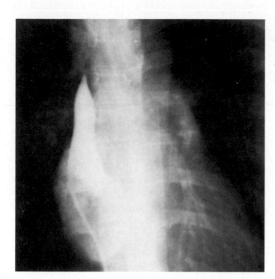

Fig C 25-7
Chronic sclerosing mediastinitis. Venogram shows smooth tapering of the lower portion of the superior vena cava. This 38-year-old woman had varicosities over her upper abdomen and lower chest.[52]

B

A

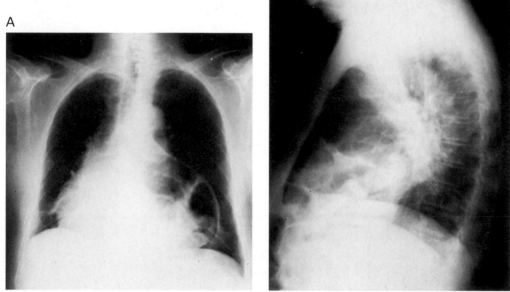

Fig C 25-8
Congenital intrapericardial hernia. (A) Frontal and (B) lateral views in an asymptomatic elderly man show loops of bowel in the chest conforming to the left pericardial border.[53]

Middle Mediastinal Lesions on Computed Tomography

Condition	Comments
Fat density (–20 to –100 H)	
Lipomatosis (Figs C 26-1 and C 26-2)	Extensive fat deposition in the mediastinum may be associated with moderate obesity, steroid therapy, Cushing's syndrome, or diabetes or may be a normal variant in nonobese patients.
Epicardial fat pad	Most common fatty mass in the thorax.
Pericardial lipoma	Localized collection of fat-density tissue (lipomas occur more commonly in the anterior mediastinum).

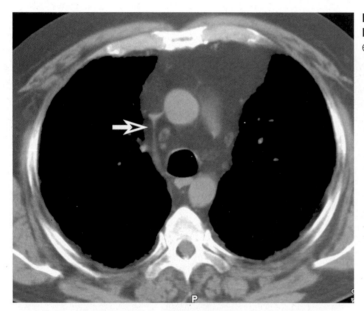

Fig C 26-1
Mediastinal lipomatosis. Diffuse fatty lesion with a mass effect on the superior vena cava and azygos vein.[54]

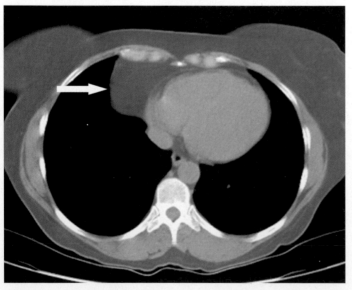

Fig C 26-2
Epicardial fat pad. Homogeneous fat attenuation (arrow) adjacent to the right border of the heart.[52]

Condition	Comments
Water density (0 to 15 H)	
Pericardial cyst (Fig C 26-3)	Smooth, thin-walled mass that most commonly occurs in the right cardiophrenic angle. Malleable lesion that may change shape when the patient is scanned in the prone or decubitus position. Easily differentiated from prominent epicardial fat pads or lipomas, which also present as cardiophrenic angle masses.
Bronchogenic cyst (Fig C 26-4)	Smooth, round, homogeneous mass that usually has a thin, imperceptible rim and does not show any change in attenuation after infusion of contrast material. May contain viscous mucoid or proteinaceous material that produces a higher attenuation in the range of a solid neoplasm.

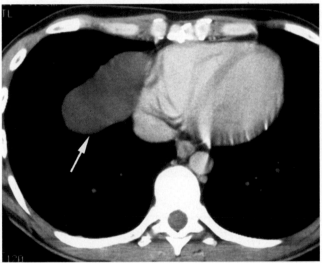

Fig C 26-3
Pericardial cyst. Contrast CT scan shows a thin-walled cyst of water attenuation (arrow).[55]

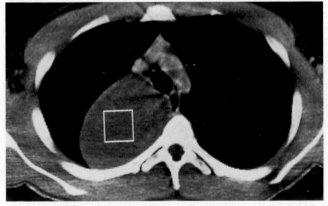

Fig C 26-4
Bronchogenic cyst. CT scan in a young man with an incidental upper respiratory infection shows a large right upper mediastinal mass extending from the right of the trachea to the posterior chest wall. The cyst had a uniform appearance and near-water density and extended vertically from the lower pole of the thyroid gland to the carina.[56]

Condition	Comments
Soft-tissue density (15 to 40 H) Lymphadenopathy (Figs C 26-5 to C 26-8)	Most commonly the result of metastases, lymphoma, granulomatous disease (tuberculosis, histoplasmosis), pneumoconiosis, or sarcoidosis.
Mediastinitis/abscess	Suggested by the presence of bubbles of gas or a discrete cavity with a thick, shaggy wall.

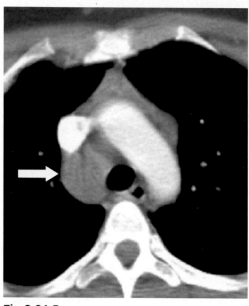

Fig C 26-5
Lymphadenopathy. The enlarged nodes (arrow) obliterate the air-soft tissue interface between the right lung and the tracheal wall (right paratracheal stripe).[52]

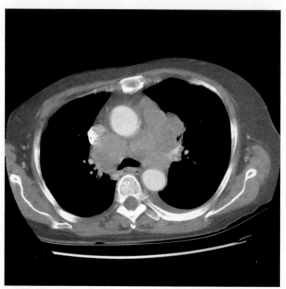

Fig C 26-6
Bronchogenic carcinoma. Soft-tissue mass within the aortopulmonary window and subcarinal space, a finding consistent with metastatic lymphadenopathy. There is also lymphadenopathy in the paratracheal region, which produced a thickened right paratracheal stripe on plain radiographs.[57]

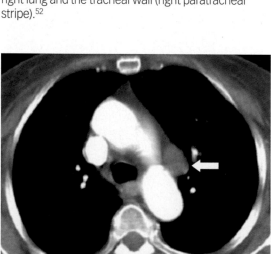

Fig C 26-7
Lymphoma. Enlarged nodes (arrow) obliterate the normal concave border of the interface between the left lung and the mediastinum constituting the aorticopulmonary window.[52]

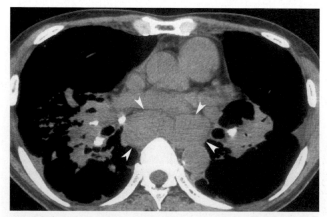

Fig C 26-8
Sarcoidosis. Diffuse bilateral mediastinal and hilar adenopathy. Calcification in the affected hilar nodes suggests a prolonged clinical course. Note the simultaneous presence of huge subcarinal nodes (arrowheads), an unusual finding in other granulomatous diseases such as tuberculosis.[58]

Condition	Comments
Mediastinitis/abscess/ infectious spondylitis (Figs C 28-7 and C 28-8)	Suggested by the presence of bubbles of gas or a discrete cavity with a thick shaggy wall. Osteolytic vertebral destruction can be seen in infectious spondylitis.
Spinal tumor (Fig C 28-9)	Primary or metastatic neoplasms can produce a paravertebral mass with osteolytic or osteoblastic vertebral changes.

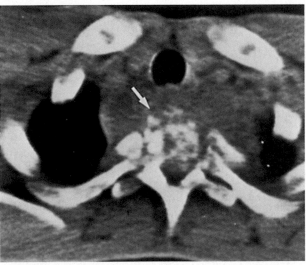

Fig C 28-7
Tuberculous spondylitis and paraspinal cold abscess.
Unenhanced scan obtained above the aortic arch shows a paravertebral mass that is destroying the vertebral body (arrow) and displacing the trachea anteriorly.[59]

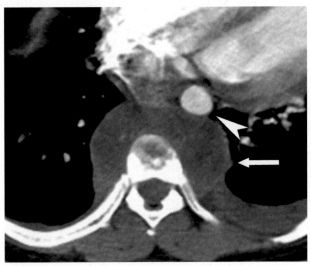

Fig C 28-8
Parspinal abscess. Soft-tissue mass (arrow) extending bilaterally that effaced the paraspinal lines (arrow). Arowhead indicates descending thoracic aorta.[52]

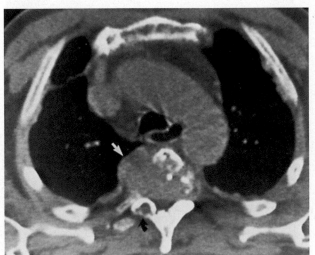

Fig C 28-9
Multiple myeloma. Unenhanced scan at the aortic arch level demonstrates a soft-tissue mass (white arrow) that is destroying the vertebral body and compromising the spinal canal. There are also associated osteolytic lesions of the posterior elements and adjacent ribs (black arrow).[59]

Condition	Comments
Mediastinal hemorrhage/ hematoma (Fig C 28-10)	Uniform, symmetric widening of the mediastinum (especially the superior portion) in a patient with a history of trauma, surgery, or a dissecting aneurysm.
Extramedullary hematopoiesis (Fig C 28-11)	Generally occurs in the paravertebral region in the lower half of the thorax. May appear as a fat-density mass.
Lymphadenopathy (Fig C 28-12)	Posterior mediastinal (paraspinal) lymph nodes are considered enlarged if they exceed 6 mm in diameter (same criteria as for retrocrural nodes in the abdomen). Enlarged paraspinal nodes must not be mistaken for the azygos or hemiazygos veins, which are clearly tubular structures seen at multiple levels.
Bronchopulmonary sequestration	Congenital pulmonary malformation in which a portion of pulmonary tissue is detached from the remainder of the normal lung and receives its blood supply from a systemic artery. Typically appears as a sharply circumscribed mass in the posterior portion of a lower lobe (usually the left) contiguous to the diaphragm. May contain air or an air-fluid level if infection has resulted in communication with the airways or contiguous lung tissue.

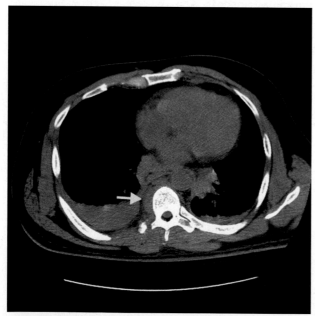

Fig C 28-10
Hematoma. Large mediastinal soft-tissue mass (arrow) from multiple right transverse process fractures of the lower thoracic spine. Note the associated right hemothorax.[63]

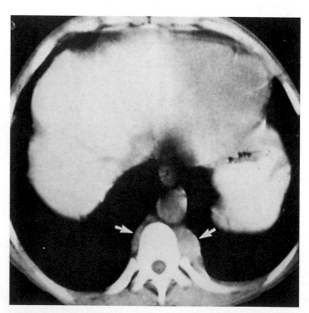

Fig C 28-11
Extramedullary hematopoiesis. Upper abdomen scan in a patient with homozygous sickle cell disease demonstrates bilateral, well-demarcated paravertebral soft-tissue masses (arrows) that are larger on the left. The diffuse increased attenuation of the liver reflects multiple blood transfusions.[59]

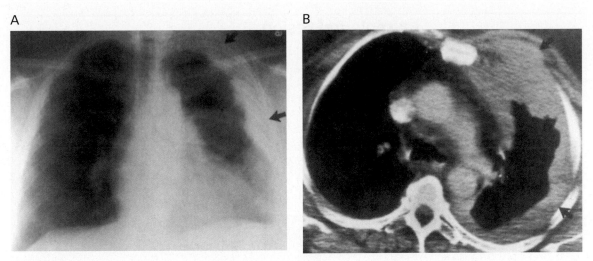

Fig C 33-8
Lymphoma. (A) Frontal chest radiographic shows irregular pleural thickening (arrows). (B) Concurrent CT scan demonstrates diffuse pleural thickening (arrows), greater than 1 cm in thickness, involving the left mediastinal and costal pleura.[64]

Extrapleural Lesion

Condition	Comments
Chest wall hematoma (Figs C 34-1 to C 34-3)	Usually a history of trauma and often evidence of a rib fracture. May also occur with sternal fractures (hematoma best seen on lateral view). Callus formation about an old rib fracture may be mistaken for a pulmonary nodule.

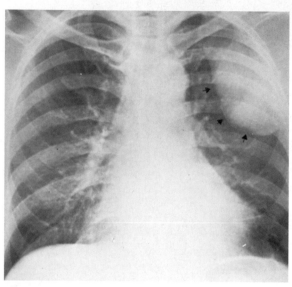

Fig C 34-1
Pulmonary hematoma. Large extrapleural density (arrows) over the left upper lobe.

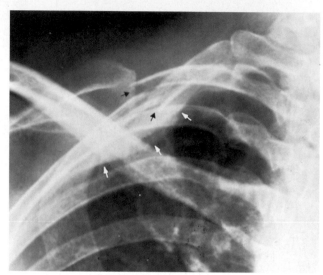

Fig C 34-2
Chest trauma. Small extrapleural hematoma (white arrows) associated with fractures of the first and second ribs (black arrows).

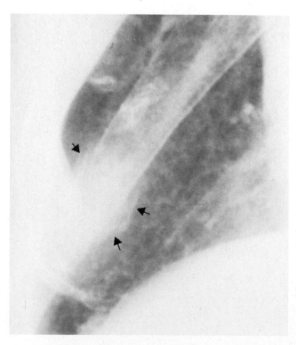

Fig C 34-3
Cough fracture. simulating a pulmonary nodule. A coned view of the right lower lung on a routine chest radiograph shows callus formation about a rib (arrows) in an asymptomatic person.

Condition	Comments
Rib neoplasm (Fig C 34-4)	Metastases and myeloma are the most common causes of an extrapleural mass associated with rib destruction in adults. Ewing's tumor and metastatic neuroblastoma are the most common causes in children.
Mediastinal, spinal, sternal, or subphrenic lesion (see Fig C 14-6)	Tumors, cysts, and inflammatory processes may produce extrapleural masses.
Chest wall infection	An extrapleural mass with rib destruction is most commonly a manifestation of actinomycosis (often with parenchymal infiltrate, pleural effusion, and even a cutaneous fistula). A similar pattern may also be due to nocardiosis, blastomycosis, aspergillosis, or, rarely, tuberculosis.
Extrapleural lipoma	Common chest wall lesion that may grow between ribs to present as both an intrathoracic and a subcutaneous mass. Characteristic fat density on CT.
Surgery or blunt trauma	Ruptured aneurysm, partial pleurectomy, sympathectomy, plombage, and mineral oil injection for the treatment of tuberculosis.
Congenital lobar agenesis	Missing lobe is often replaced by a chunk of extrapleural aureolar tissue that produces an anterior extrapleural mass paralleling the sternum. There is loss of the right heart border on frontal views.

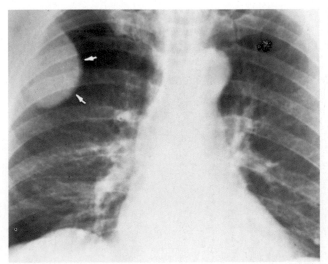

Fig C 34-4
Extramedullary myeloma. Large extrapleural mass (arrows) containing a proliferation of plasma cells.

Pleural Calcification

Condition	Imaging Findings	Comments
Organized hemothorax (Fig C 35-1)	Usually unilateral calcification of the visceral pleura (Fig C 35-1) in the form of a broad continuous sheet or multiple discrete plaques.	Typically extends from about the level of the mid-thorax posteriorly, coursing around the lateral lung margins in a generally inferior direction and roughly paralleling the major fissure. There is often evidence of healed rib fractures and a history of significant chest trauma.
Organized empyema (Fig C 35-2)	Usually unilateral calcification of the visceral pleura in the form of a broad continuous sheet or multiple discrete plaques.	Typically extends from about the level of the mid-thorax posteriorly, coursing around the lateral lung margins in a generally inferior direction and roughly paralleling the major fissure. Usually a history of severe pulmonary infection.
Old tuberculous empyema (Fig C 35-3)	Usually unilateral calcification of the visceral pleura in the form of a broad continuous sheet or multiple discrete plaques. May be bilateral (usually asymmetric).	Typically extends from about the level of the mid-thorax posteriorly, coursing around the lateral lung margins in a generally inferior direction and roughly paralleling the major fissure. Extensive apical parenchymal scarring or cavitary disease is virtually diagnostic.

A
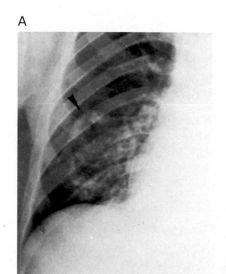

B
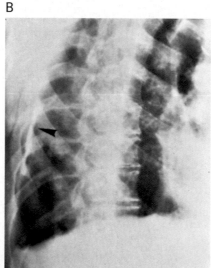

Fig C 35-1
Calcified thickened pleura. (A) The density in the lower lung (arrowhead) has a well-defined irregular border closely resembling a cavity. (B) An oblique view, however, shows a pathognomonic linear density (arrowhead) paralleling but separated from the chest wall.[65]

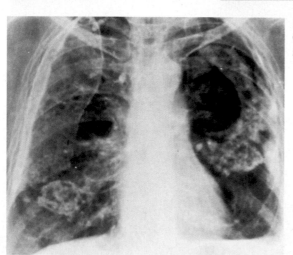

Fig C 35-2
Organized empyema. Bilateral broad continuous sheets of calcification overlie much of the lung surface.

Condition	Imaging Findings	Comments
Pneumoconiosis (Figs C 35-4 to C 35-6)	Usually bilateral plaques of calcification involving the parietal pleura, commonly along the diaphragm. There may sometimes be calcification in extensively thickened pleura along the lateral chest wall.	Most commonly caused by asbestosis. May also be due to other silicates (eg, talcosis). The diaphragmatic pleura are almost always extensively involved (unlike hemothorax or empyema). Extensive encasement of both lungs may occur. Basilar reticulonodular interstitial disease is highly suggestive, though often absent.

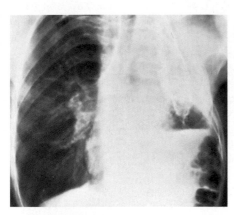

Fig C 35-3
Old tuberculous empyema. Broad sheet of calcification overlies much of the left hemithorax. Note the elevation of the left hemidiaphragm and retraction of the trachea to the left, all consistent with loss of volume due to the chronic granulomatous disease.

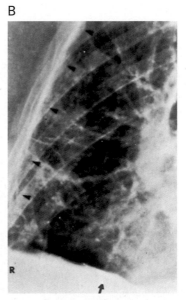

B

A

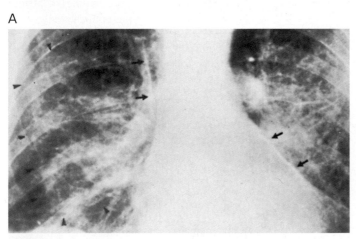

Fig C 35-4
Asbestosis. (A) Frontal view shows en face calcifications on the right (arrowheads) and linear calcifications in profile in the mediastinal reflection of the pleura on the right and in the pericardium on the left (transverse arrows). (B) A left oblique film shows linear pleural calcification in profile in the area of the central tendon of the right hemidiaphragm (arrows). The en face plaques in (A) now appear in profile as extensive linear calcifications (arrowheads) adjacent to anterior ribs.[66]

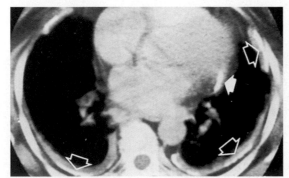

Fig C 35-5
Asbestosis. CT scan shows calcified pleural plaques along the lateral and posterior chest wall (open arrows) and adjacent to the heart (closed arrow).

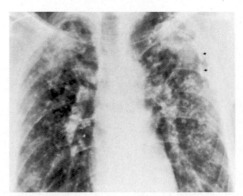

Fig C 35-6
Coal-workers' pneumoconiosis. Bilateral fibrous masses in the apices with upward retraction of the hila. Note the pleural calcification (arrows) in the left apex.

Pleural Effusion with Otherwise Normal-Appearing Chest

Condition	Imaging Findings	Comments
Tuberculosis (Fig C 36-1)	Serous exudate with low glucose content and predominantly lymphocytic reaction. Almost always unilateral.	Common manifestation of primary tuberculosis in adults (approximately 40%) but less frequent in children (10%). The patient may have a negative tuberculin test in early stages. Active pulmonary tuberculosis often develops if the effusion is not treated.
Other infections (Fig C 36-2)	Serous exudate that may be bilateral.	Bacteria, fungi (especially actinomycosis and nocardiosis), viruses, mycoplasma.
Thoracic lymphoma	Serosanguineous exudate that may be unilateral or bilateral.	Usually evidence of pulmonary or mediastinal lymph node involvement. Suggestive findings include hepatosplenomegaly and peripheral lymph node enlargement.
Metastatic carcinoma	Serous exudate with variable blood content and typically elevated glucose. Unilateral or bilateral.	Most common primary sites are breast, pancreas, stomach, ovary, and kidney. At times, a pleural effusion may be the only presenting finding.
Ovarian neoplasm (Meigs' syndrome)	Serous exudate that is more frequent on the right (may be left-sided or bilateral).	Most commonly an ovarian fibroma associated with ascites. Can also develop with other benign or malignant ovarian tumors. The effusion usually disappears after removal of the ovarian neoplasm.
Carcinoma of pancreas/ retroperitoneum	Serous exudate (pleural fluid negative for malignant cells).	Often no direct tumor involvement of the thorax. The effusion disappears after removal or treatment of the primary lesion.

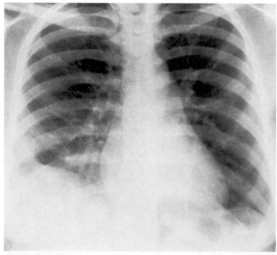

Fig C 36-1
Primary tuberculosis. Unilateral right tuberculous pleural effusion without parenchymal or lymph node involvement.

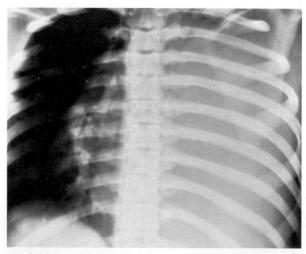

Fig C 36-2
Coccidioidomycosis. Complete homogeneous opacification of the left hemithorax. The massive pleural effusion must be associated with virtually complete collapse of the left lung as there is no contralateral shift of the mediastinal structures.

Condition	Imaging Findings	Comments
Pulmonary thromboembolic disease	Serosanguineous effusion that is most often unilateral.	Effusion is infrequently the sole manifestation of pulmonary embolism (may obscure small parenchymal abnormalities). The presence of fluid almost always indicates infarction.
Subphrenic abscess	Ipsilateral serous exudate.	More commonly associated with elevation and fixation of the hemidiaphragm and basal atelectasis (see Fig C 34-2). There may be gas or a mottled pattern of density in the subphrenic space.
Pancreatitis (Fig C 36-3)	Serous or serosanguineous exudate with a high amylase level. Predominantly left-sided (may be bilateral).	May occur in acute, chronic, or relapsing pancreatitis or with a pancreatic pseudocyst. Other manifestations include elevation of the hemidiaphragm and basal atelectasis.
Trauma	Varied composition (blood, chyle, or food after esophageal rupture).	Hemothorax complicating traumatic aortic rupture and effusion after esophageal perforation are almost always left-sided. The side of a chylothorax depends on the site of the thoracic duct rupture (see Fig C 38-1).
Abdominal surgery	Serous exudate.	Usually very small but may be detected in almost half the patients if lateral decubitus views are obtained.
Postmyocardial infarction syndrome (Dressler's syndrome)	Left-sided or bilateral transudate is the most common finding (80%) and may occur alone.	Characterized by fever and pleuropericardial chest pain that begins 1 to 6 weeks after acute myocardial infarction. Pericardial effusion or pulmonary infiltrates frequently occur (see Fig CA 22-2). Striking response to steroid therapy.

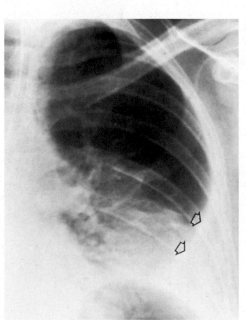

Fig C 36-3
Pancreatitis. Blunting of the normally sharp angle between the diaphragm and the rib cage (arrows) along with a characteristic upward concave border (meniscus) of the fluid level.

Condition	Imaging Findings	Comments
Cirrhosis with ascites	Transudate that is more often right-sided (may be on the left or bilateral).	Ascitic fluid probably enters the pleural space via diaphragmatic lymphatics (as in Meigs' syndrome). Usually evidence of ascites and other signs of cirrhosis.
Systemic lupus erythematosus (Fig C 36-4)	Serous exudate that is bilateral in approximately 50% of patients. The effusion is predominantly left-sided when unilateral. Tends to be small (occasionally massive).	Pleural effusion is an isolated abnormality in approximately 10% of cases. It is often associated with a pericardial effusion and usually clears without residua. Nonspecific cardiomegaly and pulmonary involvement develop in most patients.
Rheumatoid disease	Serous exudate with a predominance of lymphocytes and a low glucose level. Usually unilateral.	Occurs almost exclusively in men. May antedate the signs and symptoms of rheumatoid arthritis, but usually follows them. There is often no pulmonary evidence of rheumatoid disease.
Asbestosis	Serous or blood-tinged exudate that is usually bilateral and often recurrent.	More commonly occurs in association with pleural plaques and calcification.
Renal disease (Fig C 36-5)	Transudate or serous exudate.	Causes include nephrotic syndrome, acute glomerulonephritis, hydronephrosis, and uremic pleuritis.
Peritoneal dialysis	Serous exudate.	Probably the same underlying mechanism as with ascites. May be impossible to distinguish from a uremic effusion.

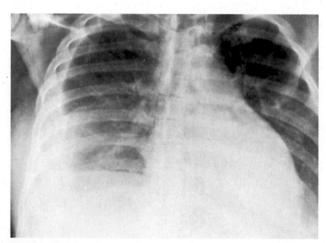

Fig C 36-4
Systemic lupus erythematosus. Large right pleural effusion in a young woman.

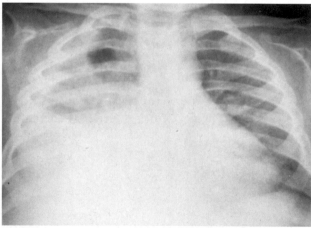

Fig C 36-5
Nephrotic syndrome. Diffuse cardiomegaly with a large right pleural effusion, which is situated both along the lateral chest wall and in a subpulmonic location.

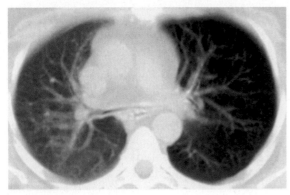

Fig C 41-18
Relapsing polychondritis. Expiratory scan shows abnormal collapse of the bronchi with air trapping in the left lung.[77]

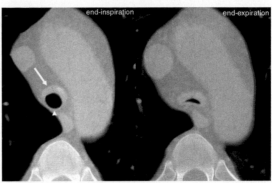

Fig C 41-19
Relapsing polychondritis. End-inspiration and end-expiration scans show dynamic collapse of the trachea with expiration (right). Note the calcification and thickening of the cartilaginous parts of the trachea (arrow), with sparing of the posterior wall (arrowhead).[82]

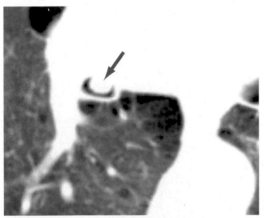

Fig C 41-20
Foreign body. Well-circumscribed mass in the bronchus intermedius (arrow).[76]

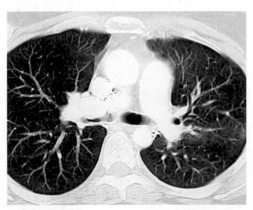

Fig C 41-21
Post-transplantation stenosis. Focal narrowing at the anastomotic site within the right lung in a patient who had undergone bilateral lung transplantation.[82]

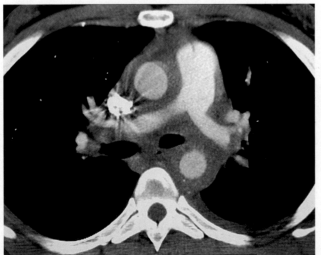

Fig C 41-22
Fibrosing mediastinitis. Mass of soft-tissue attenuation that diffusely infiltrates the mediastinum, encasing and narrowing the left main bronchus (*), ascending (A) and descending (D) aorta, proximal right (R) and left (L) pulmonary arteries, and esophagus (arrowhead).[55]

Broncholithiasis*

Condition	Comments
Erosion by and extrusion of a calcified adjacent lymph node (Figs C 42-1 and C 42-2)	By far the most common cause, it is usually associated with long-standing foci of necrotizing granulomatous lymphadenitis (especially tuberculosis). Nevertheless, the frequency of broncholithiasis complicating granulomatous infection is quite low. Broncholiths vary in size and are usually irregular, often possessing spur-like projections or sharp edges. It is thought that repeated physical impingement of calcified peribronchial lymph nodes on the bronchial wall during respiratory motion is responsible for broncholith formation. The most common sites are the proximal right middle lobe bronchus and the origin of the anterior segmental bronchus of the upper lobes because of airway anatomy and lymph node distribution.

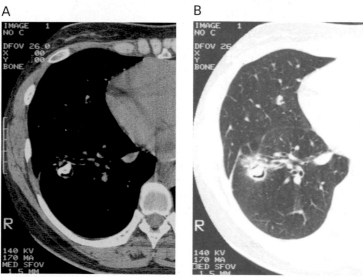

Fig 42-1
Extrusion of a calcified adjacent lymph node. CT scans with mediastinal (A) and lung (B) windows shows a calcified nodule within a dilated bronchus.[81]

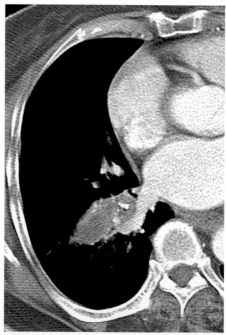

Fig 42-2
Extrusion of a calcified adjacent lymph node. Calcified nodule (arrowhead) in the anterior basal segment of the right lower lobe with secondary atelectasis.[79]

*The presence of calcified or ossified material within the bronchial lumen.

Condition	Comments
In situ calcification of aspirated foreign material/ aspiration of bone tissue (Figs C 42-3 and C 42-4)	Persistence of a noncalcified foreign body, such as a vegetable fiber, within a bronchus for a prolonged period can serve as a nidus for calcium deposition. Rarely, bone fragments or other radiopaque material may be aspirated
Erosion by and extrusion of calcified or ossified bronchial cartilage plate	Diffuse tracheobronchial calcification is commonly associated with advanced age. In rare cases, broncholithiasis can result from calcification of bronchial cartilage with subsequent sequestration of the calcified material into the bronchial lumen.
Disorders mimicking broncholithiasis Primary endobronchial infection with dystrophic calcification (Fig C 42-5)	Rarely, primary endobronchial fungus ball due to actinomycosis may calcify and result in the formation of a calcified endobronchial nodule.

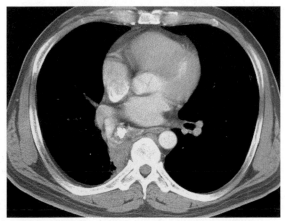

Fig 42-3
Calcification of an aspirated foreign body. The calcified nodule in the bronchus intermedius proved to be a vegetable fiber with dystrophic calcification. Note the atelectasis of the right lower lobe.[79]

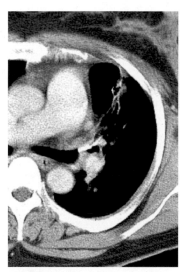

Fig 42-4
Aspiration of an opaque anchovy bone. Tubular calcified lesion at the orifice of the upper lobe bronchus (arrow).[79]

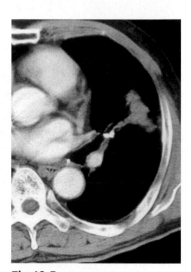

Fig 42-5
Endobronchial actinomycosis with dystrophic calcification. Calcified nodule within the bronchus of the lingular division of the left upper lobe (arrow) with peripheral atelectasis.[80]

Condition	Comments
Calcified endobronchial tumor (Figs C 42-6 and C 42-7)	Some calcification is often seen in central carcinoid tumors on CT examinations. When the tumor is totally ossified and situated within the bronchus, it simulates broncholithiasis. Although endobronchial hamartomas are rare, they can mimic broncholithiasis when they have a central cartilaginous core.
Tracheobronchial disease with mural calcification (Fig C 42-8)	Amyloid deposition may form a polypoid submucosal airway nodule with stippled calcification that mimics a broncholith. Protrusion into the lumen of a submucosal osteocartilaginous growth along the lateral wall of the trachea or main bronchus can also simulate broncholithiasis.

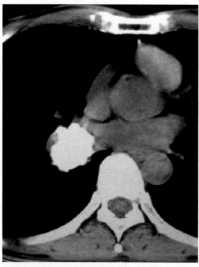

Fig 42-6
Carcinoid tumor. Sharply defined, totally ossified mass (arrow) that is centrally situated in the right lower lobe bronchus and produces abrupt bronchial obstruction.[79]

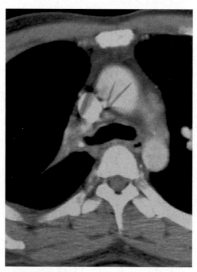

Fig 42-7
Hamartoma. Small calcified nodule obstructing the right upper lobe bronchus (arrow).[79]

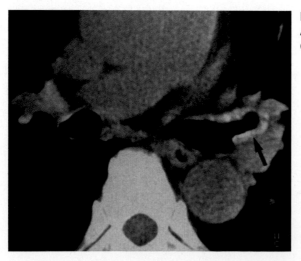

Fig 42-8
Amyloidosis. Localized thickening of the bronchial wall with calcification and partial intraluminal protrusion (arrows).[81]

Condition	Comments
Hypertrophied bronchial artery with intraluminal protrusion (Fig C 42-9)	The bronchial arteries become enlarged in such disorders as acute or chronic pulmonary infections, pulmonary thromboembolism, and chronic obstructive pulmonary disease. Protrusion of a hypertrophied bronchial artery into the lumen may mimic a broncholith on contrast-enhanced CT scans. Careful examination of images obtained above and below the abnormality or unenhanced CT may be required to confirm the vascular nature of the lesion.

A

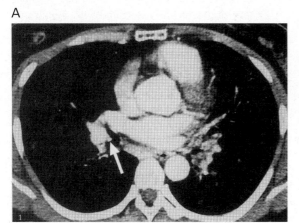

B

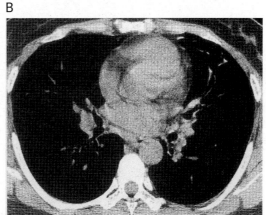

Fig 42-9
Hypertrophied bronchial artery. (A) Contrast-enhanced scan shows a high-attenuation nodular structure (arrow) at the bifurcation of the bronchus intermedius, which mimics broncholithiasis. (B) This unenhanced section scan reveals that the high-attenuation structure is not calcified.[82]

Retrotracheal Space Abnormalities

Condition	Comments
Vascular lesions	
Aberrant right subclavian artery (Fig C 43-1)	The aberrant vessel arises from the posterior portion of the aortic arch and crosses the mediastinum from left to right, posterior to the trachea and esophagus.
Aberrant left subclavian artery (Fig C 43-2)	The most common anomaly seen with a right-sided aortic arch, it is not associated with congenital heart disease. CT and MRI can differentiate this from a right-sided aortic arch with mirror-image branching, which is associated with a high prevalence of congenital heart disease.
Double aortic arch (Fig C 43-3)	One of the most common symptomatic anomalies of the aortic arch, it usually is apparent in infancy because of respiratory symptoms or difficulty in feeding related to tracheal or esophageal compression. The larger, higher, and more posterior right arch fuses with the left arch posteriorly to form a single descending aorta that is typically left-sided.
Aortic aneurysm (Fig C 43-4)	Can appear as a fusiform or saccular mass-like lesion that protrudes into the retrotracheal space. Complications include ulceration and rupture.
Esophageal lesions Atresia	Congenital incomplete formation of the tubular esophagus. It can manifest as an air-distended pouch or mass-like lesion (due to mucosal secretion) in the retrotracheal space that deforms the adjacent part of the trachea.

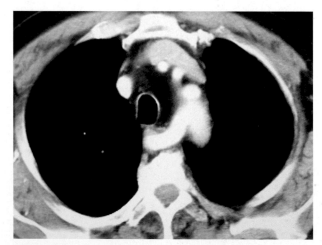

Fig C 43-1
Aberrant right subclavian artery. CT scan shows that the aberrant vessel arises as the last branch of a left-sided aortic arch posterior to the esophagus.[83]

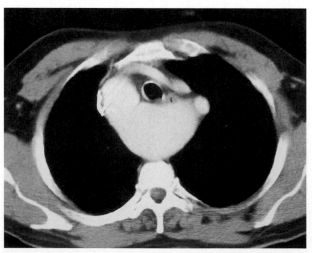

Fig C 43-2
Aberrant left subclavian artery with a right-sided aortic arch.[83]

Condition	Comments
Duplication cyst (Fig C 43-5)	Although most of these congenital lesions arise in the lower esophagus, one developing in the upper portion may appear as a mass in the retrotracheal space. Of water-attenuation on CT and with high signal intensity on T2-weighted MR images, they may have high signal intensity on T1-weighted images due to intracystic hemorrhage or proteinaceous debris.

A
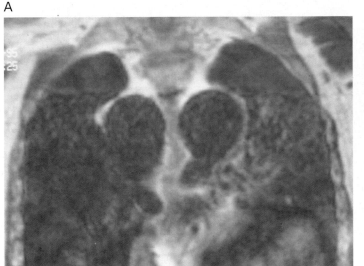

B
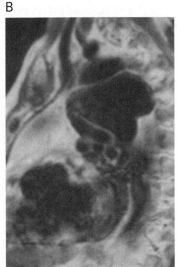

Fig C 43-3
Double aortic arch. (A) Coronal T1-weighted MR image shows the right and left aortic arches. (B) On a sagittal image, the retrotracheal space is obscured by both aortic arches.[83]

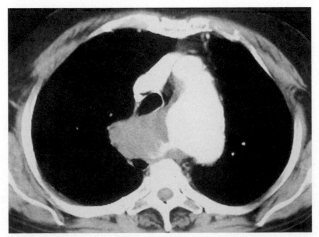

Fig C 43-4
Aneurysm of the transverse aortic arch. CT scan shows a penetrating atherosclerotic ulcer and a contained rupture or mediastinal hematoma.[83]

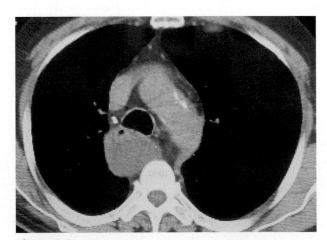

Fig C 43-5
Esophageal duplication cyst. CT scan shows a well-circumscribed mass with water attenuation adjacent to the esophagus. The appearance and location of the mass are typical for an esophageal duplication cyst in this asymptomatic young woman, in whom the lesion was an incidental finding on chest radiography.[83]

Condition	Comments
Zenker's diverticulum (Fig C 43-6)	Pulsion diverticulum in the upper esophagus that usually extends dorsally into the postcricoid area. If large, it can be detected in the retrotracheal space as a large air- or fluid-filled, mass-like lesion.
Achalasia	Dilatation of the esophagus due to inadequate relaxation of the lower esophageal sphincter can cause anterior displacement and bowing of the trachea by the fluid- or food-filled esophagus. Aspiration pneumonia is an associated complication
Tumors	Carcinoma can cause marked inhomogeneous thickening of the esophageal wall with infiltration extending to the posterior wall of the trachea. A leiomyoma can produce a smooth impression on the posterior wall of the trachea and anterior displacement of the airway.
Miscellaneous mediastinal masses Lymphatic malformation (Fig C 43-7)	Also known as lymphangioma, approximately 5% of these rare benign lesions occur in the mediastinum. Most are found in children over 2 years old (the site of 75% of lesions) and they can extend into the retrotracheal space. In adults, mediastinal lymphatic malformations are usually due to an incompletely resected childhood tumor. Although typically appearing as lobular, multicystic lesions, they may appear solid on CT or have high signal on T1-weighted MR images due to intracystic protein or hemorrhage.

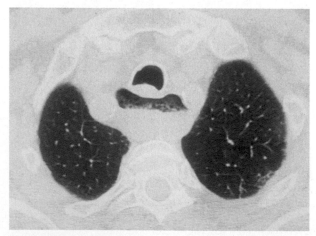

Fig C 43-6
Zenker's diverticulum. CT demonstrates a large retrotracheal diverticulum with an air-fluid level due to retained alimentary content.[83]

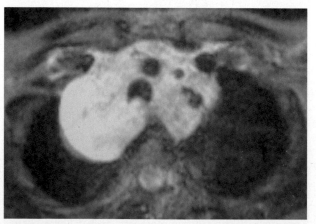

Fig C 43-7
Lymphatic malformation. Axial T2-weighted image shows a characteristic hyperintense lesion that surrounds, but does not displace, the trachea and great vessels. The tumor extends toward the anterior soft tissues of the chest wall.[83]

Condition	Comments
Hemangioma (Fig C 43-8)	Rare mediastinal tumor composed of large interconnecting vascular spaces with varying amounts of interposed stromal elements such as fat and fibrous tissue. The heterogeneous mass usually demonstrates rimlike peripheral contrast enhancement. Phleboliths are present in <10% of cases.
Thyroid goiter (Fig C 43-9)	Most thyroid masses in the mediastinum are caused by intrathoracic extension of neck masses. In approximately 20% of cases, the lesion extends posteriorly behind the esophagus and adjacent to the trachea to involve the retrotracheal space. On CT, the heterogeneous mass commonly contains areas of hemorrhage, necrosis, and calcification.
Hemorrhage (Fig C 43-10)	Complication of traumatic aortic injury or such iatrogenic procedures as placement of a central venous catheter. Posterior extension of mediastinal hemorrhage can produce a mass-like area in the retrotracheal space. In patients with aortic transaction, the trachea is typically displaced to the right.
Infection (Fig C 43-11)	Infection can spread to the retrotracheal space from contiguous structures such as the thoracic spine and paravertebral spaces, or caudad from the retropharyngeal and prevertebral spaces.
Acute mediastinitis (Fig C 43-12)	Diffuse inflammation or abscess formation in the retrotracheal space may result from rupture of the esophagus secondary to blunt thoracic trauma, foreign body impaction, or diagnostic or therapeutic endoscopic procedures. Esophageal fistulization related to esophageal carcinoma may also be a cause of mediastinal abscess

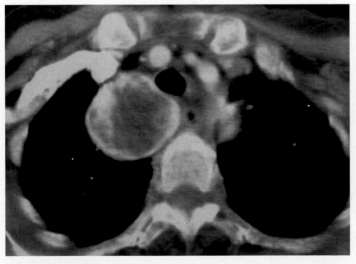

Fig C 43-8
Hemangioma. Contrast CT scan shows a well-defined mass with intense central and rim-like peripheral enhancement.[83]

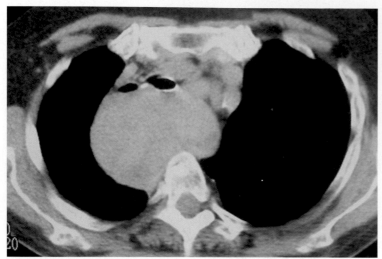

Fig C 43-9
Intrathoracic goiter. CT scan shows a well-defined, homogeneous soft-tissue mass that fills the retrotracheal space and displaces the trachea, esophagus, and supraaortic vessels anteriorly.[83]

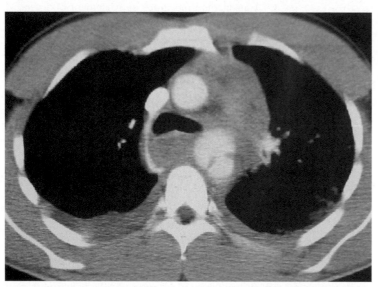

Fig C 43-10
Hematoma. Contrast CT scan shows a mediastinal hematoma in the retrotracheal space. There is a pseudoaneurysm (*) medial to the proximal descending thoracic aorta. Bilateral pleural effusions are also seen.[83]

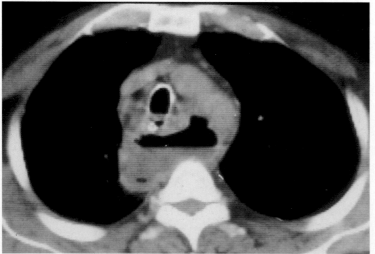

Fig C 43-11
Retropharyngeal infection with mediastinal abscess formation. CT scan shows widening of the middle mediastinum with a large abscess that fills the retrotracheal space and displaces the trachea and esophagus anteriorly. There is an air-fluid level within the abscess cavity.[83]

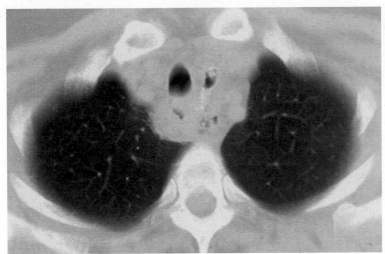

Fig C 43-12
Mediastinal abscess with fistulization. CT scan shows marked thickening of the esophageal wall. Air bubbles and a small amount of contrast material are seen within the retrotracheal space, reflecting the formation of a fistula (arrow).[83]

Upper Airway Obstruction in Children

Condition	Imaging Findings	Comments
Croup (Fig C 44-1)	Smooth tapered narrowing of the subglottic trachea.	Very common and usually mild.
Epiglottitis (Fig C 44-2)	Huge swelling of the epiglottis and aryepiglottic folds (fills the entire hypopharynx).	Much more uncommon and far more dangerous condition than croup. Caused by *Haemophilus influenzae*.
Foreign body (Fig C 44-3)	Opaque or nonopaque lesion that may involve the pharynx, larynx, or trachea.	Foreign body at the tracheal bifurcation is difficult to diagnose (causes symptoms of both upper and lower tract obstruction; prolonged and difficult inspiration and expiration on fluoroscopy).

A   B

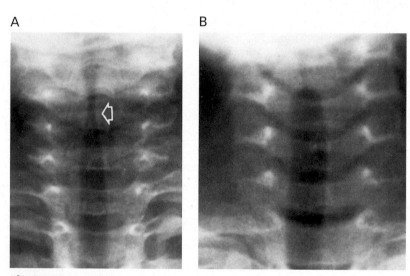

Fig C 44-1
Croup. (A) Smooth, tapered narrowing (arrow) of the subglottic portion of the trachea (gothic arch sign). (B) A normal trachea with broad shouldering in the subglottic region.

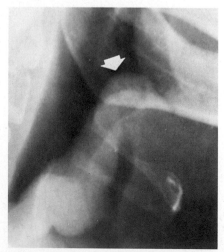

Fig C 44-2
Epiglottitis. Lateral radiograph of the neck demonstrates a wide, rounded configuration of the inflamed epiglottis (arrow).[84]

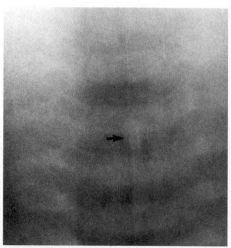

Fig C 44-3
Chicken bone in the glottis.[85]

Condition	Imaging Findings	Comments
Intrinsic mass (Fig C 44-4)	Single or multiple filling defects in the airway.	Tracheal hemangioma, fibroma, laryngeal papillomatosis, bronchial duplication cyst.
Extrinsic mass	Extrinsic impression on the airway.	Cystic hygroma, thyroglossal duct cyst, ectopic thyroid tissue, pulmonary or mediastinal mass, anomalous vessel.
Tracheal stricture	Diffuse or localized tracheal narrowing.	Posttraumatic, postoperative, postintubation. Primary congenital stenosis is exceedingly rare.
Vascular ring	Narrowing of the distal trachea.	Wide spectrum of anomalous vascular patterns (usually associated with a right-sided aortic arch). Often one or more impressions on the barium-filled esophagus.
Choanal atresia	Soft-tissue or bony obstruction. Usually no abnormality on plain radiographs.	Bilateral atresia causes severe respiratory distress in the newborn infant. The obstruction can be demonstrated after the introduction of a small amount of oily contrast material into the nostrils.
Enlarged tonsils and adenoids (Fig C 44-5)	Soft-tissue mass narrowing the airway in the nasopharynx and oropharynx.	May be gross hypertrophy without upper airway obstruction.

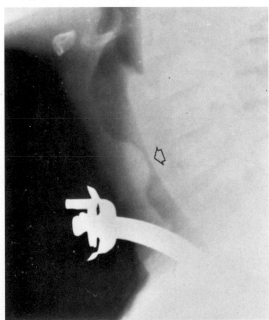

Fig C 44-4
Fibroma of the cervical trachea. Lateral view of the neck shows a sharply defined homogeneous soft-tissue density (arrow) arising from the upper anterior portion of the trachea. This 11-year-old boy had experienced dyspnea and inspiratory stridor for several years.[73]

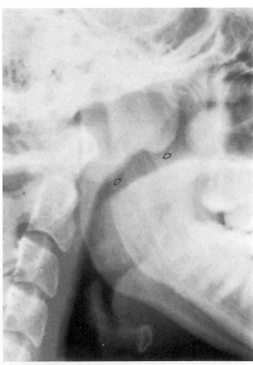

Fig C 44-5
Enlarged tonsils and adenoids. Marked impressions (arrows) on the upper airway.

Condition	Imaging Findings	Comments
Peritonsillar abscess	Soft-tissue mass in the region of the soft palate and hypopharynx.	
Pharyngeal airway obstruction by retroplaced tongue	Micrognathia associated with airway obstruction that varies between inspiratory and expiratory films.	Pierre Robin syndrome (cleft palate, micrognathia, retrodisplaced tongue); Möbius' syndrome (cranial nerve palsies often associated with micrognathia); extremely rare isolated micrognathia.
Esophageal atresia and tracheoesophageal fistula (Figs C 44-6 and C 44-7)	Blind air-filled upper esophageal pouch causing anterior displacement and compression of the tracheal air shadow.	Diagnosis confirmed by the looping of a radiopaque catheter (may inject a small amount of contrast material). Gas in the bowel indicates a distal tracheoesophageal fistula. Also H-type fistulas (cause recurrent aspiration).
Laryngomalacia	Downward displacement and buckling of the aryepiglottic folds in inspiration.	Aryepiglottic hypermobility (the larynx itself is structurally normal, but there is excessive relaxation of the supraglottic structures). The diagnosis is made fluoroscopically with the patient in the lateral position.
Tracheomalacia (Fig C 44-8)	Collapse of the trachea on expiration (may be focal or generalized).	Entity that is distinct from laryngomalacia, much less common, and due to weakening of the supporting cartilage and muscles of the trachea.
Congenital vocal cord paralysis (Fig C 44-9)	Unilateral or bilateral absence of normal movement of the vocal cords.	Life-threatening if bilateral (vocal cords tend to remain closed).

A
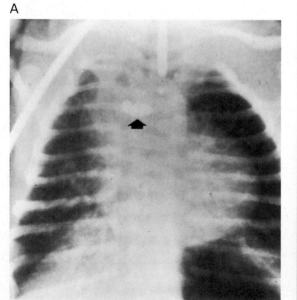

B
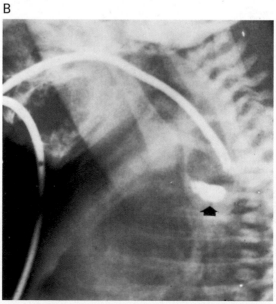

Fig C 44-6
Congenital tracheoesophageal fistula. Contrast material injected through a feeding tube demonstrates occlusion of the proximal esophageal pouch (arrows) in (A) frontal and (B) lateral projections. Note the air in the stomach.

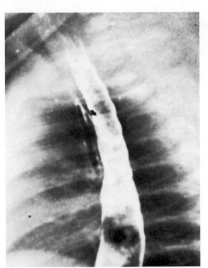

Fig C 44-7
Congenital tracheoesophageal fistula (type IV or H, fistula). Note the sharp downward course of the fistula from the trachea to the esophagus (arrow).

A

B

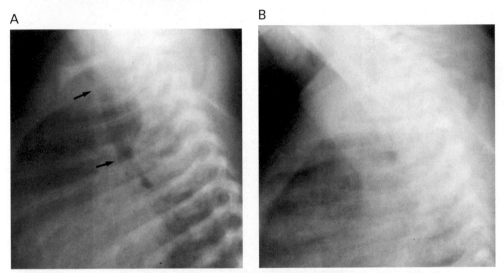

Fig C 44-8
Tracheomalacia. (A) Inspiratory view demonstrates a normal trachea (arrows). (B) On expiration, the tracheal air column is totally obliterated.[85]

A

B

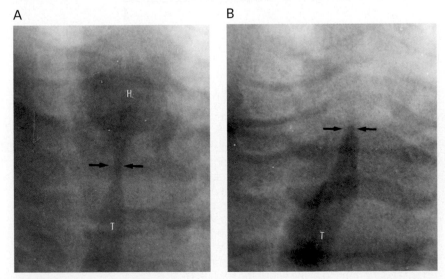

Fig C 44-9
Bilateral vocal cord paralysis. (A) Inspiratory view shows the typical midline apposition of the vocal cords (arrows). The hypopharynx (H) is overdistended. T = trachea. (B) On expiration, the vocal cords (arrows) remain in the midline, and the subglottic trachea (T) overdistends.[85]

Condition	Imaging Findings	Comments
Macroglossia	Enlarged tongue causing extrinsic impression on the airway.	May occur in hypothyroidism and in the Beckwith-Wiedemann syndrome (visceromegaly, omphalocele or umbilical hernia, pancreatic and adrenal hyperplasia, increased bone age, or neoplastic disease).
Laryngeal web (Fig C 44-10)	Narrowing of the air column.	Membranous stenosis in a glottic, supraglottic, or infraglottic position.
Diphtheria	Narrowing of the air column.	Extension of the characteristic membrane from the pharynx into the larynx, trachea, and even the bronchial tree can lead to increasing airway obstruction, cyanosis, and even death.

A

B

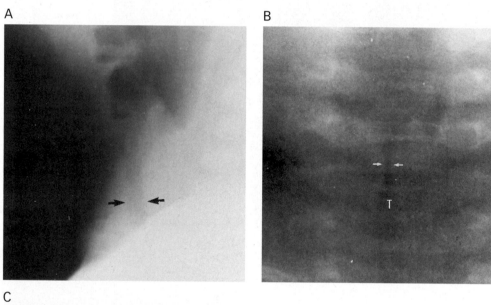

C

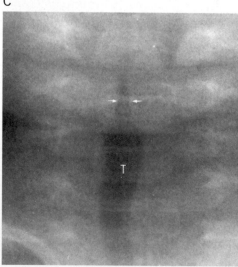

Fig C 44-10
Laryngeal web. (A) Inspiratory lateral view demonstrates an overdistended hypopharynx, an indistinct vocal cord area, and a mild paradoxically narrowed subglottic portion of the trachea (arrows). (B) Inspiratory frontal view demonstrates midline fixation of the cords (arrows) and subglottic narrowing of the entire trachea (T). (C) Expiratory view shows persistent fixation of the vocal cords (arrows) and overdistention of the subglottic trachea (T).[85]

Condition	Imaging Findings	Comments
Laryngospasm	Narrowing of the air column.	Life-threatening anaphylactic reactions occur seconds to minutes after the administration of a specific antigen (generally by injection, as with radiographic contrast material or less commonly by ingestion) and cause upper or lower airway obstruction, or both. Laryngeal edema may be experienced as a "lump" in the throat, hoarseness, or stridor, while bronchial obstruction is associated with a feeling of tightness in the chest or audible wheezing.

Widening of the Right Paratracheal Stripe
(5 Millimeters or More)

Condition	Comments
Tracheal disorders (see Fig C 40-5)	An abnormality of any of the layers of the trachea (mucosa, submucosa, cartilage rings) can widen the right paratracheal stripe. Conditions include benign and malignant tracheal tumors and diffuse tracheal narrowing (postintubation edema, tracheobronchitis, posttraumatic stenosis, relapsing polychondritis).
Causes of mediastinal widening (Fig C 45-1; see Figs C 14-4, C 14-5, and C 14-8)	Lymph node enlargement (sarcoidosis, metastases, lymphoma, tuberculosis, histoplasmosis); hemorrhage from blunt chest trauma; mediastinitis; intrathoracic goiter; and postsurgical changes from mediastinoscopy, cardiac surgery, and right radical neck dissection. Neurofibromatosis involving the right vagus nerve can also cause widening of the right paratracheal stripe.
Pleural disorders	Diseases that cause thickening of the parietal or visceral pleura or an increase in pleural fluid can widen the right paratracheal stripe. These include free or encapsulated pleural effusion, mesothelioma, and pleural thickening or fibrosis from any cause.
Miscellaneous disorders	Right upper lobe atelectasis, radiation fibrosis, polyarteritis nodosa, Wegener's granulomatosis, and desquamative interstitial pneumonia.

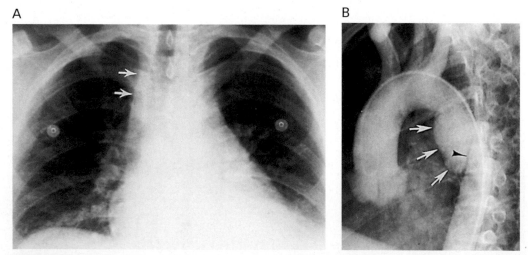

A   B

Fig C 45-1
Mediastinal hemorrhage secondary to blunt chest trauma. (A) Supine chest radiograph shows a right paratracheal stripe (arrows) measuring 1 cm in width. (B) Aortography in the same patient demonstrates a pseudoaneurysm at the level of the aortic isthmus (arrows). The arrowhead indicates an intimal flap.[86]

Elevated Diaphragm

Condition	Comments
Normal variant	Dome of the diaphragm tends to be approximately half an interspace higher on the right than on the left. In approximately 10% of individuals, the hemidiaphragms are at the same height or the left is higher than the right.
Eventration (Figs C 46-1 and C 46-2)	Unilateral hypoplasia of a hemidiaphragm (very rarely both) with the thinned, weakened musculature inadequate to restrain the abdominal viscera. Localized eventration primarily involves the anteromedial portion of the right hemidiaphragm, through which a portion of the right lobe of the liver bulges. In a posterior eventration, upward displacement of the kidney can produce a rounded mass. Total eventration occurs almost exclusively on the left. Eventrations may have paradoxical diaphragmatic motion (though more commonly seen in diaphragmatic paralysis).
Phrenic nerve paralysis (Fig C 46-3)	Unilateral or bilateral diaphragmatic elevation with characteristic paradoxical motion of the diaphragm (tends to ascend rather than descend with inspiration). Results from any process interfering with the normal function of the phrenic nerve (inadvertent surgical transection, primary bronchogenic carcinoma, or mediastinal metastases); intrinsic neurologic disease (poliomyelitis, Erb's palsy, peripheral neuritis, hemiplegia); injury to the phrenic nerve, thoracic cage, cervical spine, or brachial plexus; pressure from a substernal thyroid or aneurysm; or lung or mediastinal infection (paralysis may be temporary).

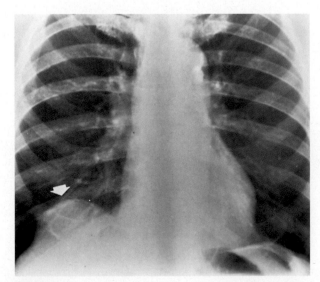

Fig C 46-1
Partial eventration. Of the right hemidiaphragm (arrow).

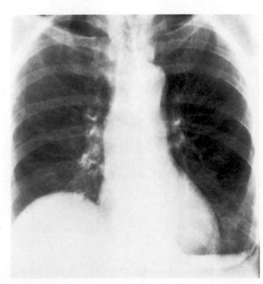

Fig C 46-2
Complete eventration. Of the right hemidiaphragm.

Condition	Comments
Increased intra-abdominal volume	Unilateral or bilateral diaphragmatic elevation in patients with ascites, obesity, or pregnancy.
Intra-abdominal inflammatory disease	Unilateral or bilateral diaphragmatic elevation. Most commonly due to subphrenic abscess. Also perinephric, hepatic, or splenic abscess; pancreatitis; cholecystitis; and perforated ulcer.
Intra-abdominal mass (Fig C 46-4)	Unilateral or bilateral diaphragmatic elevation caused by enlargement of the liver or spleen; abdominal tumor or cyst of the liver, spleen, kidneys, adrenals, or pancreas; or distended stomach or splenic flexure (left hemidiaphragm).

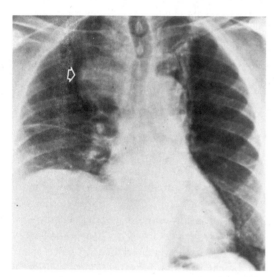

Fig C 46-3
Phrenic nerve paralysis. Primary bronchogenic carcinoma (arrow) involving the phrenic nerve causes paralysis of the right hemidiaphragm.

A   B

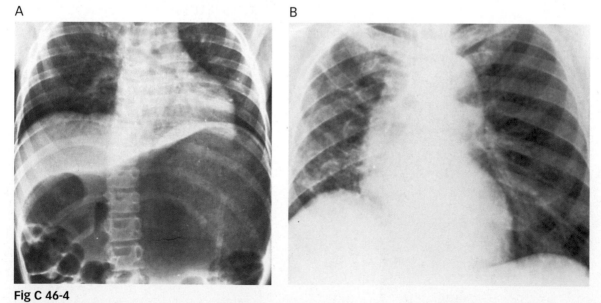

Fig C 46-4
Intra-abdominal mass. (A) Acute gastric dilatation causes diffuse elevation of both leaves of the diaphragm. (B) Huge syphilitic gumma of the liver produces elevation of the right hemidiaphragm.

Condition	Comments
Acute intrathoracic process (splinting of diaphragm) (Fig C 46-5)	Unilateral or bilateral diaphragmatic elevation due to chest wall injury, atelectasis, pulmonary infarct, or pleural disease (fibrosis, acute pleurisy).
Tumor or cyst of diaphragm	Very rare lesion that simulates unilateral diaphragmatic elevation.
Subpulmonic effusion (Fig C 46-6)	Closely simulates an elevated hemidiaphragm. On frontal views, the peak of the pseudodiaphragmatic contour is lateral to that of a normal hemidiaphragm (situated near the junction of the middle and lateral thirds rather than near the center).
Altered pulmonary volume	Unilateral or bilateral diaphragmatic elevation due to atelectasis (associated pulmonary opacity); postoperative lobectomy or pneumonectomy (rib defects, sutures, shift of the heart and mediastinum); hypoplastic lung (crowded ribs, mediastinal shift, absent or small pulmonary artery, sometimes the scimitar syndrome).
Diaphragmatic hernia (Figs C 46-7 and C 46-8)	Mimics unilateral diaphragmatic elevation on frontal views. Lateral views show the characteristic anterior location of Morgagni's hernia or the posterior position of Bochdalek's hernia.
Traumatic rupture of diaphragm (Figs C 46-9 and C 46-10)	Mimics unilateral diaphragmatic elevation. Injury to the right side causes herniation of the soft-tissue density of the liver into the right hemithorax. On the left, air-containing stomach and bowel herniate into the chest (may mimic diaphragmatic elevation if the bowel loops are filled with fluid).

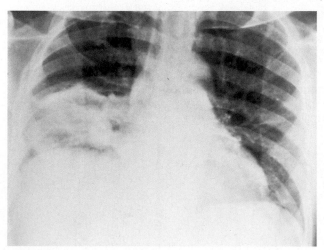

Fig C 46-5
Acute pneumonia. Elevation of the right hemidiaphragm due to splinting secondary to a right lower lung infiltrate.

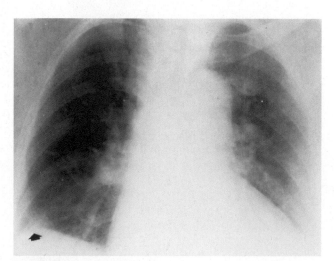

Fig C 46-6
Subpulmonic effusion. The peak of the pseudodiaphragmatic contour (arrow) is lateral to that of a normal hemidiaphragm.

A

B

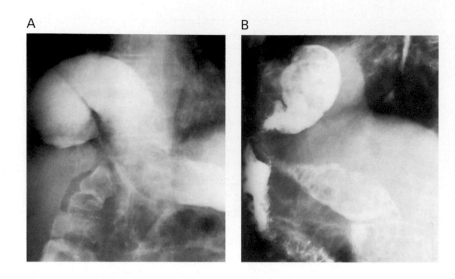

Fig C 46-7
Morgagni hernia. (A) Frontal and (B) lateral views demonstrate barium-filled bowel in a hernia sac that lies anteriorly and to the right.

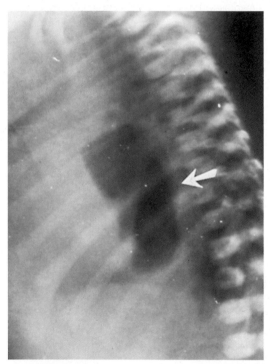

Fig C 46-8
Bochdalek hernia. Gas-filled loop of bowel (arrow) is visible posteriorly in the thoracic cavity.

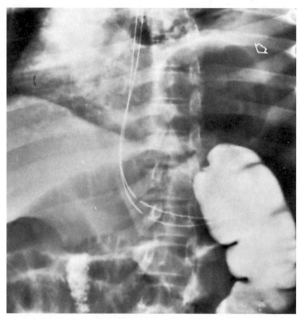

Fig C 46-9
Traumatic rupture of the diaphragm. Herniation of a portion of the splenic flexure (arrow), with obstruction to the retrograde flow of barium.

A

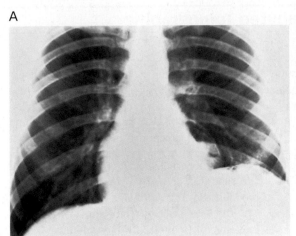

B

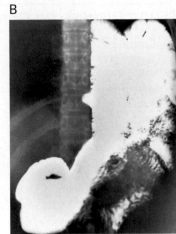

Fig C 46-10
Traumatic rupture of the diaphragm. (A) On a frontal projection, the radiographic appearance simulates eventration or paralysis of the left hemidiaphragm. (B) The administration of barium clearly demonstrates the herniation of bowel contents into the chest.

Interstitial Lung Disease on Computed Tomography*

Condition	Imaging Findings	Comments
Usual interstitial pneumonia (UIP) (Fig C 47-1)	Fine or coarse reticular opacities in the subpleural regions of the lung bases. Irregular pleural, vascular, and bronchial interfaces with normal parenchyma.	Most commonly seen in patients who have idiopathic pulmonary fibrosis (fibrosing alveolitis). Also occurs in patients with asbestosis and collagen vascular diseases, particularly rheumatoid arthritis and scleroderma.
Desquamative interstitial pneumonia (DIP) (Fig C 47-2)	Similar to UIP, although the fibrosis tends to be less severe.	Because the pathologic patterns of both UIP and DIP can often be seen in the same patient, it is probable that DIP represents the early stage and UIP the late stage of the same disease. The predominant pattern of ground-glass (rather than reticular) opacities is seen in nearly all patients, reflecting the presence of intra-alveolar macrophages and interstitial inflammation.
Cryptogenic organizing pneumonia (COP) (Fig C 47-3)	Patchy, unilateral or bilateral air-space consolidation and small nodular opacities with a predominantly subpleural distribution. Typical peribronchial thickening.	May be seen in several conditions, including viral and bacterial pneumonia, extrinsic allergic alveolitis, chronic eosinophilic pneumonia, and collagen vascular diseases. In most patients, however, no cause is found and the condition is referred to as *idiopathic* or *cryptogenic*.

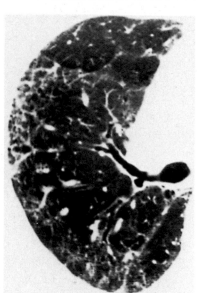

Fig C 47-1
Usual interstitial pneumonia. Scan at the level of the right upper lobe bronchus in a woman with idiopathic pulmonary fibrosis shows a reticular pattern and irregular interfaces predominantly in the subpleural lung regions.[87]

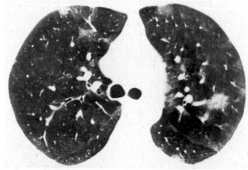

Fig C 47-2
Desquamative interstitial pneumonia. Scan at the carinal level shows patchy areas of air-space opacification ("ground-glass" density).[87]

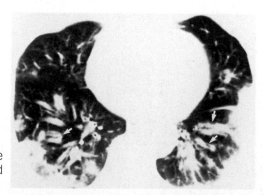

Fig C 47-3
Cryptogenic organizing pneumonia. Air-space consolidation in the subpleural regions associated with peribronchial thickening (arrows).[87]

*Thickening of the interlobular septa producing a reticular, fine nodular, or reticulonodular pattern. Also thickening of fissures and visceral pleural surfaces. In late stages, coarse thickening around dilated cystic spaces (honeycombing).

Condition	Imaging Findings	Comments
Lymphangitic carcinomatosis (Fig C 47-4)	Uneven thickening of bronchovascular bundles and interlobular septa producing a virtually pathognomonic "beaded-chain" pattern.	Filling and expansion of lymphatics by tumor cells that is most common in carcinomas of the breast, lung, stomach, and colon. CT can demonstrate characteristic findings in patients with normal chest radiographs.
Pulmonary edema (Fig C 47-5)	Smooth thickening of interlobular septa.	Usually most evident in the lung periphery, where the septa appear as lines running perpendicular to the pleura.
Sarcoidosis (Fig C 47-6)	Irregular nodules or interstitial thickening along the bronchovascular bundles.	In late stages, fibrosis typically radiates from the hila to the middle and upper lung zones. Fibrotic distortion of lung parenchyma may be seen on CT before it is apparent on plain chest radiographs.
Asbestosis (Figs C 47-7 to C 47-9)	Interstitial abnormalities (parenchymal bands, thickened interlobular septa, and honeycombing) that typically have a subpleural distribution.	In patients with combined asbestos–cigarette smoke exposure, CT can play a major role in distinguishing emphysematous lung destruction from the peripheral interstitial changes of asbestosis. CT also may detect focal lung masses (cancer, round atelectasis) that are not visible on plain chest radiographs.

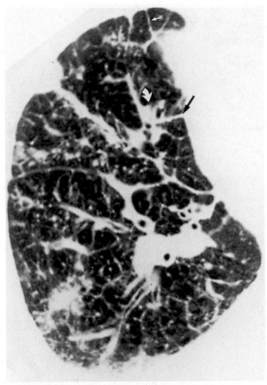

Fig C 47-4
Lymphangitic carcinomatosis. Scan through the right lower lung shows extensive abnormalities with thickening of the interlobular septa (straight arrows), major fissure, and bronchovascular bundles (curved arrow). There is also a pleural effusion.[87]

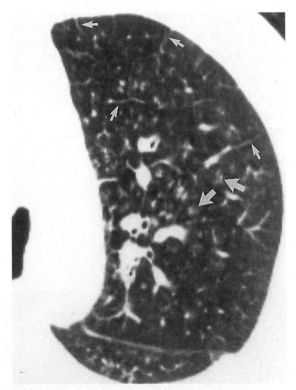

Fig C 47-5
Pulmonary edema. Thickening of the interlobular septa (small arrows) and ill-defined centrilobular opacities (large arrows). Note also the thickening of the peribronchovascular interstitium, with peribronchial cuffing.[88]

A

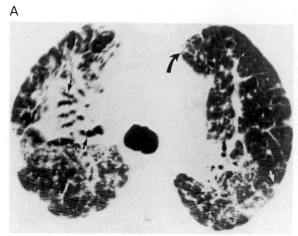

B

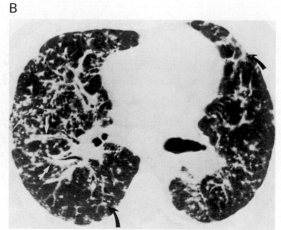

Fig C 47-6
Sarcoidosis. (A) Scan at the carinal level shows central conglomeration of fibrosis and ectatic bronchi (straight black arrows). Nodular thickening of the interlobular septa (curved arrow) and subpleural granulomas (white arrows) are also identified. (B) Scan through the lower lung zones demonstrates nodular thickening of the bronchovascular bundles (straight arrows) and interlobular septa (curved arrows).[87]

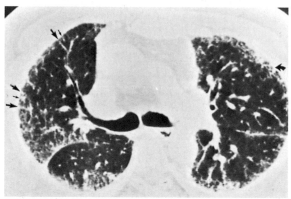

Fig C 47-7
Asbestosis. Supine scan shows moderate thickening of interlobular septal (arrows) and peribronchial (arrowheads) structures in the nondependent subpleural parenchyma. On the left, there is a suggestion of subpleural honeycombing (curved arrow). The interlobar fissures are thickened, and there is serration of the lung-pleural interface at sites of interstitial fibrosis, changes indicative of visceral pleural fibrosis.[89]

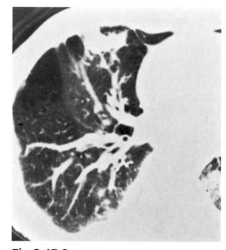

Fig C 47-8
Asbestosis. Scan through the right middle lobe shows an irregular mass with aerated lung interposed between it and the adjacent pleural thickening. A focal band of soft tissue can be seen in contact with the pleura. The mass was stable on serial radiographs and thus was considered to represent a variant of round atelectasis.[89]

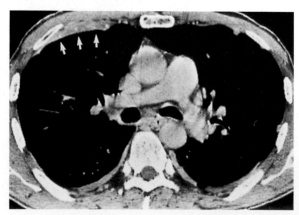

Fig C 47-9
Asbestosis. Moderate bilateral paraspinous and costal pleural thickening. Scattered calcifications are visible in the right anterior costal plaque (arrows).[89]

Condition	Imaging Findings	Comments
Other pneumoconioses (Fig C 47-10)	Fine nodular opacifications (1–10 mm) that usually are most numerous in the posterior aspect of the upper lung zones.	Silicosis, coal-workers' pneumonia, graphite pneumoconiosis, and talcosis. In severe disease, there is an increased number and size of the nodules with confluence.
Extrinsic allergic alveolitis (Fig C 47-11)	Fine nodular or reticulonodular pattern in the subacute stage. Bilateral areas of hazy increased density (ground-glass opacification) with preservation of underlying vascular markings may occur.	Hypersensitivity disease of the lungs caused by inhalation of antigens contained in certain organic dusts. In the acute stage, there is diffuse air-space consolidation that resolves to an interstitial pattern within a few days. Repeated exposure to the antigen may lead to acute and subacute changes superimposed on chronic fibrosis.
Pulmonary Langerhans cell histiocytosis (Fig C 47-12)	Small irregular nodules and cystic air spaces that diffusely involve the upper two-thirds of the lungs but characteristically spare the lower lung zones and the tips of the lingula and middle lobe.	Histologically an infiltrative lung disease of Langerhans cells. CT is better than plain chest radiographs in showing the structure and distribution of lung abnormalities. Nodules are typical of the early stages; cystic air spaces represent the late stage of disease.

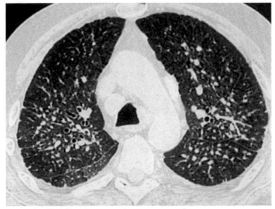

Fig C 47-10
Silicosis. Upper lobe distribution of small nodules.[90]

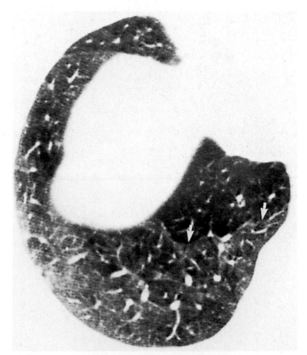

Fig C 47-11
Extrinsic allergic alveolitis. Bird-breeder's lung. Scan at the level of the right hemidiaphragm shows patchy areas of hazy interstitial density ("ground-glass" density; arrows) that typically do not obscure the underlying vascular markings.[87]

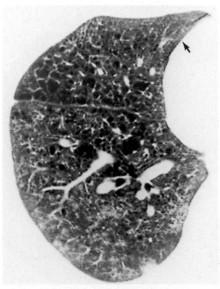

Fig C 47-12
Pulmonary Langerhans cell histiocytosis. Scan through the right lower lung zone shows cystic air spaces with thin walls. Characteristically the tip of the middle lobe (arrow) is spared.[87]

Condition	Imaging Findings	Comments
Lymphangiomyomatosis (Fig C 47-13)	Numerous thin-walled cystic air spaces of various sizes surrounded by relatively normal lung parenchyma.	Rare disease characterized by progressive proliferation of smooth muscle in the walls of bronchi, bronchioles, alveolar septa, pulmonary vessels, lymphatics, and pleura that leads to air trapping and the development of cystic air spaces. Seen only in women, almost all of whom are of childbearing age.
Radiation fibrosis (Fig C 47-14)	Reticular pattern. Often associated with volume loss, traction bronchiectasis, and pleural thickening that results in a sharp demarcation between normal and irradiated lung.	Late stage of radiation-induced lung injury, which develops gradually in patients with radiation pneumonitis when complete resolution does not occur. It evolves within the previously irradiated field, 6–12 months after radiation therapy, and usually becomes stable within 2 years after treatment.

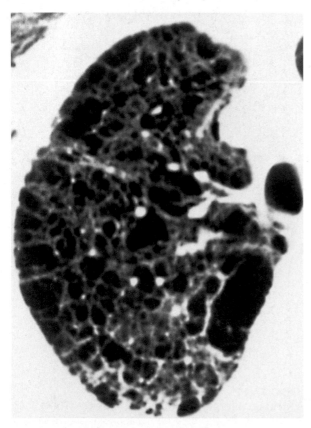

Fig C 47-13
Lymphangiomyomatosis. Scan through the right upper lobe shows numerous thin-walled cystic air spaces of various sizes. The patient also had pneumomediastinum and extensive subcutaneous emphysema.[5]

Condition	Comments
Atypical mycobacterial and fungal infections (Figs C 48-3 to C 48-5)	May produce a pattern indistinguishable from that of tuberculosis, though without the upper lobe predominance.

A   B

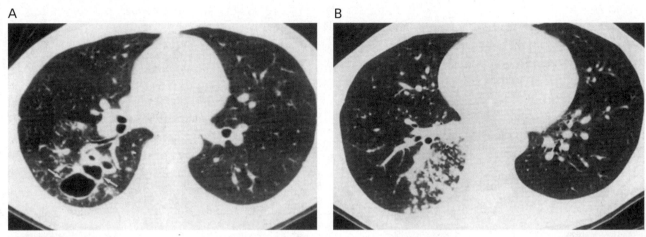

Fig C 48-3
Mycobacterium kansasii. (A) Cavitary lesions in the right upper lobe (arrows). (B) More inferior image shows the "tree-in-bud" pattern of endobronchial spread of infection. (B reprinted from ref. 56.)

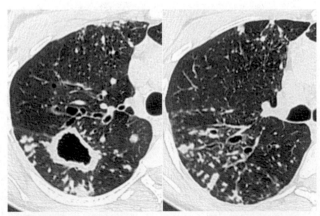

Fig C 48-4
***Mycobacterium avium-intracellulare* complex**. Multiple peripheral small nodules connected to branching linear opacities and a thick-walled cavity in the superior segment of the lower lobe. Note the thickening of the bronchial walls, bronchial dilatation, and mucus impaction.[91]

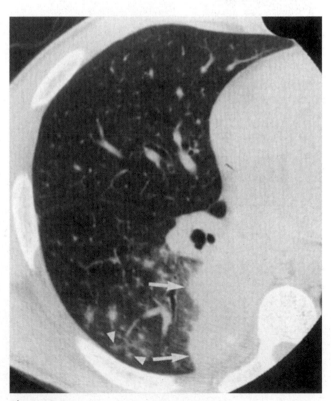

Fig C 48-5
Blastomycosis. Pulmonary consolidation (arrows) associated with endobronchial spread of fungus ("tree-in-bud," arrowheads) in the right lower lobe.[92]

Condition	Comments
Other bacterial infections (Fig C 48-6)	*Staphylococcus aureus* and *Haemophilus influenzae bronchiolitis* also can produce the "tree-in-bud" pattern.
Invasive pulmonary aspergillosis (Fig C 48-7)	Should be suggested when this pattern occurs in combination with a "halo" of ground-glass opacity in a patient with leukemia.
Viral infection (Figs C 48-8 and C 48-9)	Cytomegalovirus infection, which typically occurs in immunocompromised individuals, can cause thickening of the bronchovascular bundles and the "tree-in-bud" pattern. In infants and young children, this appearance may be due to bronchial wall thickening and dilatation related to respiratory syncytial virus.

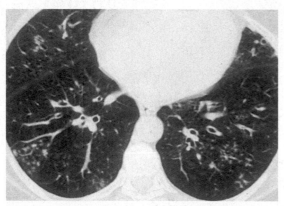

Fig C 48-6
***Staphylococcus aureus* bronchiolitis.** Small peripheral centrilobular nodules and branching linear opacities in a patient with acquired human immunodeficiency syndrome.[91]

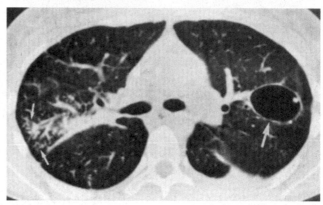

Fig C 48-7
Aspergillosis. Thin-walled cavity in the left upper lobe (large arrow) and "tree-in-bud" pattern in the right upper lobe (small arrows).[93]

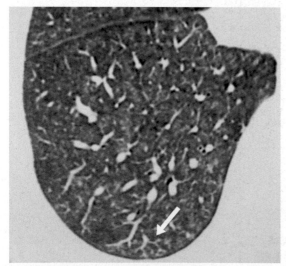

Fig C 48-8
Cytomegalovirus pneumonia. Centrilobular ground-glass opacities in addition to nodules and "tree-in-bud" opacities in a patient with chronic myelogenous leukemia who underwent bone marrow transplantation.[91]

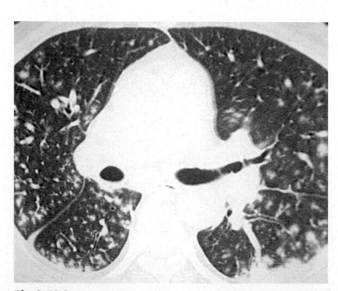

Fig C 48-9
Respiratory syncytial virus. Peripheral poorly defined centrilobular nodules and "tree-in-bud" opacities bilaterally in a patient with leukemia. Note the scattered lung nodules surrounded by halos of ground-glass attenuation.[91]

Condition	Comments
Allergic bronchopulmonary aspergillosis (Fig C 48-10)	Immune reaction results in damage to the bronchial wall, central bronchiectasis, and the formation of mucous plugs that contain fungus and inflammatory cells, producing the "finger-in-glove" sign of large airway impaction. Involvement of small airways causes the "tree-in-bud" pattern. Indirect signs of small airway disease include a mosaic pattern of lung attenuation and air trapping on expiratory scanning.
Cystic fibrosis (Fig C 48-11)	Abnormally low water content of airway mucus is at least partially responsible for decreased clearance of mucus, mucous plugging of small and large airways, and an increased incidence of bacterial airway infection. Bronchial wall inflammation progressing to bronchiectasis is eventually seen on HRCT, along with bronchial wall and peribronchial thickening and air trapping on expiratory scanning. Large amounts of bronchiolar secretions result in the "tree-in-bud" pattern.

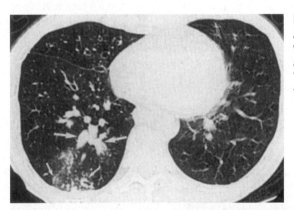

Fig C 48-10
Allergic bronchopulmonary aspergillosis. This woman with a history of asthma shows impaction of dilated large airways, producing the "finger-in-glove" sign (large arrows). There is also impaction of dilated small airways, producing the "tree-in-bud" pattern (small arrows).[93]

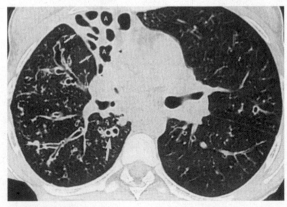

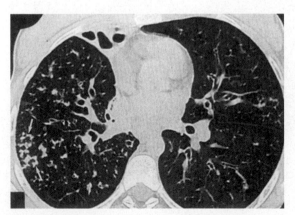

Fig C 48-11
Cystic fibrosis. (A) Dilated, thick-walled bronchi (large arrow), as well as collapse of the right middle lobe (small arrows), which contains dilated airways (A). (B) More inferior image shows the "tree-in-bud" pattern (arrows).[92]

Condition	Comments
Dyskinetic cilia syndromes (Fig C 48-12)	In these inherited abnormalities of ciliary structure and function, recurrent bronchial infections lead to bronchiectasis. Airway damage can extend to the smaller airways, resulting in bronchiolectasis, centrilobular opacities ("tree-in-bud" pattern), and air trapping.
Juvenile laryngotracheobronchial papillomatosis	Bronchiolar involvement by neoplasms is uncommon, but has been described with juvenile laryngotracheobronchial papillomatosis. Most frequently seen in adults, this condition is thought to be related to infection with the human papillomavirus. Papillomas may spread from the larynx to the bronchi and bronchioles and result in centrilobular nodules and the "tree-in-bud" appearance.
Aspiration (Fig C 48-13)	Aspiration of infected oral secretions or other irritant material can cause bronchiolar disease. In acute cases, extensive exudative bronchiolar disease may develop and result in a "tree-in-bud" pattern. Predisposing factors include structural abnormalities of the pharynx, esophageal disorders (achalasia, Zenker's diverticulum, hiatal hernia and reflux, esophageal carcinoma), neuorologic defects, and chronic illness.

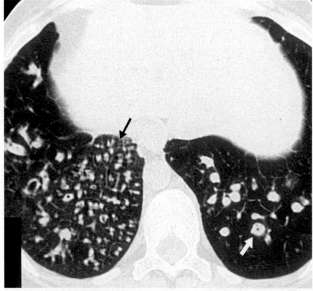

Fig C 48-12
Primary cilial dyskinesia. Bronchial (white arrow) and bronchiolar thickening with mucoid impaction and the "tree-in-bud" pattern (black arrow). Note the air trapping in the left lower lobe.[91]

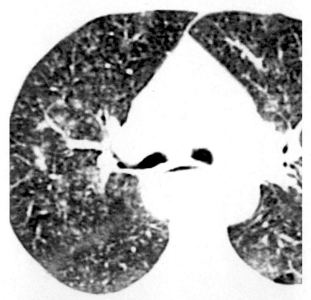

Fig C 48-13
Diffuse peribronchiolitis. Recurrent aspiration of foreign particles in a patient with achalasia. Multiple centrilobular areas of increased attenuation with a characteristic "tree-in-bud" appearance. Note the esophageal dilatation with an air-fluid level.[91]

Condition	Comments
Connective tissue disease (Fig C 48-14)	Rheumatoid arthritis and Sjögren syndrome may affect the small airways and produce the "tree-in-bud" pattern
Pulmonary intravascular tumor emboli (Figs C 48-15 and C 48-16)	Pulmonary intravascular tumor emboli are most commonly associated with cancers of the breast, liver, kidney, stomach, prostate and ovary. The "tree-in-bud" pattern due to tumor emboli may be caused either by filling of the centrilobular arteries with tumor cells or by a rare thrombotic microangiopathy, in which widespread fibrocellular intimal hyperplasia of small pulmonary arteries (carcinomatous arteritis) is initiated by tumor microemboli. Patients with pulmonary tumor emboli present with progressive dyspnea, cough, and signs of hypoxia and pulmonary hypertension.
Idiopathic Diffuse panbronchiolitis (Fig C 48-17)	Inflammatory lung disease of unclear etiology that is prevalent in Asia and represents a transmural infiltration of lymphocytes and plasma cells, with mucus and neutrophils filling the lumen of affected bronchioles. In addition to the "tree-in-bud" pattern appearance, there may be nodules, bronchiectasis, or large cystic opacities accompanied by dilated proximal bronchi.

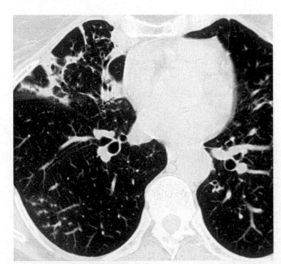

Fig C 48-14
Sjögren syndrome. Peripheral "tree-in-bud" patterns in the right lower lobe. Note the bronchial dilatation, bronchial wall thickening, and consolidation.[91]

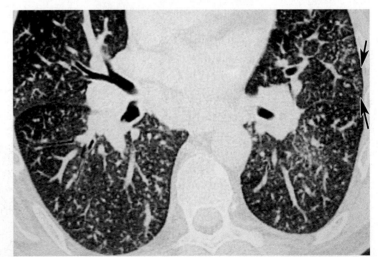

Fig C 48-15
Pulmonary intravascular tumor embolism. Multiple centrilobular nodules and branching lines with the "tree-in-bud" appearance (arrows), caused by tumor emboli from gastric adenocarcinoma.[91]

Condition	Comments
Cryptogenic organizing pneumonia (Fig C 48-18)	Irreversible fibrosis of small airway walls that narrows or obliterates the lumen. A common sequela of lung transplantation (representing chronic rejection) and bone marrow transplantation (in which it reflects chronic graft versus host disease), it also can result from collagen vascular disorders, inhalation of toxic fumes, and infection.

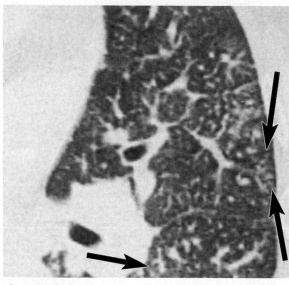

Fig C 48-16
Tumor emboli. Coned view at level of the left basal trunk shows multifocal "tree-in-bud" appearance (arrows) due by tumor emboli (thrombotic microangiopathy caused by metastatic gastric carcinoma).[35]

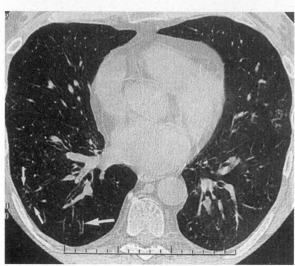

Fig C 48-17
Diffuse panbronchiolitis. Relatively mild case of dilated bronchioles (large arrow) and the "tree-in-bud" pattern (small arrows).[92]

A

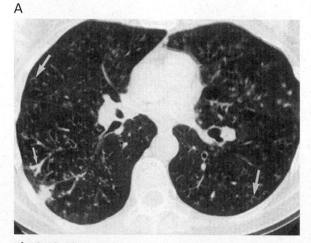

B

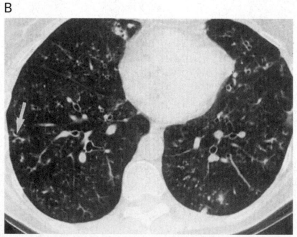

Fig C 48-18
Cryptogenic organizing pneumonia. (A) Nodular and linear branching opacities in a bronchiolar distribution (large arrows), as well as a "V-shaped" area of bronchiolar impaction (small arrow). (B) More inferior image shows the "tree-in-bud" pattern (arrow).[93]

Condition	Comments
Asthma (Fig C 48-19)	Diffuse obstructive lung disease with hyperactivity of the airways to a variety of stimuli and a high degree of reversibility (either spontaneously or as a result of treatment). In addition to the "tree-in-bud" pattern, HRCT findings include bronchiectasis, bronchial wall thickening, and areas of hyperlucency (resulting from decreased lung perfusion secondary to reflex vasoconstriction in hypoventilated areas as well as air trapping).

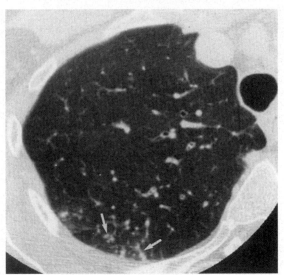

Fig C 48-19
Asthma. "Tree-in-bud" pattern in the posterior segment of the right upper lobe (arrows).[92]

Alveolar Lung Disease on Computed Tomography*

Condition	Imaging Findings	Comments
Bacterial pneumonia (Fig C 49-1)	Nonspecific alveolar pattern.	Although CT cannot suggest a specific organism, it can demonstrate that the pneumonia is more extensive than shown on plain chest radiographs. CT also can reveal a central tumor as the cause of pneumonia; show evidence of necrosis or abscess formation at an early stage; and detect pleural complications, such as pneumothorax, effusion, empyema, and bronchopleural fistula. In immunocompromised patients, CT may detect an early opportunistic infection of the lungs when plain chest radiographs are negative.
Tuberculosis Primary (Fig C 49-2)	Focal consolidation, often with hilar or mediastinal adenopathy and pleural effusion.	CT can show or confirm lymphadenopathy and subtle cavitation that is not visible on plain radiographs. It also can serve to guide bronchoscopy or biopsy.
Secondary (Fig C 49-3)	In addition to an alveolar pattern, cavitation is common. Atelectasis, lung scarring, and calcification often develop. Endobronchial dissemination of infection from rupture of a tuberculous cavity into the airway produces scattered ill-defined nodules or areas of more confluent opacifications surrounding small airways.	CT is of special value in patients with widespread abnormalities on plain radiographs, in whom it can detect cavities, identify areas of bronchiectasis, and distinguish pleural from adjacent parenchymal disease. In endobronchial dissemination, CT may reveal the cavity from which the infection spread into the airways.
Pneumocystis carinii pneumonia (Fig C 49-4)	Bilateral patchy consolidation or ground-glass pattern that often has a sharp demarcation between diseased and normal lung tissue.	Approximately 20% of patients have a more reticular pattern of disease. Thin-walled, air-filled lung cysts (especially apical and subpleural) occur in about 40% of patients and may cause a pneumothorax; thick-walled cavities usually indicate superinfection.

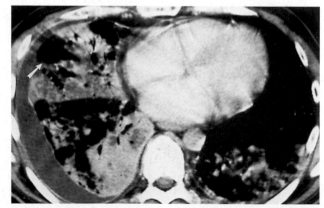

Fig C 49-1
***Legionella* pneumonia.** Central air bronchograms, abscess formation anteriorly (arrow), and accompanying pleural effusions.[94]

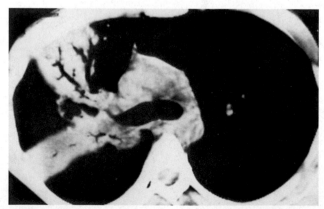

Fig C 49-2
Tuberculous pneumonia. Air bronchograms and accompanying hilar lymphadenopathy. (Courtesy of Junpei Ikezoe, MD.)[94]

*Rounded, often poorly defined nodules that are the same size as acini (6–10 mm) and can later coalesce to form larger lesions. Initially, there may be a ground-glass pattern (homogeneous slight increase in lung attenuation without obscuration of underlying vessels) as a small amount of fluid tends to layer against the alveolar walls and is indistinguishable from alveolar wall thickening in interstitial disease.

Condition	Imaging Findings	Comments
Invasive pulmonary aspergillosis (Fig C 49-5)	Single or multiple ill-defined nodules. Characteristic "halo sign" in which a zone of intermediate attenuation (hemorrhage and coagulative necrosis) surrounds a central dense fungal nodule.	More common in patients who are immunocompromised as a result of chemotherapy for lymphoma or leukemia or undergoing immunosuppressive therapy for organ transplantation than in those with AIDS. An "air-crescent" sign may develop late in the course of infection when the host's immune function begins to recover.
Other fungal infections	Various patterns of cavitary pneumonia or nodular disease.	Most frequently, *Cryptococcus neoformans*, which tends to disseminate to the brain and meninges.

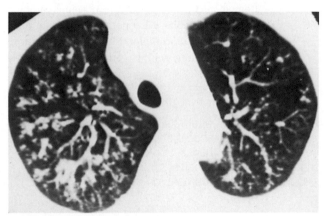

Fig C 49-3
Endobronchial spread of tuberculosis. Note the patchy peribronchial and peribronchiolar distribution of the nodular opacities. (Courtesy of Junpei Ikezoe, MD.)[94]

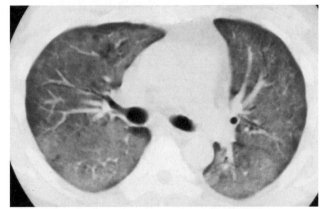

Fig C 49-4
***Pneumocystis carinii* pneumonia in AIDS.** Diffuse, bilateral ground-glass opacities with minimal peripheral sparing.[95]

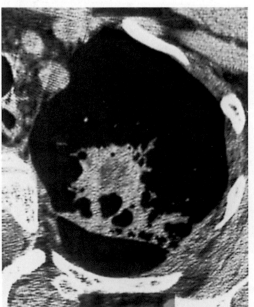

Fig C 49-5
Aspergillosis. Scan performed at the time of bone marrow recovery in a neutropenic chemotherapy patient shows a low-attenuation center that probably reflects early necrosis. The air-filled spaces near the lower border represent uninvolved emphysematous air spaces.[94]

Condition	Imaging Findings	Comments
Radiation pneumonitis (Fig C 49-6)	In early stages, a pattern of patchy opacifications that progresses to discrete and solid consolidation.	Usually limited to the radiation port, with a straight border between the irradiated opacified area and normal lung. Eventually leads to pulmonary fibrosis.
Pulmonary thromboembolism (Fig C 49-7)	Classically, a wedge-shaped peripheral opacification abutting the pleura with its apex directed toward the hilum.	May produce multiple peripheral nodules. A common and important finding is the presence of a feeding vessel leading to the lesion. Although this indicates the vascular origin of the process, a similar appearance can be seen with septic emboli and metastases.
Septic emboli (Fig C 49-8)	Multiple peripheral nodules, often with an evident feeding vessel.	Result from infectious particles reaching the lung from an infected heart valve, intravenous catheter, or injected debris. Persons at risk include drug abusers, immunocompromised patients, and those with indwelling venous catheters or prosthetic heart valves.

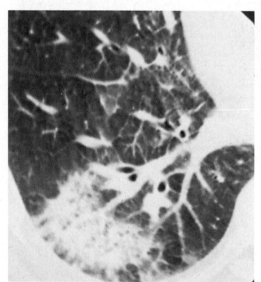

Fig C 49-6
Radiation pneumonitis. Two months after radiation therapy for tracheal carcinoma, localized air-space consolidation has developed in the right lower lobe. There is also interstitial disease that produces thickened intralobular septa centrally. Later scans showed the development of dense scarring.[94]

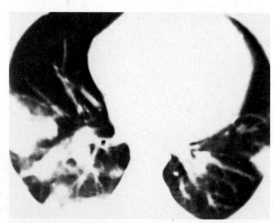

Fig C 49-7
Pulmonary thromboembolism. There are multiple rounded subpleural opacities, some of which have lung vessels leading to them. (Courtesy of Robert D. Tarver, MD.)[94]

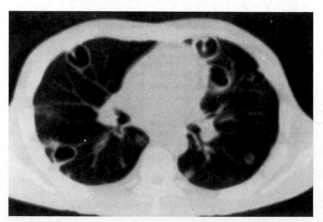

Fig C 49-8
Septic emboli. Multiple peripheral cavitating opacities. The vascular connections, particularly in the right middle lobe, indicate their hematogenous origin.[96]

Condition	Imaging Findings	Comments
Chronic eosinophilic pneumonia (Fig C 49-9)	Peripheral distribution of bilateral patchy consolidation.	Typically presents with subacute systemic and respiratory symptoms and blood eosinophilia.
Löffler's syndrome	Peripheral distribution of bilateral patchy consolidation.	Also associated with blood eosinophilia, though it differs from chronic eosinophilic pneumonia in that the air-space abnormalities are transient, resolving in some areas and reappearing in others over days.
Alveolar proteinosis (Fig C 49-10)	Bilateral, patchy, but usually symmetric air-space disease. Air bronchograms are surprisingly uncommon.	Plain radiographs may be strikingly abnormal despite the mild degree of respiratory impairment. There may be superimposed interstitial thickening that resolves after bronchopulmonary lavage and thus probably represents edema and cellular debris rather than fibrosis.

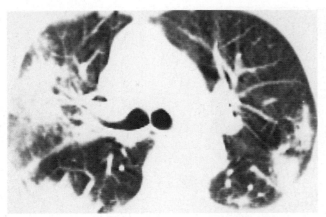

Fig C 49-9
Eosinophilic pneumonia. Bilateral patchy infiltrates with a peripheral distribution.[94]

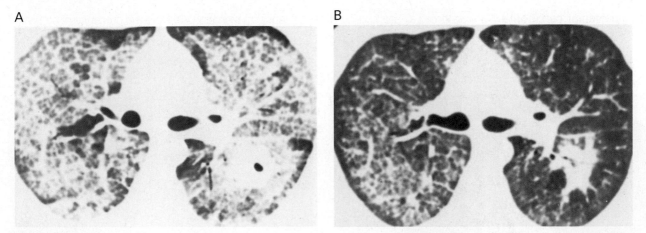

A

B

Fig C 49-10
Alveolar proteinosis. (A) Widespread air-space disease and superimposed reticular interstitial thickening. Note the nocardial abscess in the left lower lobe. (B) After bronchoalveolar lavage, the air-space and interstitial components have diminished.[97]

Condition	Imaging Findings	Comments
Bronchioloalveolar (alveolar cell) carcinoma (Fig C 49-11)	Widespread air-space disease that is often associated with prominent air bronchograms. CT attenuation in the affected lobe is typically less than that caused by pneumonia, reflecting the mucin content of the malignant cells and the air spaces.	Results from spread of tumor through the bronchioalveolar tree. Can involve an entire segment or lobe and even spread to the contralateral lung. After injection of contrast material, vessels within the affected lobe stand out against the low-attenuation background, producing the "angiogram sign" (not specific as it also can be seen in pulmonary edema, pulmonary infarction, and lipoid pneumonia).
Lipoid pneumonia (Fig C 49-12)	Posterior or lower lobe opacifications that may have low attenuation (reflecting aspiration of lipid material).	Results from chronic aspiration or inhalation of petroleum-based compounds or animal or vegetable oils (eg, in patients who use mineral oil as a laxative or who apply an oily compound to their lips or nose before going to bed).

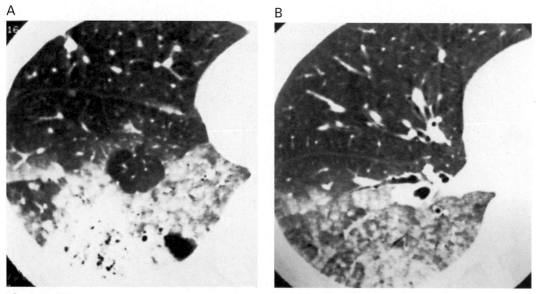

Fig C 49-11
Bronchioloalveolar carcinoma. (A) Widespread air-space filling with geographic margination. (B) Note the presence of air bronchograms. (Courtesy of David P. Naidich, MD.)[94]

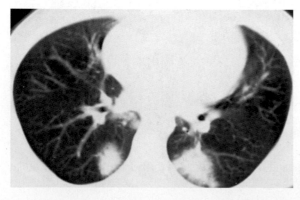

Fig C 49-12
Lipoid pneumonia. Characteristic dependent location of the consolidation.[94]

Condition	Imaging Findings	Comments
Alveolar sarcoidosis (Fig C 49-13)	Ill-defined opacifications that may be discrete or form larger areas of segmental consolidation. The pattern resembles an acute inflammatory process and may contain an air bronchogram.	Coalescence of small granulomas that results in encroachment on alveolar spaces that mimics air-space disease. More commonly a diffuse reticulonodular pattern and typical bilateral enlargement of hilar and paratracheal lymph nodes (see Figs C 13-6 and C 14-8).
Pulmonary contusion (Fig C 49-14)	Air-space consolidation that may be associated with rib or spine fractures, mediastinal or chest wall hematoma, and pneumothorax or hemothorax.	Most common chest injury resulting from blunt chest trauma. The shearing action on alveolar and capillary walls results in focal collections of hemorrhage and edema.
Pulmonary edema (Fig C 49-15)	Ground-glass, low-grade lung opacification or frank air-space consolidation.	Both cardiogenic and noncardiogenic edemas are reported to have a predominantly central distribution.

A

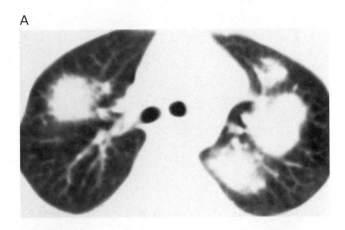

B

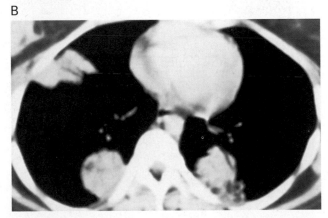

Fig C 49-13
Alveolar sarcoidosis. (A) Large central masses with partially well-defined and partially ill-defined margins. (B) More peripheral lesions with air bronchograms.[94]

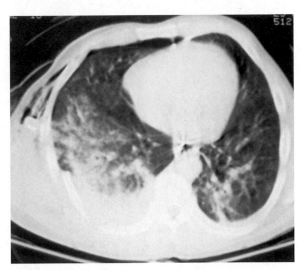

Fig C 49-14
Pulmonary contusion. There are accompanying hemothorax, rib fractures, subcutaneous emphysema, and pleural drain.[94]

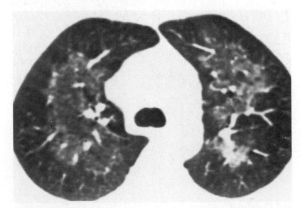

Fig C 49-15
Pulmonary edema. Central "ground-glass," low-grade lung opacification persists 3 weeks after myocardial infarction.[94]

Condition	Imaging Findings	Comments
Cocaine abuse/crack lung (Figs C 49-16 and C 49-17)	Variable degree of cardiomegaly, airspace disease and consolidation, interlobular septal thickening, and peribronchovascular edema.	Acute cardiac pulmonary edema, noncardiogenic edema due to increased permeability of damaged pulmonary capillary endothelium, and pulmonary eosinophilia.
Nontraumatic pulmonary hemorrhage (Fig C 49-18)	Widespread bilateral air-space consolidation.	May occur in patients with bleeding diatheses, idiopathic pulmonary hemosiderosis, Goodpasture's syndrome, polyarteritis nodosa, or Wegener's granulomatosis. There is usually clearing 2 to 3 days after a single bleeding episode, though reticular changes may persist much longer.

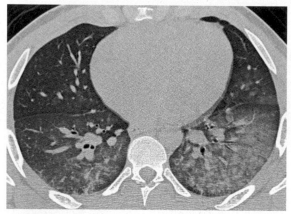

Fig C 49-16
Cocaine abuse. Acute pulmonary edema with bilateral heterogeneous opacities.[11]

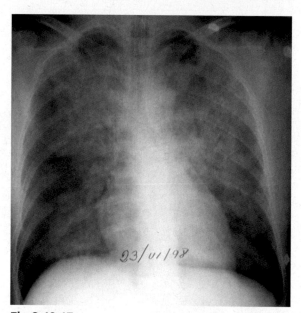

Fig C 49-17
Crack lung with pulmonary eosinophilia. Extensive bilateral heterogeneous central and peripheral opacities.

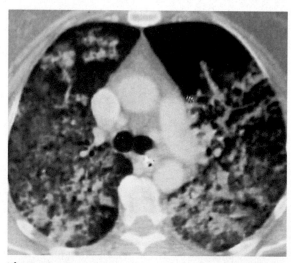

Fig C 49-18
Pulmonary hemorrhage. Widespread, patchy, and geographic air-space filling in this patient with necrotizing vasculitis.[94]

Condition	Imaging Findings	Comments
Metastases (Fig C 49-19)	Multiple, typically subpleural masses that are spherical or ovoid.	Identification of a pulmonary vascular connection to the nodule helps confirm its hematogenous origin. On CT, partial volume effects (creating the appearance of a connection with an adjacent vessel) can make a granuloma mimic a metastatic lesion if thin sections are not obtained.
Lymphoma (Fig C 49-20)	Nodular or patchy air-space disease that sometimes contains air bronchograms.	Seeding of the lung may result in a pattern indistinguishable from that of fungal infection. Lymphoma also can invade the lung directly from mediastinal or hilar lymph nodes.

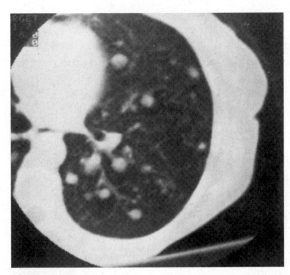

Fig C 49-19
Metastases. Multiple pulmonary nodules with vascular connections indicating their hematogenous origin.[96]

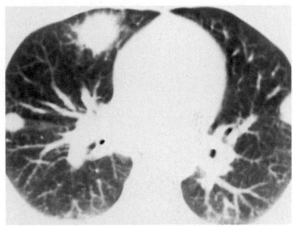

Fig C 49-20
Lymphoma. Multiple nodular opacities, some with well-defined and some with ill-defined margins. The major differential diagnostic consideration is fungal infection in this patient with Hodgkin's disease.[94]

Condition	Imaging Findings	Comments
Pulmonary lymphangitic carcinomatosis (Fig C 50-1)	Smooth or nodular thickening of the peribronchovascular interstitium and interlobular septa, with preservation of normal lung architecture at the lobular level. Hilar lymphadenopathy in approximately 50% of cases.	Tumor growth in the lymphatic system of the lungs occurs most commonly in patients with carcinomas of the breast, lung, stomach, pancreas, prostate, cervix, or thyroid. Although usually resulting from hematogenous spread to the lung, with subsequent interstitial and lymphatic invasion, it can occur because of direct lymphatic spread of tumor from mediastinal and hilar lymph nodes. Characteristic HRCT findings can be seen in patients with normal chest radiographs (which do not clearly visualize the peripheral lung regions where involvement tends to occur). In a patient with a known tumor and symptoms of dyspnea, HRCT findings typical of pulmonary lymphangitic carcinomatosis are usually considered diagnostic, and in clinical practice a lung biopsy is usually not performed.
Hematogenous metastases (Fig C 50-2)	Small discrete nodules that have a peripheral and basal predominance when limited in number, but a uniform distribution when there are innumerable lesions. Some nodules may appear to be related to small branches of pulmonary vessels.	Although HRCT may be used to characterize the distribution and morphology of lung nodules visible on chest radiographs in patients with hematogenous pulmonary metastases, conventional CT with contiguous slices is more valuable for detecting pulmonary metastases in patients with normal chest radiographs.

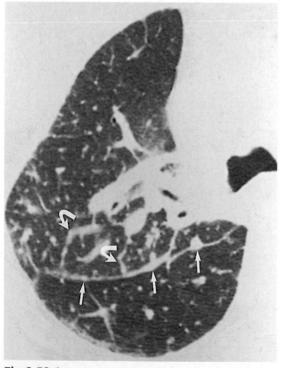

Fig C 50-1
Pulmonary lymphangitic carcinomatosis. Nodular thickening of the interlobular septa (curved arrows) and interlobar fissure (straight arrows).[88]

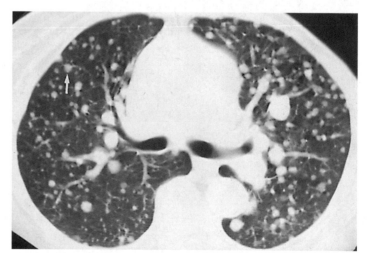

Fig C 50-2
Hematogenous metastases. Sharply defined nodules. Although some nodules (arrow) appear to be related to small vascular branches, most nodules lack a specific relationship to lobular structures and appear to be random in distribution. Note the subpleural nodules and lack of septal thickening.[88]

Condition	Imaging Findings	Comments
Bronchioloalveolar carcinoma (Fig C 50-3A, B)	Diffuse, patchy, or multifocal areas of consolidation that are peribronchovascular and contain air-bronchograms or air-filled cystic spaces. There may be extensive centrilobular air-space nodules or diffuse small nodules mimicking the appearance of hematogenous metastases.	Because fluid and mucus produced by the tumor is of low attenuation, bronchioalveolar carcinoma may demonstrate the "CT angiogram sign" (contrast-enhanced pulmonary vessels appearing denser than surrounding opacified lung). CT plays a crucial role in the initial evaluation of patients, as it can detect diffuse disease (indicating unresectability) in those who appear to have limited and potentially resectable lesions based on plain radiographs.
Kaposi's sarcoma (Fig C 50-4)	Irregular ("flamed-shaped") and ill-defined peribronchovascular nodules combined with peribronchovascular and interlobular septal thickening, pleural effusions, and lymphadenopathy.	Approximately 15% to 20% of patients with AIDS (almost all occurring in homosexual or bisexual men) develop Kaposi's sarcoma. Of these, pulmonary involvement occurs in about 20%. In most patients, the presence of typical nodules on CT and a parahilar distribution of abnormalities allow Kaposi's sarcoma to be distinguished from other thoracic complications of AIDS.

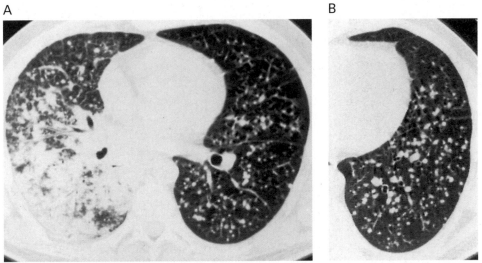

Fig C 50-3
Bronchioloalveolar carcinoma. (A) Areas of consolidation in the right lower lobes, ill-defined nodules (some of which appear to be centrilobular), and multiple small, well-defined nodules. (B) Targeted view of the left lung shows numerous small nodules, at least some of which show a random distribution similar to hematogenous metastases. Note the presence of subpleural nodules.[88]

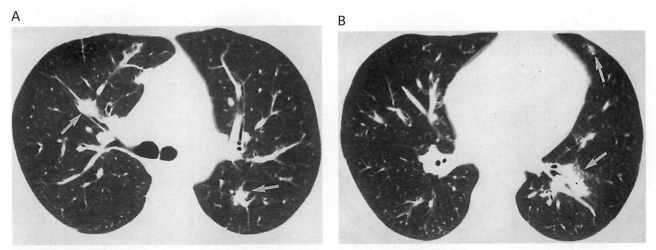

Fig C 50-4
Kaposi's sarcoma. (A, B) Ill-defined nodules (arrows) in the parahilar and peribronchovascular regions.[88]

Condition	Imaging Findings	Comments
Sarcoidosis (Fig C 50-5)	Small, sharply defined nodules that may be found in the peribronchovascular regions (adjacent to parahilar vessels and bronchi), adjacent to the major fissures, in the costal subpleural regions, within the interlobular septa, and in the centrilobular regions.	Nodules generally represent coalescent groups of microscopic granulomas, though they can reflect nodular areas of fibrosis. They may be numerous and distributed throughout both lungs, or be more localized to small areas in one or both lungs (often with an upper lobe predominance).
Inhalation disorders (Fig C 50-6)	Multiple small nodules in a centrilobular and subpleural location that are diffusely scattered throughout both lungs. In mild disease, they may be seen only in the upper lobes and have a posterior predominance.	Primarily silicosis and coal-workers' pneumoconiosis. Nodules infrequently occur in relation to thickened interlobular septa (as in pulmonary lymphangitic carcinoma or sarcoidosis). The development of irregular conglomerate masses (progressive massive fibrosis), indicating the presence of complicated disease, is always associated with a background of small nodules visible on HRCT.

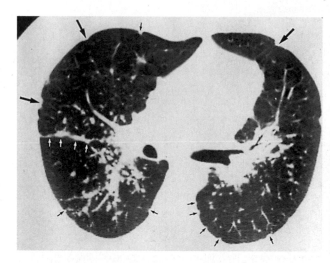

Fig C 50-5
Sarcoidosis. "Perilymphatic" distribution of numerous small nodules in relation to the parahilar, bronchovascular interstitium. The bronchial walls appear irregularly thickened. Subpleural nodules (small arrows) are seen bordering the costal pleural surfaces and right major fissure. This appearance is virtually diagnostic of sarcoidosis. Clusters of subpleural granulomas (large arrows) have been termed pseudoplaques.[88]

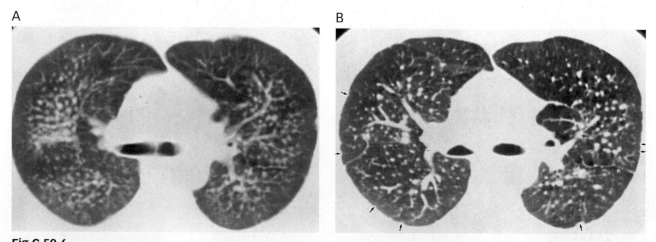

A

B

Fig C 50-6
Silicosis. (A) Conventional CT scan shows numerous lung nodules bilaterally, with relative sparing of the lung periphery. (B) HRCT at the same level more clearly defines the presence of subpleural nodules (small arrows). The nodules are smoothly marginated and sharply defined. The profusion of nodules is more easily evaluated on the conventional CT.[88]

Condition	Imaging Findings	Comments
Tuberculosis (Figs C 50-7 and C 50-8)	Ill-defined air-space nodules (reflecting endobronchial spread of infection) or small, well-defined nodules resulting from miliary or hematogenous spread of the disease.	Hilar and mediastinal lymph node enlargement is commonly seen in patients with active tuberculosis. HRCT may detect the presence of diffuse lung involvement when corresponding chest radiographs are normal or show only minimal or limited disease.
Atypical (nontuberculous) mycobacterial infections (Fig C 50-9)	Small or large nodules with areas of bronchiectasis, or patchy unilateral or bilateral air-space consolidation.	The presence of small nodules in areas of lung distant to the dominant focus of infection probably represents endobronchial spread of infection.

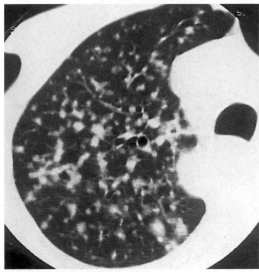

Fig C 50-7
Tuberculosis (endobronchial spread in reactivation disease). Typical appearance of numerous, diffuse, poorly defined nodules, some of which are perivascular and centrilobular.[88]

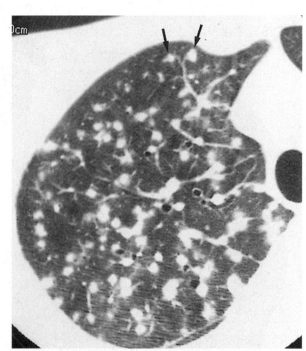

Fig C 50-8
Tuberculosis (miliary). Numerous well-defined 1–2-mm nodules diffusely distributed through the right lower lobe. Some nodules appear septal (arrows) or subpleural, whereas others appear to be associated with small feeding vessels, suggesting a hematogenous origin.[88]

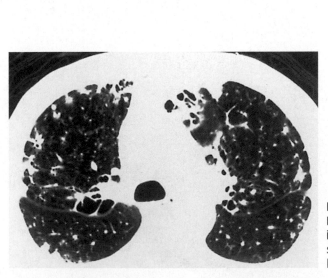

Fig C 50-9
Mycobacterium avium-intracellulare complex (MAC) infection. Characteristic findings of bronchiectasis and small nodules and clusters of nodules in the peripheral lung.[54]

Condition	Imaging Findings	Comments
Invasive pulmonary aspergillosis (Fig C 50-10)	"Halo" or ground-glass opacity surrounding focal dense parenchymal nodules.	The halo and central nodule are reported to reflect, respectively, a rim of coagulation necrosis or hemorrhage surrounding a central fungal nodule or infarct.
Septic embolism (Fig C 50-11)	Bilateral peripheral nodules in varying stages of cavitation.	Cavitary pulmonary nodules presumably result from septic occlusion of small peripheral arterial branches, resulting in the development of metastatic lung abscesses. A characteristic appearance is the finding of feeding vessels in association with the peripheral nodules.

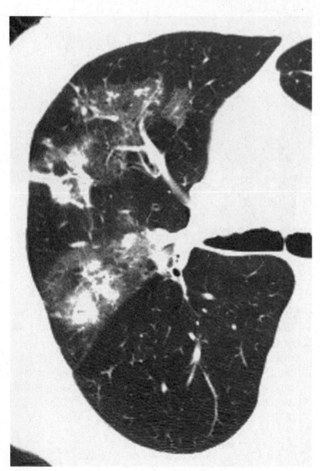

Fig C 50-10
Invasive pulmonary aspergillosis. Multiple pulmonary nodules are associated with the halo sign.[88]

A   B

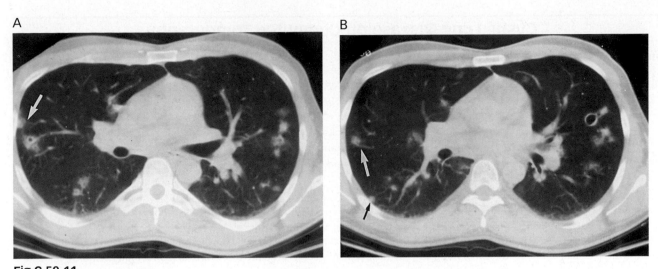

Fig C 50-11
Septic pulmonary emboli. (A, B) Scattered, mostly peripheral, poorly defined foci of air-space consolidation, many of which contain varying degrees of cavitation. Note that a number of these appear to be associated with "feeding" vessels (arrows), suggesting a hematogenous origin.[88]

Cystic Lung Disease on Computed Tomography

Condition	Imaging Findings	Comments
Emphysema (Figs C 51-1 and C 51-2)	Initially, scattered low-attenuation areas within the lung, easily separable from surrounding normal parenchyma despite the absence of clearly definable walls. With progression, whole zones of the lung become lucent, and there is often a decrease in the number and caliber of associated blood vessels.	Secondary findings that are frequently present include subpleural blebs and bullae and hyper-inflated lungs. Large bullae can compress and distort the underlying parenchyma, sometimes into bizarre configurations. CT is of special value in detecting otherwise unsuspected blebs and bullae in select high-risk populations, such as those with suspected α_1-antitrypsin deficiency or those who present with recurrent pneumothoraces.
Bronchiectasis (Fig C 51-3)	Dilated, thick-walled airways extending toward the lung periphery. With increasing severity, bronchi may become beaded and resemble a "string of pearls." In its most severe form, there may be discrete pulmonary cysts and the grouping of dilated bronchi to produce a "cluster of grapes" pattern.	The CT appearance varies depending on whether the bronchi course in a predominantly horizontal or vertical plane. When horizontal, dilated bronchi are seen along their length and produce parallel or "tram" lines. When vertical, dilated bronchi appear as thick-walled circular lucencies, almost always accompanied by adjacent pulmonary artery branches, which combine to produce a characteristic "signet ring" pattern.

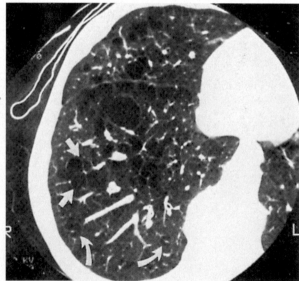

Fig C 51-1
Emphysema. There are scattered low-density cysts without clearly definable walls. Many appear to be aligned adjacent to peripheral vessels corresponding to lobular anatomy (straight arrows). Note that residual lobular vessels can still be identified within the center of some of these cysts (curved arrows).[98]

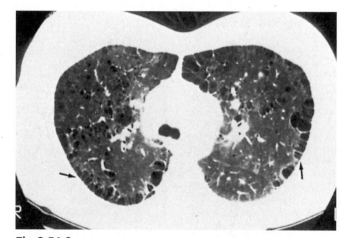

Fig C 51-2
Emphysema. Innumerable peripheral blebs and bullae diffusely involve both lungs. Septa separate individual bullae, resembling a stacked-coin appearance. These septa presumably account for the finding of prominent linear opacifications within the lungs ("dirty lung"). In addition to peripheral bullae, discrete areas of markedly low tissue attenuation without clearly definable walls also can be identified within the lung parenchyma. Note that the intervening lung parenchyma is normal and that the intrapulmonary vessels are well defined and have smooth contours.[98]

Condition	Imaging Findings	Comments
Usual interstitial pneumonia (UIP) (Fig C 51-4)	In severe disease, cystic spaces (measuring 2–4 mm) develop. In the final stages of disease, lung volume markedly decreases, and a characteristic pattern of honeycombing can be defined.	Most commonly related to idiopathic pulmonary fibrosis, a similar pattern can be seen in collagen vascular diseases (especially scleroderma and rheumatoid arthritis), pulmonary infections, and exposure to industrial inhalants (primarily asbestos).
Swyer-James syndrome (Fig C 51-5)	Diffuse emphysema (severe decreases in density of atelectatic involved lung segments), bronchiectasis, but patent central bronchi.	Presumably caused by an acute, possibly viral, bronchiolitis acquired in infancy or childhood that damages the terminal and respiratory bronchioles, so that subsequent normal development of the lung is impaired.

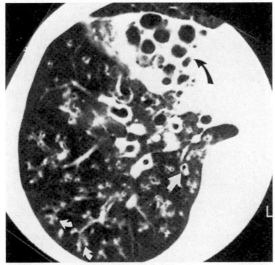

Fig C 51-3
Cystic bronchiectasis. Dilated, thick-walled bronchi lie adjacent to peripheral pulmonary artery branches, producing a signet ring appearance (arrows). Dilated bronchi within the atelectatic middle lobe resemble a cluster of grapes (curved arrow). Small, poorly defined centrilobular opacities seen peripherally represent fluid-filled distal airways (curved arrows).[98]

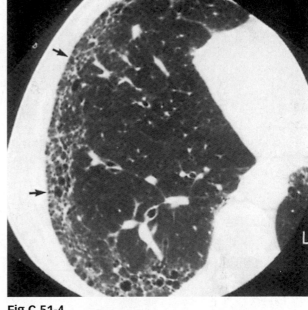

Fig C 51-4
Idiopathic pulmonary fibrosis. Coarse reticulation with variable-sized, thick-walled cysts producing a honeycombed appearance.[98]

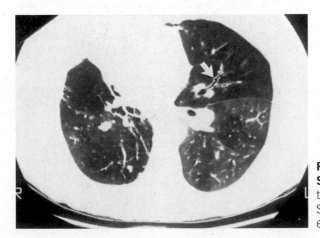

Fig C 51-5
Swyer-James syndrome. Diffuse emphysematous changes throughout both lungs associated with dilated bronchi (arrow). Sections through the central airways (not shown) showed no evidence of a central endobronchial lesion.[98]

Condition	Imaging Findings	Comments
Pulmonary Langerhans cell histiocytosis (Fig C 51-6)	Thin- and thick-walled irregular cystic spaces. With increasing severity, these cysts may develop bizarre, branching configurations mimicking bronchiectasis.	One study reported a predictable pattern of progression from small nodules, which cavitated to thick-walled cysts, and then to thin-walled cysts with eventual confluence.
Lymphangioleiomyomatosis (Fig C 51-7)	Multiple thin-walled cysts, varying in size from a few millimeters to 5 cm, that progress to become almost uniformly distributed throughout the lungs.	Rare disease of women of childbearing age that is characterized by disordered proliferation within the pulmonary interstitium of benign-appearing smooth muscle. Patients typically present with progressive dyspnea or hemoptysis (or both), with either recurrent pneumothoraces (caused by rupture of peripheral dilated air spaces secondary to air trapping from obstructed airways) or chylous effusion (secondary to dilated and obstructed lymphatics).
Pneumocystis carinii pneumonia (Fig C 51-8)	Predictable evolution of CT pattern that begins as small, thin-walled cysts localized to focal areas of pulmonary consolidation. The cysts may coalesce to more multiseptated, bizarre thick-walled cysts that frequently abut the pleural space.	Even after the underlying infection has been adequately treated, residual cysts may still be seen long after all evidence of parenchymal consolidation has disappeared. In time, most of these cysts will regress, although underlying parenchymal damage may remain.
Tuberculosis (Fig C 51-9)	Mostly thick-walled cavities, although thin-walled lesions are frequently seen in patients undergoing treatment.	Extensive pleural abnormalities are usually also present. There is no correlation between the CT (or radiographic) appearance of tuberculous cavities and disease activity.

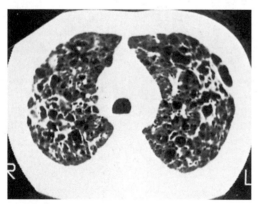

Fig C 51-6
Pulmonary Langerhans cell histiocytosis.
Innumerable thick-walled cysts of various sizes, many with bizarre, branching configurations.[98]

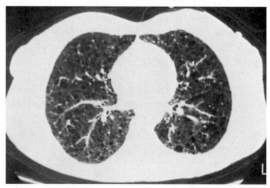

Fig C 51-7
Lymphangioleiomyomatosis. Innumerable thin-walled cysts of approximately equal size that are uniformly distributed throughout both lungs.[98]

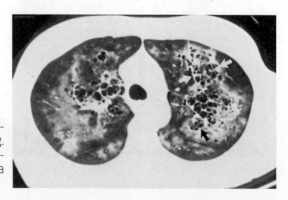

Fig C 51-8
***Pneumocystis carinii* pneumonia.** Discrete thin- and thick-walled cysts occurring in association with consolidated lung. Coalescence of cysts results in the formation of a few bizarre-shaped cysts (arrows). Note that the intervening parenchyma appears grossly normal.[98]

Condition	Imaging Findings	Comments
Septic emboli (Fig C 51-10)	Peripheral nodules in varying stages of cavitation, presumably caused by showers of infected material reaching the lungs at various times.	When seen in cross section, a characteristic "feeding" vessel can often be identified.
Metastases (Fig C 51-11)	Single or multiple cavitary lesions that often are associated with an adjacent feeding pulmonary artery.	Cavitary metastases are rare, occurring in less than 5% of cases. They most often result from primary squamous cell carcinomas (especially from the head and neck, cervix, and bladder). Less frequent causes are primary adenocarcinomas, especially those arising in the gastrointestinal tract, and primary extrathoracic sarcomas.
Sarcoidosis (Fig C 51-12)	Cystic changes in a distinctive subpleural and especially peribronchovascular distribution.	Cystic changes in sarcoidosis are usually attributed to interstitial fibrosis, leading to honeycombing, bronchiectasis, and emphysema with resultant bullae and blebs. These "pseudocavities" are lined with dense fibrous tissue, not granulomas. Indeed, true cavitation of sarcoid nodules due to necrosis is extremely rare.

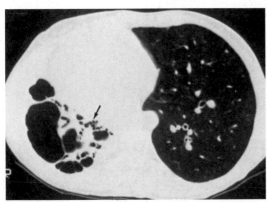

Fig C 51-9
Tuberculosis. Essentially complete replacement of the right lower lobe by cavities and bronchiectasis (arrow). Note that dilated bronchi appear to extend into some of these cavities.[98]

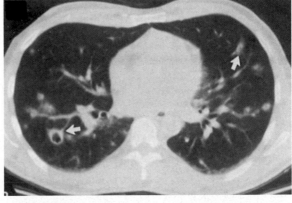

Fig C 51-10
Septic emboli. Scattered nodules in varying stages of cavitation in a patient with staphylococcal endocarditis. Many of the cavities are clearly related to adjacent vessels (arrows).[98]

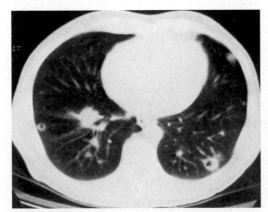

Fig C 51-11
Metastases. In this patient with colon cancer, there are scattered cavitary nodules bilaterally. As in Fig C 43-10, many of the cavities are clearly related to adjacent vessels.[98]

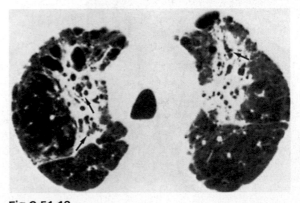

Fig C 51-12
Sarcoidosis. Characteristic pattern of bullae associated with central scarring and bronchiectasis. Note the scattered, poorly marginated nodules, some of which appear to have a perivascular distribution.[98]

Mosaic Pattern on Chest Computed Tomography*

Condition	Imaging Findings	Comments
Primary small airway disease (Fig C 52-1)	Decreased size and number of vessels in lucent lung compared with higher attenuation lung. Air trapping as evidenced by no increase in attenuation or decrease in volume of the lucent lung on expiratory scans.	Small airway diseases that result in focal or poor ventilation of lung parenchyma are the most common causes of the mosaic pattern. Areas of poorly ventilated lung are poorly perfused because of reflex vasoconstriction or because of a permanent reduction in the pulmonary capillary bed. The inciting pathologic processes can be permanent (eg, obliterative bronchiolitis) or reversible (eg, asthma).
Pulmonary vascular disease (Fig C 52-2)	Decreased size and number of vessels in lucent lung compared with higher attenuation lung. No air trapping on expiratory scans.	Can reflect pulmonary thromboembolic disease or pulmonary arterial hypertension. Regions of hyperemic (higher attenuation) lung mimic ground-glass infiltrates when seen adjacent to oligemic (lower attenuation) regions of lung.

A   B

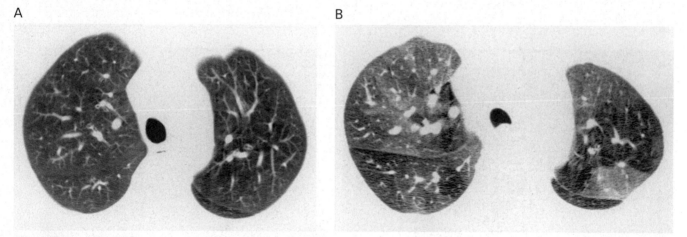

Fig C 52-1
Asthma. (A) CT scan obtained at suspended full inspiration shows normal findings, including a normal gradient of attenuation. (B) Repeat study obtained at suspended full expiration shows patchy diffuse air trapping with typical mosaic pattern of lung attenuation.[99]

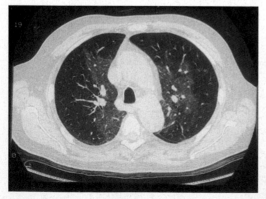

Fig C 52-2
Chronic pulmonary emboli and resulting pulmonary artery hypertension. Mosaic pattern of lung attenuation with perihilar ground-glass attenuation and oligemic peripheral lung. Note that the caliber of vessels in regions of higher attenuation is greater than that in lower attenuation oligemic lung.[99]

*Regional differences in lung perfusion that result in variable lung attenuation in a lobular or multilobular distribution. Vessels in the lucent regions of the lung typically appear smaller than those in denser areas.

Condition	Imaging Findings	Comments
Primary parenchymal disease (Fig C 52-3)	Similar size and number of vessels in both regions of the lung. No air trapping on expiratory scans.	Infiltrative processes with the interstitium of the lung or partial filling of the air spaces by fluid, cells, or fibrosis results in an increase in the CT attenuation of the affected lung compared with that of the normal parenchyma. Diseases that can produce the mosaic pattern include *Pneumocystis carinii* pneumonia, chronic eosinophilic pneumonia, hypersensitivity pneumonia, bronchiolitis obliterans organizing pneumonia, and pyogenic pneumonia.

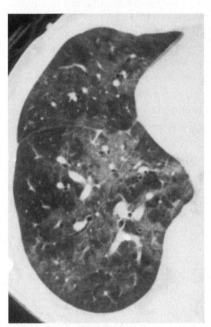

Fig C 52-3
***Pneumocystis carinii* pneumonia in AIDS.** Mosaic pattern is produced by ground-glass infiltrate that spares single lobular and multilobular regions.[99]

Crazy-Paving Pattern on Computed Tomography*

Condition	Comments
Pneumocystis carinii pneumonia (Fig C 53-1)	Common pulmonary infection in the severely immunocompromised patient. Symptoms include dry cough, dyspnea, and low-grade fever. Plain radiographs show bilateral, perihilar reticular opacifications that often progress to alveolar consolidation within a few days.
Bronchioloalveolar (alveolar cell) carcinoma (Fig C 53-2)	The tumor typically spreads through the airways and air spaces with preservation of the lung architecture. A characteristic, though infrequent, clinical feature is bronchorrhea, the expectoration of large quantities of sputum.
Alveolar proteinosis (Fig C 53-3)	Filling of the alveoli by a proteinaceous material that is positive at periodic acid-Schiff staining, associated with an inflammatory response in the adjacent interstitium. Most common between ages 20–50, it typically produces bilateral, symmetric alveolar consolidation, particularly in a perihilar or hilar distribution resembling pulmonary edema.

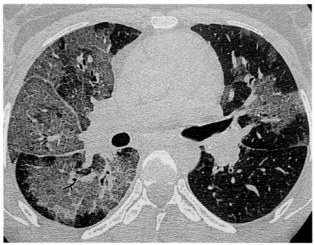

Fig C 53-1
***Pneumocystis carinii* pneumonia.** Ground-glass attenuation with intralobular lines in a young man with acquired immunodeficiency syndrome.[100]

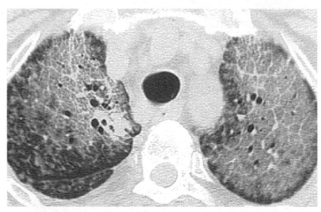

Fig C 53-2
Bronchioloalveolar carcinoma. Bilateral crazy-paving pattern and centrilobular nodules.[100]

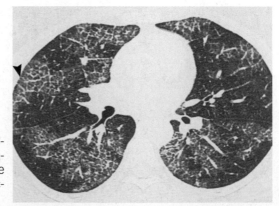

Fig C 53-3
Alveolar proteinosis. Diffuse geographic ground-glass attenuation with superimposed intra- and interlobular septal thickening (arrowhead). Note the polygonal appearance, which represents the secondary pulmonary lobule.[100]

*Scattered or diffuse ground-glass attenuation with superimposed interlobular septal thickening and interlobular lines.

Condition	Comments
Sarcoidosis (Fig C 53-4)	Systemic disorder characterized by the development of noncaseating granulomatous inflammation. More common findings include irregular thickening of the bronchovascular bundles and small nodules along vessels, as well as the typical bilateral hilar and mediastinal lymphadenopathy.
Nonspecific interstitial pneumonia (Fig C 53-5)	Clinical presentation similar to interstitial pulmonary fibrosis, but associated with a much better prognosis. Involvement is usually bilateral and symmetric, predominantly affecting the basal and subpleural regions.
Organizing pneumonia	Also known as cryptogenic organizing pneumonia, this chronic inflammatory process is characterized by focal plugs of granulation tissue in distal small airways and responds well to steroid therapy. Although most cases are idiopathic, there is an association with collagen vascular disease, drug toxicity, and infection.
Lipoid pneumonia (Fig C 53-6)	Pulmonary disorder resulting from chronic aspiration or inhalation of animal, vegetable, or petroleum-based oils or fats. Imaging findings include bilateral lower lobe air-space consolidation, mixed alveolar and interstitial opacities, and even poorly defined mass-like lesions mimicking pulmonary neoplasms. On CT, the lesion typically has low attenuation, indicating the presence of lipid deposition.

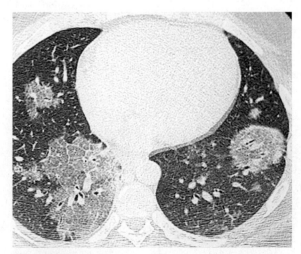

Fig C 53-4
Sarcoidosis. Scattered bilateral areas of ground-glass attenuation associated with inter- and intralobular lines in a young asymptomatic man.[101]

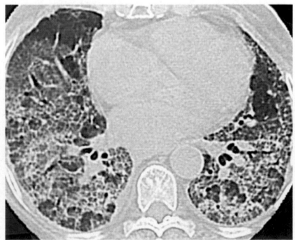

Fig C 53-5
Nonspecific interstitial pneumonia. Bilateral diffuse ground-glass attenuation and inter- and intralobular lines in a patient on Amiodarone therapy. Note the traction bronchiectasis.[100]

Condition	Comments
Adult respiratory distress syndrome (ARDS) (Figs C 53-7 and C 53-8)	Form of pulmonary edema characterized by refractory hypoxemia and respiratory distress. Underlying causes include shock, contusion, infection, sepsis, aspiration, drug abuse, and the inhalation of noxious substances. Chest radiographs typically show bilateral homogeneous pulmonary opacities.
Pulmonary hemorrhage (Fig C 53-9)	Causes include idiopathic pulmonary hemosiderosis, Goodpasture syndrome, collagen vascular disease, drug-induced coagulopathy, and hemorrhage associated with malignancy.

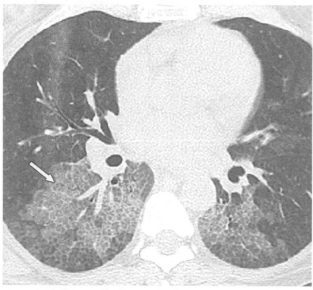

Fig C 53-6
Lipoid pneumonia. Geographic ground-glass attenuation associated with interlobular thickening and inralobular lines (arrow).[100]

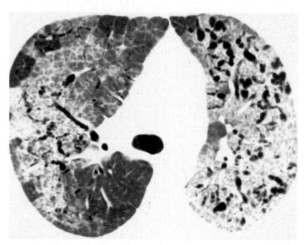

Fig C 53-7
Acute respiratory distress syndrome. Scattered ground-glass attenuation and thickening of the intra- and interlobular septa. In this young man who developed barotraumas, note the air within the areas of interlobular thickening, a finding indicative of pulmonary interstitial emphysema.[102]

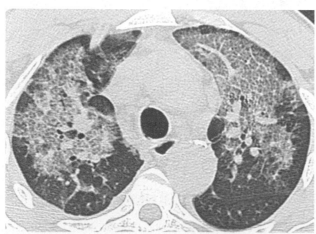

Fig C 53-8
Cocaine abuse. Diffuse bilateral reticular opacities with superimposed thickening of inter- and intralobular interstitium.[11]

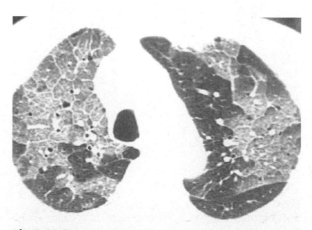

Fig C 53-9
Diffuse pulmonary hemorrhage. In this patient with systemic lupus erythematosus and massive hemoptysis, there are geographic areas of ground-glass attenuation with interlobular septal thickening.[101]

Condition	Comments
Severe acute respiratory syndrome (SARS) (Fig C 53-10)	Atypical pneumonia of unknown etiology, possibly due to a coronavirus. Beginning in Hong Kong, where it initially affected mainly medical personnel, the disease rapidly spread to nearby countries, Europe, North America, and Australia.

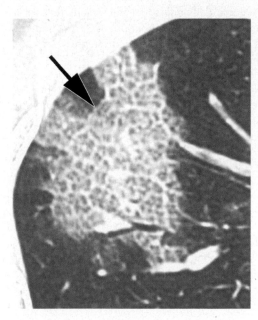

Fig C 53-10
SARS. Ground-glass opacification and thickened interlobular septa (arrow) and intralobular interstitium produce the crazy-paving pattern.[103]

Upper Zone–Predominant Disease

Condition	Comments
Postprimary tuberculosis (Fig C 54-1)	Cavitary disease with patchy areas of consolidation and bronchial wall thickening that primarily involves the apical posterior segment of the upper lobes.
Sarcoidosis (Fig C 54-2)	Predominantly interstitial abnormality that has a bronchovascular distribution on CT. Adenopathy is common, though it usually regresses as the interstitial lung disease worsens.
Pulmonary Langerhans cell histiocytosis (Fig C 54-3)	Nodules evolving into bizarre-shaped cysts that are seen almost exclusively in young smokers and probably represent an allergic reaction to some component of cigarette smoke.
Silicosis/coal-workers' pneumoconiosis (Fig C 54-4)	Nodular interstitial thickening that may progress to pulmonary massive fibrosis (PMF) resulting from long-term exposure to occupational dusts.
Centrilobular emphysema (Fig C 54-5)	Destruction of lung parenchyma, classically near the central arteriole and bronchiole of the secondary pulmonary lobule, with well-defined margins between normal and abnormal lung.

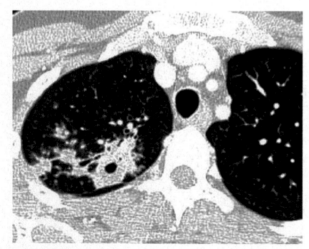

Fig C 54-1
Postprimary tuberculosis. Large cavitary lesion with surrounding consolidation involves the apical posterior segment of the right upper lobe. (Courtesy of Diana Litmanovich, M.D., Boston)

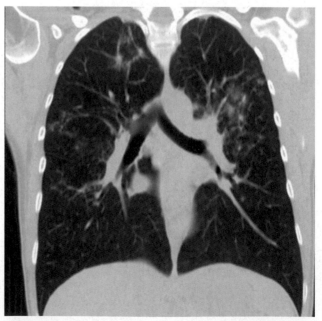

Fig C 54-2
Sarcoidosis. Coronal projection shows that the interstitial abnormalities in a bronchovascular distribution primarily involve the upper lung zones. (Courtesy of Diana Litmanovich, M.D., Boston)

Condition	Comments
Chronic eosinophilic pneumonia (Fig C 54-6)	Peripheral lung consolidation that produces the "photographic negative" of the central "bat-wing" pattern of cardiogenic pulmonary edema. Rapid response to steroid therapy.
Chronic hypersensitivity pneumonitis	Group of allergic lung diseases with various patterns caused by the inhalation of a variety of organic and chemical antigens. The most common types are farmer's lung and bird fancier's lung.

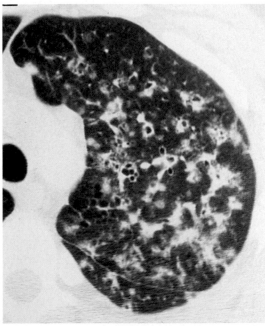

Fig C 54-3
Pulmonary Langerhans cell histiocytosis. Irregular nodules and thick-walled cysts in the upper lung. Lower sections (not shown) showed relative sparing of the lung bases.[104]

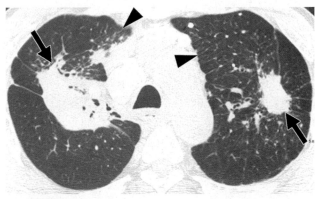

Fig C 54-4
Silicosis. Scan obtained at the level of the aortic arch shows large symmetric bilateral opacities with irregular margins (arrows) indicative of progressive massive fibrosis, as well as numerous small nodules and septal thickening (arrowheads).[105]

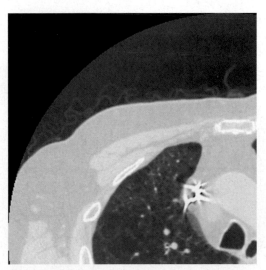

Fig C 54-5
Centrilobular emphysema. Section through the upper lobes shows subtle areas of lung destruction limited to individual secondary pulmonary lobules. The structure of these lobules, including the central core structures, is intact. Such subtle emphysema will often remain undetected on chest radiography. (Courtesy of Diana Litmanovich, MD, Boston)

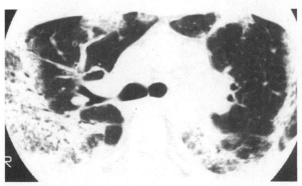

Fig C 54-6
Chronic eosinophilic pneumonia. Air-space consolidation primarily involves the peripheral lung.[106]

Condition	Comments
Cystic fibrosis (Fig C 54-7)	Bronchiectasis that is more severe in the upper lobes, especially the right. Autosomal recessive gene disorder that produces thick viscous secretions
Allergic bronchopulmonary aspergillosis (Fig C 54-8)	Central bronchiectasis with peripheral sparing, typically developing as a hypersensitivity reaction in patients with a history of asthma. The condition also occurs as a complication of cystic fibrosis.
Neurogenic pulmonary edema (Fig C 54-9)	Edema due to hydrostatic changes and capillary leak that develops within minutes to hours of any central nervous system insult that acutely raises intracranial pressure.

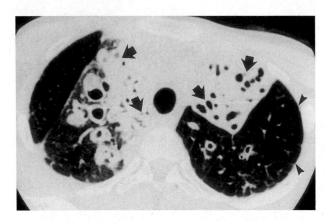

Fig C 54-7
Cystic fibrosis. Scan obtained at the level of the upper lobes demonstrates severe signs of bronchiectasis partly filled with mucus, moderate signs of bronchial wall thickening, multiple areas of consolidation (arrows) with air bronchograms, and emphysema (arrowheads).[107]

A   B

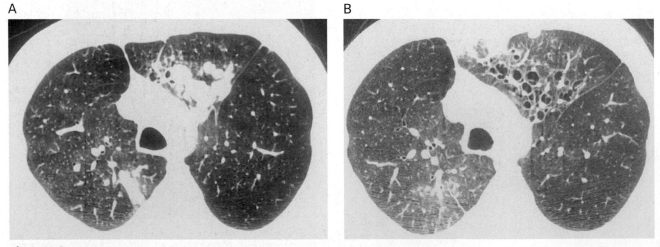

Fig C 54-8
Allergic bronchopulmonary aspergillosis. (A) Initial scan shows multiple tubular areas of increased attenuation in the left upper lobe. (B) Repeat study 2 months later shows cystic bronchiectasis in the region.[46]

Condition	Comments
Lipoma (Fig C 56-3)	Although the most common benign neoplasm, involvement of the lung parenchyma is rare. Lipoma is typically detected as an incidental finding on plain chest radiographs as a solitary pulmonary nodule in the periphery surrounded by normal lung tissue. CT shows homogeneous fat attenuation.
Lipoid pneumonia (Fig C 56-4)	Uncommon condition resulting from chronic aspiration of animal, vegetable, or mineral oil into the lung. Plain chest radiographs can show air-space consolidation, an irregular mass-like lesion, or a reticulonodular pattern that most often involves the dependent portions of the lung. The characteristic CT finding is lung consolidation with fat attenuation.

Mediastinal lesions

Condition	Comments
Lipoma/lipomatosis (Fig C 56-5)	Lipomas are well-circumscribed mesenchymal tumors that grow slowly and typically are detected incidentally on routine chest radiographs. They may produce symptoms due to the mass compressing of the primary bronchi, esophagus, veins, or phrenic or vagus nerves. CT and MRI can show the extent and fatty nature of the lesion. Mediastinal lipomatosis is diffuse, unencapsulated infiltrative deposition of fat that is commonly associated with obesity or steroid therapy.
Thymolipoma	Rare, slow-growing, benign tumor of the anterior-superior mediastinum that contains a mixture of thymic parenchyma and mature adipose tissue. The demonstration of a connection between the tumor and the superior mediastinum strongly suggests this diagnosis.

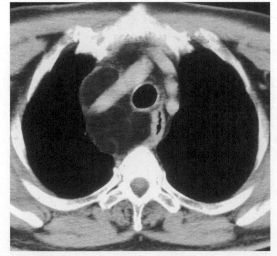

Fig C 56-3
Lipoma. CT scan shows a well-demarcated fatty mass surrounding the right brachiocephalic artery.[59]

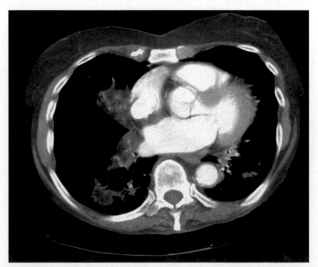

Fig C 56-4
Lipoid pneumonia. CT scan shows bilateral consolidation with low attenuation (arrows).[59]

Condition	Comments
Teratoma/teratocarcinoma (Fig C 56-6)	Teratomas are germ cell neoplasms that typically occur in young patients and appear as spherical, lobulated, encapsulated multicystic masses that predominantly involve the anterior mediastinum. On CT, the lesion appears as a heterogeneous mass containing varying amounts of soft tissue, fluid, fat, and calcification. Fat-suppressed MR imaging sequences can confirm the fat content of the mass. Malignant teratomas are usually more nodular or poorly defined, contain fat less often, and may have a thick capsule that demonstrates contrast enhancement.
Cardiac lesions Lipoma (Fig C 56-7)	Representing about 10% of all primary tumors of the heart and pericardium, a lipoma typically appears on CT as an oval, nonpedunculated mass with fat attenuation.

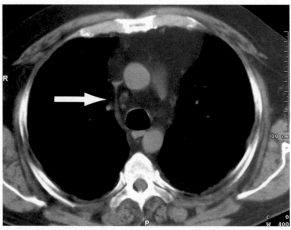

Fig C 56-5
Lipomatosis. CT demonstrates a fatty lesion with mass effect on the superior vena cava and azygos vein. Initial chest radiographs demonstrated upper mediastinal widening with soft-tissue opacity at the level of the aorticopulmonary window.[59]

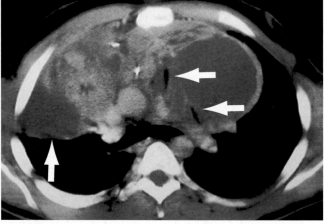

Fig C 56-6
Teratoma. CT scan shows a cystic mass with soft tissue, fluid (arrow), fat (arrowheads), and calcium attenuation.[59]

Fig C 56-7
Lipoma. Large, fat-attenuation lesion that surrounds and elevates the left anterior descending artery, a finding consistent with a sub-pericardial lipoma.[59]

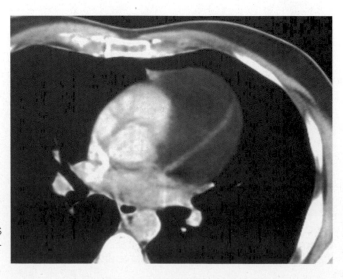

Condition	Comments
Liposarcoma (Fig C 56-8)	Primary cardiac liposarcomas, which usually originate from the right side of the heart, are very rare. They may invade locally, infiltrate the heart, or metastasize to the lungs. MRI can best demonstrate the extent and fatty nature of the lesion.
Lipomatous hypertrophy of the interatrial septum (Fig C 56-9)	Benign accumulation of fat linked to increasing patient age and obesity. On CT, this process appears as a smooth, nonenhancing, well-marginated, fat-containing lesion in the interatrial septum that characteristically has a dumbbell shape with relative sparing of the oval fossa.
Pleural and extrapleural lesions Lipoma (Fig C 56-10)	Soft, encapsulated fatty tumor that demonstrates slow growth and may become extremely large. On CT, it appears as a homogeneous mass with fat attenuation. Extrapleural fat may produce a soft-tissue shadow that can be confused with pleural thickening on plain chest radiographs. Unlike pleural plaques, extrapleural fat is typically bilateral and symmetric and does not calcify. The demonstration of low attenuation on CT confirms the diagnosis.
Diaphragmatic hernias (Figs C 56-11 to C 56-13)	Fat within herniated abdominal contents can be found in hiatal and paraesophageal hernias, as well as hernias through the foramina of Morgagni (anterior) and Bochdalek (posterior).

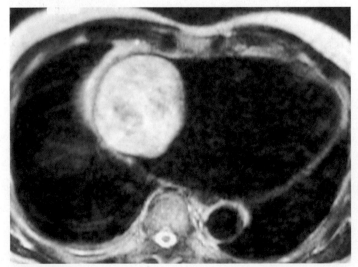

Fig C 56-8
Liposarcoma. Axial T1-weighted MR image shows a lobulated high-signal-intensity mass along the right border of the heart. (Case courtesy of Mark J. Kransdorf, MD, Mayo Clinic, Jacksonville, Fla.).[59]

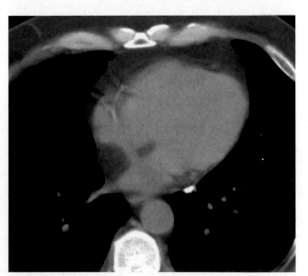

Fig C 56-9
Lipomatous hypertrophy of the interatrial septum.
CT scan shows the smooth, well-marginated fat-containing lesion.[59]

A

B

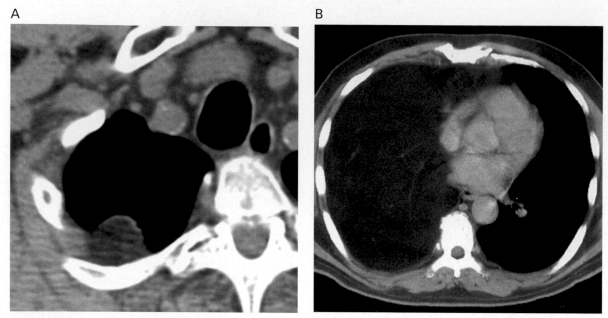

Fig C 56-10
Pleural lipoma. (A) CT scan with mediastinal windowing shows a smoothly marginated mass with fat attenuation in the apex of the right lung. (B) In another patient, there is an extensive mass of low attenuation in the right lung. (B, courtesy of James Pike, MD, Metholdist Hospital, Indianapolis, IN).[59]

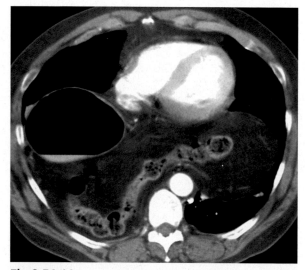

Fig C 56-11
Hiatal hernia. CT scan shows herniation of the stomach and bowel posterior to the heart.[59]

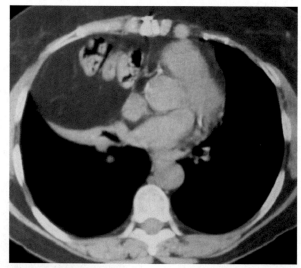

Fig C 56-12
Morgagni hernia. CT scan shows a retrosternal hernia that includes the omentum and colon.[59]

Condition	Comments
Juxtacaval fat (Fig C 56-14)	A focal collection of fat can often be observed medially, adjacent to the lumen of the inferior vena cava (IVC) near the hepatic venous confluence. It is essential to differentiate juxtacaval fat from an intracaval thrombus or tumor. Reformatted sagittal or coronal CT images may be necessary to show the true relationship between the fat collection and the lumen of the IVC.

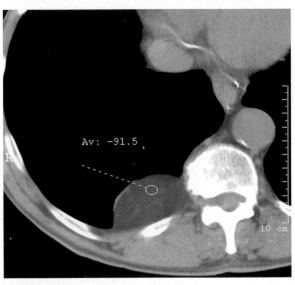

Fig C 56-13
Bochdalek hernia. CT scan shows a posterior paraspinal fat-containing lesion.[59]

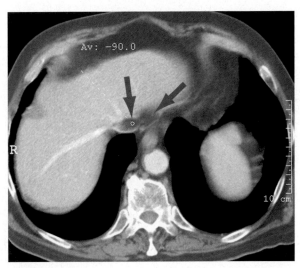

Fig C 56-14
Juxtacaval fat. CT scan shows a fat-containing lesion that appears to be within the lumen of the IVC near the hepatic vein confluence. Continuity between the juxtacaval fat (arrowhead) and paraesophageal fat (arrow) can often be seen.[59]

Filling Defect in Pulmonary Artery on Computed Tomography

Condition	Comments
Acute pulmonary embolism (Fig C 57-1)	Intraluminal clot related to an acute embolism is by far the most common cause of a filling defect within an opacified pulmonary artery on CT. Peripheral filling defects due to acute pulmonary embolism typically form acute angles with the arterial wall. A large occluding embolus prevents any enhancement of the lumen of the artery, which may be enlarged when compared with adjacent patent vessels.
Chronic pulmonary embolism (Figs C 57-2 and C 57-3)	One manifestation is a peripheral, crescent-shaped intraluminal defect that forms obtuse angles with the vessel wall. Other signs include complete occlusion of a vessel that is smaller than adjacent patent vessels, a web or flap within a contrast-filled artery, and extensive bronchial or other systemic collateral vessels. The main pulmonary artery is typically enlarged, reflecting the presence of associated pulmonary arterial hypertension. Chronic pulmonary emboli may show contrast enhancement.
Technical or patient-related artifact (Fig C 57-4)	Among the numerous CT artifacts that can be misinterpreted as pulmonary embolus are respiratory-motion, flow-related, streak, lung-algorithm, and partial-volume artifacts, image noise in large patients, vascular bifurcations, and misidentification of pulmonary veins.

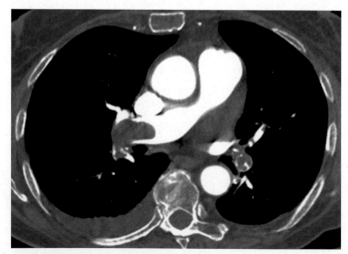

Fig C 57-1
Acute pulmonary embolus. CT pulmonary angiogram demonstrates a large filling defect within the right main and left interlobar pulmonary arteries.[113]

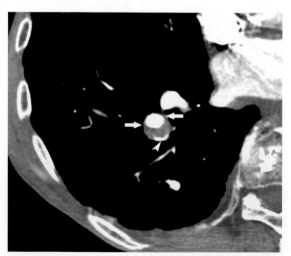

Fig C 57-2
Chronic pulmonary embolus. An eccentrically located thrombus forms obtuse angles with the vessel wall (arrows). Note the dilated collateral bronchial artery (arrowhead).[113]

Condition	Comments
Mucous plug artifact (Fig C 57-5)	A mucous plug within a bronchus, which may also demonstrate peripheral wall enhancement related to inflammation, can mimic acute pulmonary embolism. Detection of an accompanying pulmonary artery that shows normal filling with contrast material should provide a clue to the presence of this artifact. Its true nature can also be understood by viewing the bronchus on contiguous images.

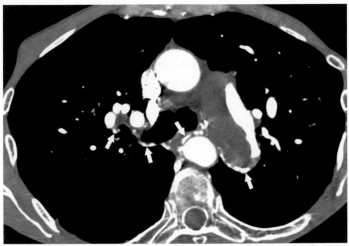

Fig C 57-3
Chronic pulmonary embolus. Extensive collateral bronchial arteries (arrows) associated with the large embolus in the main and left pulmonary arteries (arrowhead).[113]

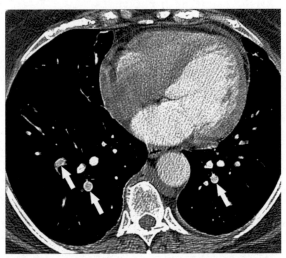

Fig C 57-4
Lung algorithm artifact mimicking pulmonary embolus. Bright rings around normal pulmonary arteries (arrows) produce an appearance mimicking multiple pulmonary emboli.[113]

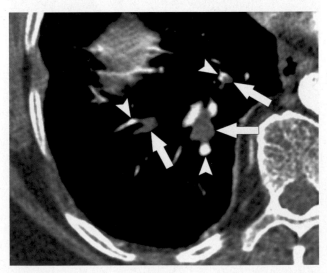

Fig C 57-5
Mucous plugs. Filling defects (arrows) that mimic acute pulmonary emboli. The posterobasal segment of the right lower lobe bronchus is dilated as well as filled with mucus. Identification of the normal accompanying pulmonary arteries (arrowheads) allows the correct interpretation of this finding.[133]

Condition	Comments
Pulmonary artery stump in situ thrombosis (Fig C 57-6)	Thrombus formation can be secondary to vessel injury, disturbance of blood flow, and hyper-coagulability, all of which are present in patients who have undergone resection for lung cancer. Intraluminal thrombosis can occasionally be identified in a pulmonary artery stump. The proper diagnosis can be made if thrombus is only seen at the surgical site and all other remote pulmonary vessels are clear.
Primary sarcoma of the pulmonary artery (Fig C 57-7 and C 57-8)	Rare cause, which appears on CT as a unilateral, lobulated, heterogeneously enhancing mass. Un-like acute pulmonary embolism, pulmonary artery sarcoma shows contrast enhancement. Chronic pulmonary embolism also can enhance, but it forms obtuse angles with the vessel wall unlike pulmonary artery sarcoma, which is lobulated and forms acute angles with the wall of the artery.
Tumor emboli (Fig C 57-9)	Large emboli in the main, lobar, and segmental pulmonary arteries can cause intravascular filling defects that mimic acute pulmonary embolism. A rare cause of this appearance, these tumor emboli result from direct invasion of the inferior vena cava or its major branches by various primary neoplasms.

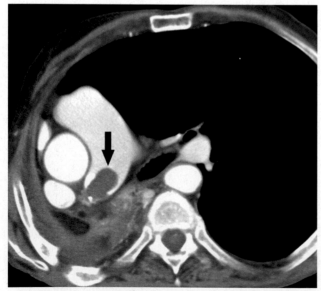

Fig C 57-6
Pulmonary artery stump. In situ thrombosis in the right pulmonary artery stump of an elderly man who had undergone a previous right pneumonectomy for lung cancer.[113]

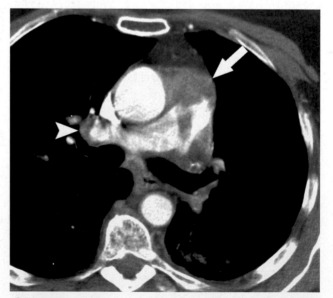

Fig C 57-7
Pulmonary artery sarcoma. Contrast scan shows a heterogeneously enhancing, lobulated mass within the main pulmonary artery (arrow). A metastatic deposit is noted within the right pulmonary artery (arrowhead).[113]

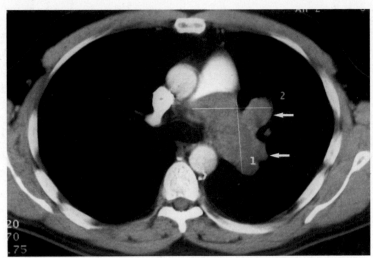

Fig C 57-8
Pulmonary artery leiomyosarcoma. Contrast scan shows a homogeneous mass that fills the left main pulmonary artery and extends into the left upper and lower lobe pulmonary arteries (arrows).[114]

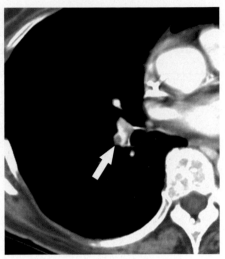

Fig C 57-9
Tumor embolus. Large tumor embolus within the right lower lobe pulmonary artery (artery) from a primary endometrial stromal sarcoma that had invaded the inferior vena cava.[113]

Computed Tomography of Blunt Chest Trauma

Condition	Imaging Findings	Comments
Aortic injury		
Acute aortic injury (Fig C 58-1)	Blood within the mediastinum, deformity of the aortic contour, intimal flap, thrombosis of debris protruding into the aortic lumen, or abrupt tapering of the diameter of the descending aorta compared with the ascending aorta ("pseudocoarctation").	A normal chest radiograph has a 98% negative predictive value for aortic injury, but an abnormal film has a low positive predictive value. Only 10% to 15% of aortograms obtained to evaluate patients with abnormal radiographic findings demonstrate an aortic tear. Approximately 90% of all injuries visible at CT occur at or just above the level of the ligamentum arteriosum. CT may demonstrate that mediastinal widening seen at chest radiography results not from an aortic injury, but rather from either a hematoma secondary to sternal or vertebral body fracture or such causes as mediastinal lipomatosis, tortuous vessels, vascular anomalies, lymphadenopathy, or pleural fluid.
Chronic pseudoaneurysm (Fig C 58-2)	Frequently calcified mass, typically located at the ligamentum arteriosum.	Only 2% of patients with untreated traumatic aortic injury survive long enough to develop a chronic pseudoaneurysm.
Pulmonary and bronchial injury		
Pneumothorax (see Fig C 58-6)	Extrapulmonary, intrathoracic collection of air that typically collects in the nondependent portion of the chest.	Pneumothorax occurs in 30% to 40% of cases of blunt chest trauma. CT is far more sensitive than plain chest radiography for detecting pneumothorax, especially in the supine trauma patient.

A

B

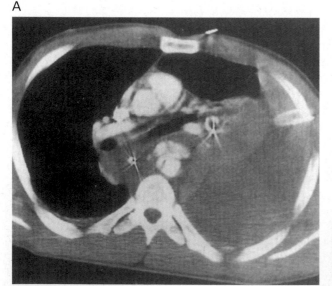
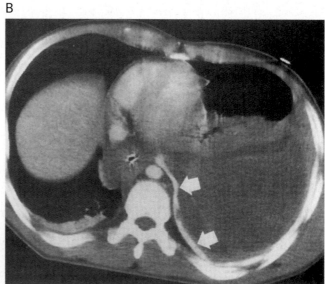

Fig C 58-1
Aortic rupture with active hemorrhage. (A) Gross disruption of the proximal descending aorta with periaortic hematoma. Note the large hemothorax. (B) Scan obtained 7 cm caudad demonstrates active bleeding with extravasation of contrast material into the left pleural space (arrows).[115]

Condition	Imaging Findings	Comments
Pulmonary parenchymal injury		Focal parenchymal injury consisting of edema and interstitial and alveolar hemorrhage, seen in approximately 30% to 70% of patients with blunt chest trauma.
Contusion (see Fig C 58-3)	Poorly defined local area of consolidation, usually in the lung periphery adjacent to the area of trauma.	Traumatic disruption of alveolar spaces with formation of a cavity filled with blood or air. Small lacerations are visible on CT in the majority of patients in whom only contusion is evident at chest radiography.
Laceration (Fig C 58-3)	Localized air collection in an area of consolidation. May be single or multiple, unilateral or bilateral.	Traumatic blood-filled lung cyst. Can persist and result in a traumatic pneumatocele as the hemorrhage resolves.

A

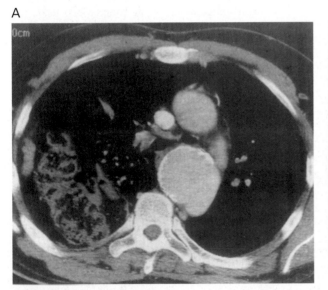

B

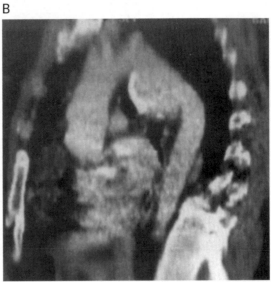

Fig C 58-2
Chronic pseudoaneurysm. The patient had been involved in a motor vehicle accident 32 years earlier. (A) Axial scan shows a large calcified pseudoaneurysm of the proximal descending aorta. Note also the ruptured right hemidiaphragm with herniation of large bowel into the chest. (B) Sagittal reformatted image shows the calcified pseudoaneurysm in the characteristic location just distal to the left subclavian artery.[115]

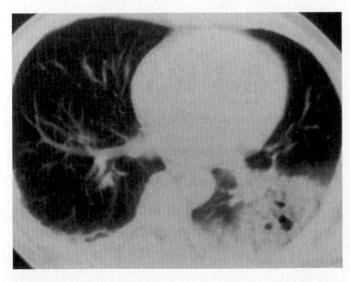

Fig C 58-3
Pulmonary laceration. Multiple small cavities within an area of pulmonary contusion.[115]

Condition	Imaging Findings	Comments
Hematoma (Fig C 58-4)	Well-circumscribed, round area of increased attenuation.	A major clue to tracheal tears on both radiographs and CT is abnormality in the appearance or position of the endotracheal tube. This includes overdistention of the cuff of the tube, protrusion of the tube wall beyond the expected margins of the tracheal lumen, and extraluminal position of the tip of the tube.
Tracheal tear (Fig C 58-5)	Tracheal transactions in the cervical region produce extensive subcutaneous air, and elevation of the hyoid bone (above the level of the C3 vertebral body) or the greater cornu (<2 cm from the angle of the mandible).	Uncommon injury that tends to occur within 2.5 cm of the carina, most often on the right. Associated fractures of the upper thorax, including the first three ribs, clavicle, sternum, and scapula, are seen in about 40% of patients with tracheobronchial injuries. Fallen lung sign is thought to be caused by disruption of the normal hilar attachments of the lung, which leads the collapsed lung to droop peripherally rather than centrally adjacent to the spine.

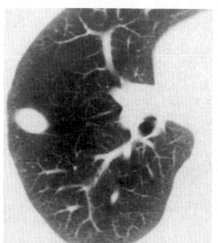

Fig C 58-4
Pulmonary hematoma. Focal, well-circumscribed nodular opacity in the right upper lobe.[115]

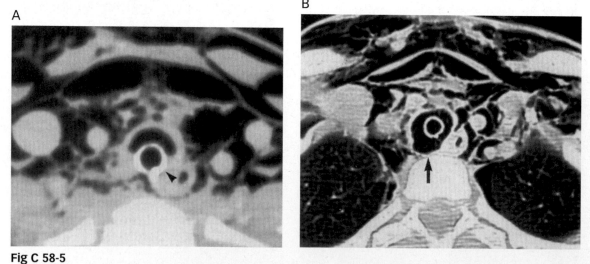

Fig C 58-5
Tracheal tear. (A, B) Eccentric placement of an endotracheal tube with respect to the tracheal ring (arrowhead in A) and disruption of the posterior wall of the trachea (arrow in B). There is extensive subcutaneous air in A, and a small left pneumothorax in B. At surgery, there were three ruptured cartilage rings and a long tear in the posterior tracheal wall.[116]

Condition	Imaging Findings	Comments
Bronchial tear (Fig C 58-6)	Persistent pneumothorax despite adequate placement of one or more chest tubes, massive and increasing subcutaneous emphysema and pneumomediastinum, focal peribronchial collections of air, discontinuity of the bronchial wall, and the "fallen lung" sign (collapsed lung or lobe falling away from the hilum).	Disruption of the diaphragm occurs in 1% to 8% of patients who survive major blunt injury to the chest or abdomen. Chest radiographic findings are abnormal in more than 75%, but are so nonspecific that the diagnosis is initially missed in the majority of cases. The mortality rate in unrecognized cases is 30%, with death occurring from delayed herniation of abdominal viscera and bowel strangulation. Sagittal and coronal reformatted images are superior to axial scans for detecting a diaphragmatic tear and herniation of abdominal contents into the thorax.
Diaphragmatic tear (Figs C 58-7 through C 58-9)	Focal discontinuity of the diaphragm (usually posterolateral, with 75–90% on the left); herniation of peritoneal fat, bowel, or abdominal organs into the chest; focal constriction of bowel or stomach as it projects through the diaphragm ("collar sign"); inability to visualize the diaphragm ("absent diaphragm sign").	More than 80% occur in the cervical and upper thoracic esophagus, most likely secondary to compression of the esophagus between the sternum and spinal column. Distal esophageal tears generally occur just above the gastroesophageal junction along the posterolateral wall on the left, with a mechanism probably similar to that in spontaneous rupture (Boerhaave syndrome) when esophageal pressures rise against a closed glottis. High mortality rate due to rapidly developing mediastinitis, unless the esophageal injury is recognized and treated within 24 hours.

A   B

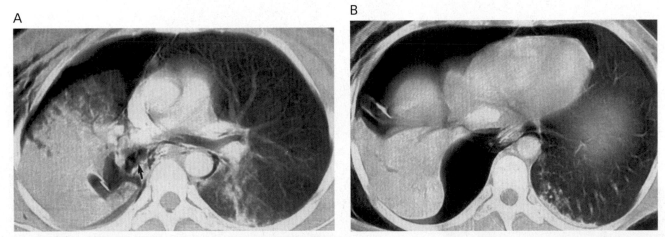

Fig C 58-6
Bronchial tear. (A) Extensive right lung contusion and a large pneumothorax despite multiple chest tubes. The tip of the right chest tube is intraparenchymal. Abnormal focal air collections are noted around the bronchus intermedius, and the wall of the bronchus is disrupted (arrow). (B) Scan obtained at a lower level demonstrates the fallen lung sign. The large right pneumothorax and small left pneumothorax are seen.[116]

Condition	Imaging Findings	Comments
Esophageal rupture	Focal extraluminal air at the site of the tear and hematoma in the mediastinum or in the esophageal wall.	Also plain chest radiographic findings of large left pneumothorax, extensive pneumomediastinum, subcutaneous emphysema, left pleural effusion and lower lobe atelectasis, and the "V sign" of Naclerio (extrapleural air within the lower mediastinum and between the parietal pleura and the diaphragm, which forms a V shape, usually on the left).
Fracture 　Rib 　(Fig C 58-10)	Best seen on bone window settings and images reformatted with an edge-enhancing algorithm. Often, associated hemothorax, pneumothorax, subcutaneous emphysema, pulmonary contusion, and soft-tissue hematomas (indicating an underlying rib injury).	Occur in approximately 60% of victims of blunt chest trauma, though only about 20% are detected on portable chest films. A fracture of the first rib indicates severe blunt chest trauma and may be associated with an aortic or bronchial tear and injury to the subclavian vessels. Fractures of five or more ribs in a row or three or more segmental rib fractures (ie, two fractures in one rib) is defined as a flail chest, which must be recognized promptly as respiratory failure may develop because of paradoxical movement of the flail segment.

A

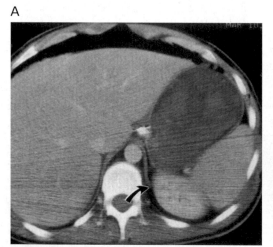

B

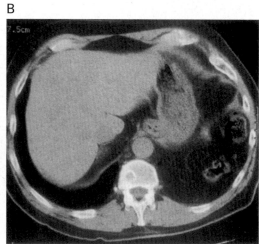

Fig C 58-7
Diaphragmatic tear. (A) Abrupt discontinuity of the left hemidiaphragm (arrow). (B) Absence of the left hemidiaphragm.[115]

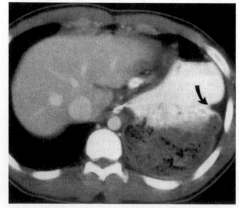

Fig C 58-8
Diaphragmatic tear (collar sign). Focal indentation of the greater curvature of the stomach (arrow).[115]

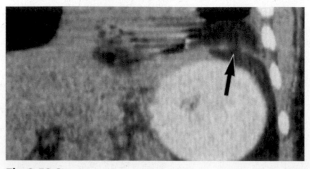

Fig C 58-9
Diaphragmatic tear. Coronal reformatted image demonstrates omental fat herniated through a diaphragmatic defect (arrow).[115]

Condition	Imaging Findings	Comments
Sternum (Fig C 58-11)	Fracture is often associated with a retrosternal mediastinal hematoma with preservation of the fat plane between the hematoma and the aorta (implying that it is not aortic in origin).	Most fractures occur within 2 cm of the manubrial-sternal junction. The fracture usually is not evident on AP portable chest radiographs but obvious at CT.
Thoracic spine (Fig C 58-12)	Paraspinal hematoma associated with disruption or fracture of the vertebral body, pedicle, or spinous process. Mediastinal hematoma confined to the posterior mediastinum is a valuable clue.	Most vulnerable portion is at the thoracoabdominal junction (T9-T11 vertebral bodies). An anterior wedge compression is usually stable, whereas a burst fracture is not. A high percentage of patients with thoracic spine fractures have spinal cord injuries, and many have associated sternal fractures. Only half of thoracic spine fractures are identified on the initial chest radiographs. Compression fractures may be easily overlooked on axial CT scans unless they are displayed with bone windows; sagittal and reformatted images can confirm a simple compression.

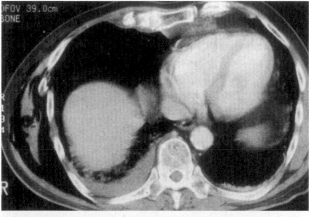

Fig C 58-10
Rib fracture. Displaced fracture with extensive subcutaneous emphysema. There is also a sternal fracture with associated retrosternal hematoma.[115]

Fig C 58-11
Sternal fracture. Midline sternal fracture with an adjacent anterior mediastinal hematoma. Note the preserved fat plane between the hematoma and the great vessels.[115]

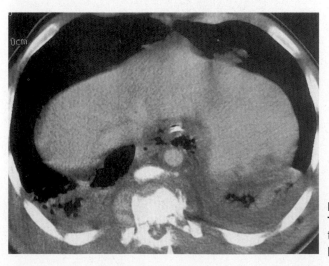

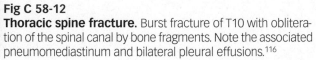

Fig C 58-12
Thoracic spine fracture. Burst fracture of T10 with obliteration of the spinal canal by bone fragments. Note the associated pneumomediastinum and bilateral pleural effusions.[116]

Abnormality of the Cardiophrenic Space on Computed Tomography or Magnetic Resonance Imaging

Condition	Comments

Normal variant
  Cardiac fat pad
  (Fig C 59-1)
	Large collection of pericardial fat can simulate a neoplastic mass. Recent studies have related the volume of pericardial fat to a possible increase in the risk of cardiovascular disease. The absence of soft-tissue components aids in differentiating prominent fat from benign or malignant fat-containing tumors.

Congenital absence of the pericardium	Infrequent, asymptomatic condition that can be associated with congenital heart disease. When there is associated agenesis of the sternopericardial ligament, the space between the heart and the chest wall can be larger than normal.

Fat-containing lesions
  Diaphragmatic hernia
  (Fig C 59-2)
	Related to a traumatic, postoperative, or congenital (the most common) origin, herniated fat and other abdominal structures can simulate a tumor in the cardipphrenic space. The presence of air within herniated intestinal loops is pathognomonic. If only omental fat has herniated, it may be difficult to differentiate from lipoma or liposarcoma. The detection of linear opacities corresponding to omental vessels favors the diagnosis of diaphragmatic hernia.

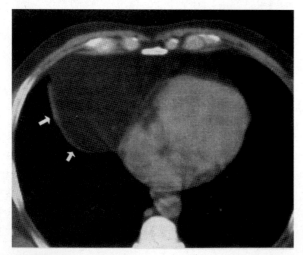

Fig C 59-1
Pericardial fat pad. CT scan shows a large pericardial fat pad (arrows) that simulated a cardiophrenic mass on plain radiographs.[117]

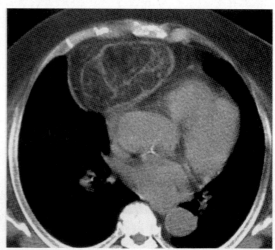

Fig C 59-2
Morgagni hernia. CT scan shows a well-defined fatty mass with numerous omental vessels and fatty infiltration.[117]

Condition	Comments
Pericardial fat necrosis (Fig C 59-3)	Uncommon benign condition that manifests as acute pleuritic chest pain in a previously healthy person. On CT, it appears as an encapsulated fatty lesion with inflammatory changes such as dense strands and thickening of the adjacent pericardium. Follow-up studies show spontaneous improvement or resolution of the findings. Like the pathologically similar fat necrosis in epiploic appendagitis, conservative treatment is indicated for this benign, self-limiting process.
Tumor (Fig C 59-4)	Lipoma and liposarcoma are uncommon tumors in this region and tend to simulate Morgagni hernia. At times, these entities can only be differentiated by demonstrating the diaphragmatic defect associated with the hernia. Thymolipoma may occasionally descend along the mediastinum and occupy the cardiophrenic space. The demonstration of an anatomic connection to the thymic bed may be required to differentiate this from a teratoma.
Cystic lesions Pericardial cyst (Fig C 59-5)	Fluid-filled lesion with well-defined borders, smooth walls, and no contrast enhancement. This asymptomatic and benign condition is usually detected as an incidental finding on plain chest radiographs.
Thymic tumor	Although usually a solid lesion, it infrequently has predominantly cystic contents.
Hydatid cyst (Fig C 59-6)	An echinococcal cyst of the liver can rarely herniate through the foramen of Morgagni.

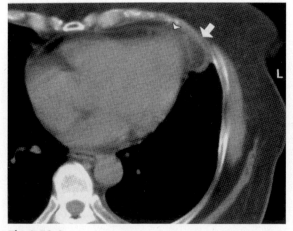

Fig C 59-3
Pericardial fat necrosis. CT scan shows an encapsulated fatty lesion with mild stranding in the left cardiophrenic space (arrow). Arrowhead = associated local pericardial thickening.[117]

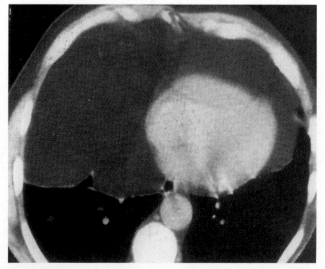

Fig C 59-4
Thymolipoma. CT scan shows a large fatty mass that wraps around the heart.[117]

Condition	Comments
Solid lesions	
Lymphoma (Fig C 59-7)	Most frequent cause of lympadenopathy in this location, which is often overlooked on chest radiographs. The peridiaphragmatic region has a rich lymphatic drainage system, and small (<8 mm) physiologic lymph nodes can normally be visualized in the cardiophrenic space.
Lymphatic metastases (Figs C 59-8 and C 59-9)	In most cases, lymphadenopathy is a sign of distant dissemination from primary tumors located either above or below the diaphragm. Involvement of lymph nodes in the internal mammary chain suggests a metastatic origin regardless of the size. Lung cancer and pleural mesothelioma are the chest tumors that most commonly affect the cardiophrenic space by lymphatic dissemination.

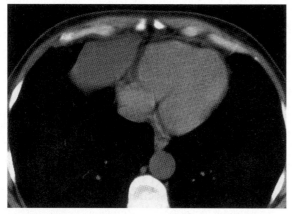

Fig C 59-5
Pleuropericardial cyst. Thin-walled, sharply defined, oval, homogeneous mass with attenuation near that of water.[117]

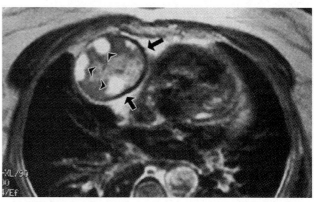

Fig C 59-6
Herniated hydatid cyst. T2-weighted MR image shows a well-defined lesion with a partially calcified wall (arrows) and small cystic lesions within it (arrowhead).[117]

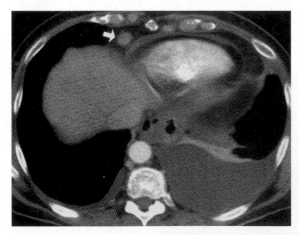

Fig C 59-7
Lymphoma. Lymph node (arrow) in the right cardiophrenic space. Note the associated pericardial and pleural effusions.[117]

Condition	Comments
Thymoma (Fig C 59-10)	Both benign and malignant thymic tumors can be located at the base of the heart and appear as solid or mixed lesions in the cardiphrenic space. The demonstration of a connection between the lesion and the superior mediastinum strongly suggests this diagnosis.
Miscellaneous lesions Abscess	In addition to herniated intestinal loops, the presence of gas within a lesion in the cardiophrenic space may be a manifestation of an abscess caused by a gas-producing microorganism.
Esophageal surgery (Fig C 59-11)	Colonic interposition for esophageal cancer may appear as a gas-containing structure at the base of the anterior mediastinum.

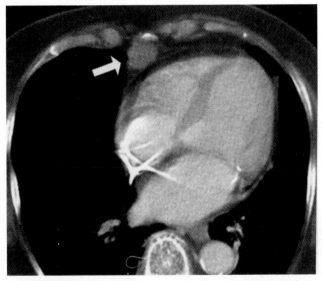

Fig C 59-8
Lymphatic metastases. Lymph node in the right cardiophrenic space from a primary ovarian carcinoma.[117]

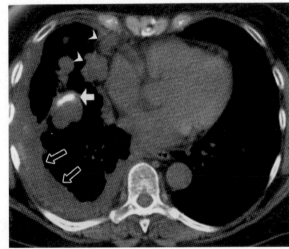

Fig C 59-9
Lymphatic metastases. Multiple nodes in the cardiophrenic space (arrowheads) secondary to metastases from pleural mesothelioma. Note the pleural thickening (open arrows). The pleural calcifications in the right major fissure (solid arrow) are due to previous asbestos exposure.[117]

Condition	Comments
Vascular disorder (Fig C 59-12)	In patients with portal hypertension, collateral circulation may result in cardiophrenic space varices that appear as tortuous tubular structures. Normal vessels in this region may also become substantially dilated secondary to occlusion of the superior vena cava and azygos vein.

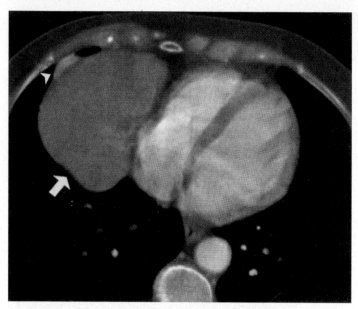

Fig C 59-10
Thymoma. Well-defined mass of soft-tissue attenuation (arrow) in the anterior mediastinum. Note the adjacent compressed lung (arrowhead).[117]

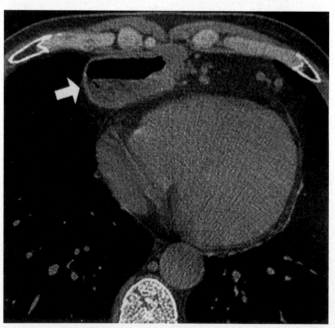

Fig C 59-11
Colonic interposition. The interposed colon (arrow) in the right cardiophrenic space represents a postoperative appearance following surgery for esophageal cancer.[117]

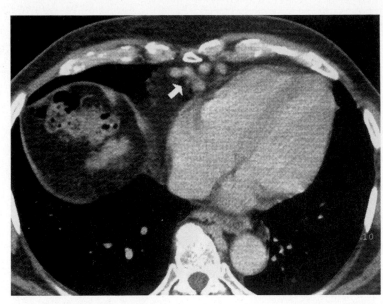

Fig C 59-12
Varices. In this patient with cirrhosis and portal hypertension, varices (arrow) in the right cardiophrenic space simulate lymph nodes.[117]

Axillary Masses on Computed Tomography

Condition	Comments
Breast cancer (Fig C 60-1)	Almost half of the women with breast cancer have axillary metastases when first seen. After primary therapy, up to 20% have local recurrence involving the chest wall; about 5% develop axillary recurrences.
Lymphoma (Fig C 60-2)	Axillary lymph node involvement has been reported in almost half of patients with non-Hodgkin's lymphoma and one-quarter of those with Hodgkin's disease. Even after apparently complete clinical remission, CT may show residual disease, especially in the apex of the axilla.
Metastases (Fig C 60-3)	Primary tumors of the head and neck, lung, and kidney may metastasize to axillary lymph nodes and simulate primary tumors or lymphoma.
Primary malignancy (Fig C 60-4)	Although rare, primary malignant neoplasms of fibrous tissue, muscle, or fat do occur in the axilla. These tumors characteristically do not respect soft tissue or muscle planes and may extend to the apex (producing symptoms of brachial plexus involvement) or spread along the chest wall.
Sarcoidosis (Fig C 60-5)	Unusual manifestation that, when combined with hilar and mediastinal adenopathy, can mimic lymphoma.

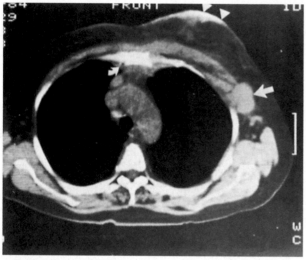

Fig C 60-1
Breast cancer. Left axillary nodes (arrow) and bilateral internal mammary nodes (curved arrows) are seen in this woman with an extensive malignancy of the left breast and involvement of the skin surface (arrowheads).[118]

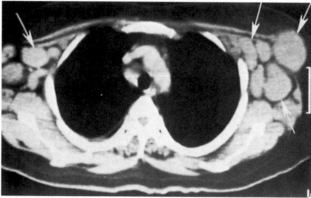

Fig C 60-2
Lymphoma. Extensive bilateral axillary adenopathy with enlarged nodes (arrows) surrounding the neurovascular bundles, but not invading them.[118]

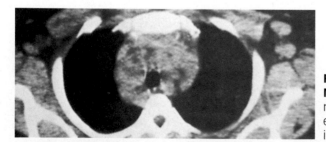

Fig C 60-3
Metastases. Extensive involvement of the left axillary nodes in a young man with neuroblastoma. Note the extension of adenopathy high into the apex of the axilla beneath the pectoralis minor muscle medially.[118]

A

B

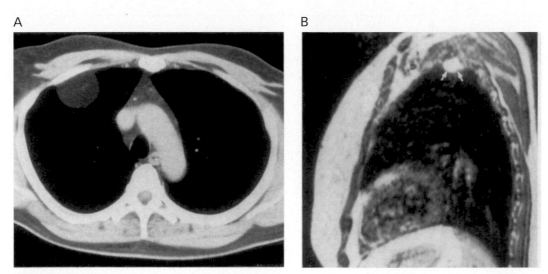

Fig C 61-6
Lipoma. (A) CT scan demonstrates extension of a chest wall lipoma into the intrathoracic extrapleural space. (B) Sagittal T1-weighted MR image in another patient shows a small apical extrapleural lipoma (arrows).[120]

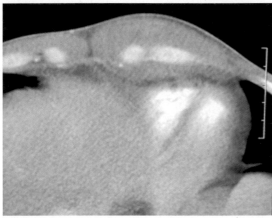

Fig C 61-7
Costochondritis. Soft-tissue mass centered around one of the lower left costochondral junctions (arrows) in an intravenous drug abuser.[10]

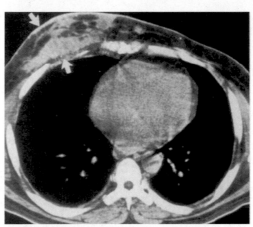

Fig C 61-8
Actinomycosis. CT scan shows extensive chest wall infection.[119]

A

B

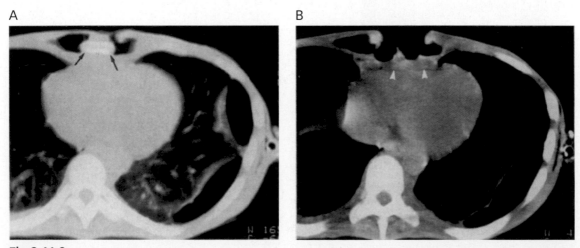

Fig C 61-9
Necrotizing infection in AIDS. CT scans obtained with lung (A) and mediastinal (B) windows show that the infection has eaten through the chest wall and extended around the sternum (arrows in A) and down to the pericardium (arrowheads in B). A pneumothorax and chest tube are present on the left.[120]

Condition	Imaging Findings	Comments
Sternoclavicular septic arthritis (Fig C 61-10)	CT and MRI show destructive changes as well as abscess formation, which is a complication in about 20% of cases.	Insertion of contaminated needles into and around the internal jugular vein may account for the increased frequency of sternoclavicular septic arthritis in intravenous drug abusers.
Paget's disease (Fig C 61-11)	Cortical thickening and bone enlargement are distinctive features, as in other bones.	Relatively uncommon in the ribs and usually an incidental finding noted during the chronic sclerotic phase of the disease.
Hematoma (Fig C 61-12)	Extrapleural mass with a CT attenuation greater than that of soft-tissue, compatible with the presence of blood.	Perivascular hematomas may develop about the subclavian artery or vein. Trauma may result in chest wall hematomas of considerable size.

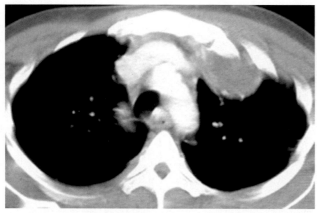

Fig C 61-10
Sternoclavicular septic arthritis. CT shows a low-attenuation collection deep to the left sternoclavicular joint (arrow), which represents an abscess extending from infection of the joint in an intravenous drug abuser.[10]

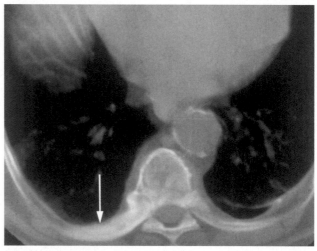

Fig C 61-11
Paget's disease. Bone enlargement with cortical thickening (arrow) involving the right posterior eighth rib.[121]

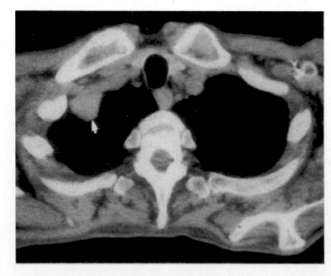

Fig C 61-12
Hematoma. Extrapleural mass (arrow) with attenuation greater than soft tissue, a finding compatible with the presence of blood.[120]

Condition	Imaging Findings	Comments
Lymphangioma (Fig C 61-13)	On CT, a well-defined cystic mass of homogeneous near-water attenuation. The fluid content appears as low signal intensity on T1-weighted MR images and high signal intensity on T2-weighted studies.	Congenital malformation representing sequestered lymphatic sacs that are isolated from the rest of the lymphatic drainage system. Most frequently seen as neck masses, they may extend to involve the mediastinum, chest wall, and axilla.

Malignant
Muscular

Condition	Imaging Findings	Comments
Leiomyosarcoma	Large spindle-shaped mass that frequently contains areas of necrosis or cystic change causing a pattern of peripheral contrast enhancement. Often displaces or distorts adjacent vessels.	Frequently painful and typically occurring in adulthood, it is usually a solitary lesion (multiplicity suggests metastases from another site).
Rhabdomyosarcoma	On MR, areas of necrosis with low signal intensity that do show contrast enhancement alternate with ring-like areas of high signal intensity and marked enhancement.	High-grade malignancy that generally affects patients younger than 45 years of age. This rapidly growing lesion causes bone invasion in more than 20% of cases.

Vascular

Condition	Imaging Findings	Comments
Angiosarcoma	On MR, a large, ill-defined heterogenous mass with strong contrast enhancement. Feeding vessels are often seen in the periphery of the tumor.	In the chest wall, angiosarcomas primarily occur in the breast, most often in association with lymphedema or radiation therapy of breast cancer.

Fibrous

Condition	Imaging Findings	Comments
Aggressive fibromatosis	Ill-defined mass with signal intensity similar to muscle or lower on T1-weighted images and heterogeneous enhancement.	Most commonly affecting adolescents and young adults, a common neoplastic disease accounting for more than half of low-grade sarcomas of the chest wall. Shoulder involvement is the most common complication.
Malignant fibrous histiocytoma (Fig C 61-14)	Large extraparenchymal mass that usually arises from the musculature of the chest wall. On MRI, heterogeneous signal intensity and marked enhancement are characteristic features.	Most common soft-tissue sarcoma in adults, although a thoracic origin is infrequent. The tumor can be associated with previous bone lesions, including Paget's disease and bone infarcts, and it is the most common sarcoma to develop after irradiation. Its origin within the musculature helps distinguish this tumor from osteosarcoma or chondrosarcoma.

B

A

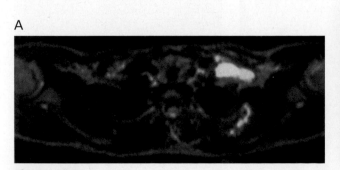
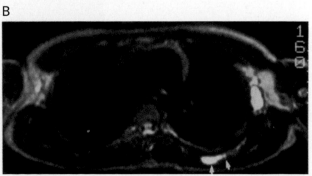

Fig C 61-13
Lymphangioma. Axial T1-weighted MR images, with (A) obtained at a higher level than (B), shows a mass that has high signal intensity because of its high water content. The mass can be traced from the neck into the axilla, where it insinuates between the muscles of the posterior chest wall (arrows in B).[120]

Condition	Imaging Findings	Comments
Peripheral nerves (Fig C 61-15)	Heterogeneous mass with ill-defined contours and heterogeneous contrast enhancement related to areas of necrosis. Primitive neuroectodermal tumors can be associated with adjacent rib destruction, pleural thickening or effusion, and focal invasion of the lung.	Neuroblastoma, ganglioneuroblastoma, malignant peripheral nerve sheath tumor. They usually arise in preexisting neurofibromas of the intercostals nerves or spinal nerve roots or in the brachial plexus.

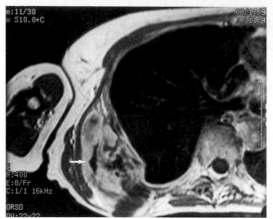

Fig C 61-14
Malignant fibrous histiocytoma. Axial T1-weighted contrast image shows a large extraparenchymal mass in the right upper hemithorax with marked enhancement. Focal areas of low signal intensity (arrow) are consistent with necrosis and fluid. The origin of the lesion within the chest wall musculature helps distinguish this tumor from osteosarcoma or chondrosarcoma.[134]

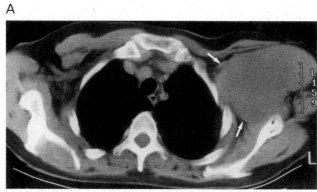

A

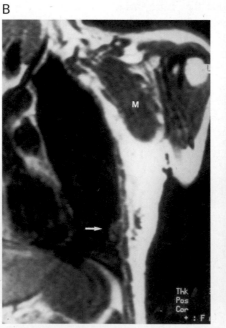

B

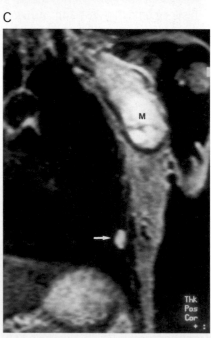

C

Fig C 61-15
Neurofibrosarcoma. (A) Unenhanced CT scan shows a large, homogeneous mass in the left axilla (arrows). Note the absence of rib destruction. On coronal MR images, the mass (M) is well-circumscribed and demonstrates low signal intensity on a T1-weighted image (B) and high signal intensity on a T2-weighted sequence (C). Note the small neurofibroma with similar signal intensity in the lower lateral aspect of the left hemithorax (arrow).[134]

Condition	Imaging Findings	Comments
Lung apex and pleura		
Pancoast tumor (Fig C 61-28)	Coronal and sagittal MR imaging is more accurate than CT in demonstrating chest wall invasion and involvement of the brachial plexus and adjacent blood vessels.	Superior sulcus tumor, most commonly a primary lung cancer, which invades through the apical fat to involve the brachial plexus and sympathetic stellate ganglion of the upper mediastinum and lower neck. The Pancoast syndrome consists of the clinical triad of ipsilateral arm pain, wasting of the muscles of the hand, and Horner syndrome
Mesothelioma (Fig C 61-29)	Coronal and sagittal MR imaging can directly evaluate the longitudinal extent of the tumor, as well as the degree of chest wall invasion and involvement of the diaphragm.	Typically related to asbestos exposure and often associated with a large pleural effusion that may obscure the underlying neoplasm on chest radiographs.

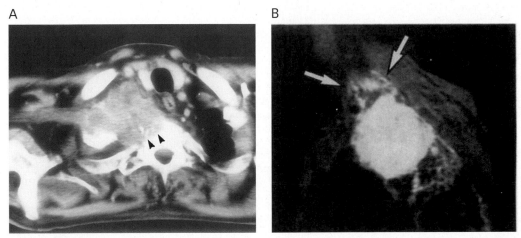

Fig C 61-28
Pancoast tumor. (A) CT scan shows a mass in the apex of the right lung that destroys the first rib and invades the adjacent T2 vertebral body (arrows).[2] (B) In another patient, a sagittal T2-weighted MR image shows a large mass arising in the apex of the right lung that has abnormal high signal intensity and infiltrates the supraclavicular fossa and surrounding brachial plexus.[120]

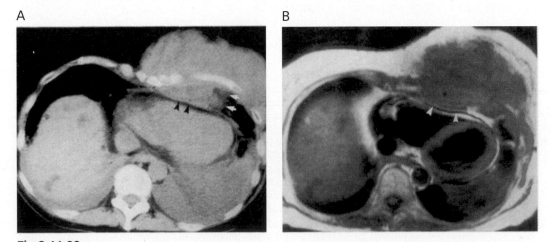

Fig C 61-29
Mesothelioma. (A) CT scan shows a huge mass involving the anterior chest and abdominal wall with growth of tumor (arrows) beneath the xiphoid process and lower ribs. The tumor appears to be contiguous to the pericardium (arrowheads) and it is difficult to determine whether this structure has been invaded. (B) Corresponding axial T1-weighted MR image shows the intact black line of the pericardium (arrowheads), indicating no invasion.[120]

Sources

1. Reprinted with permission from "Spherical Pneumonias in Children Simulating Pulmonary and Mediastinal Masses" by RW Rose and BH Ward, *Radiology* (1973;106:179–182), Copyright ©1973, Radiological Society of North America Inc.

2. Reprinted with permission from "Gram-negative Pneumonia" by JD Unger, HD Rose, and GF Unger, *Radiology* (1973;107:283–291), Copyright ©1973, Radiological Society of North America Inc.

3. Reprinted with permission from "Experience with *Hemophilus influenzae* Pneumonia" by M Vinick, DH Altman, and RE Parks, *Radiology* (1966;86:701–706), Copyright ©1966, Radiological Society of North America Inc.

4. Reprinted with permission from "Pulmonary Blastomycosis" by RA Halvorson et al, *Radiology* (1984;150:1–5), Copyright ©1984, Radiological Society of North America Inc.

5. Reprinted with permission from "The Melting Sign in Resolving Transient Pulmonary Infarction" by ME Woesner, I Sanders, and GW White, *American Journal of Roentgenology* (1971;111:782–790), Copyright ©1971, American Roentgen Ray Society.

6. Restrepo CS, Martinez S, Lemos JA. Imaging Manifestations of Kaposi Sarcoma. *RadioGraphics* 2006;26:1169–1185.

7. Reprinted from *Diagnosis of Diseases of the Chest* by RG Fraser and JAP Pare with permission of WB Saunders Company, ©1979.

8. Reprinted with permission from "The FBI Sign" by WW Wenzel, *Colorado Medicine*, formerly *Rocky Mountain Medical Journal* (1972; 69:71–72), Copyright ©1979.

9. Reprinted with permission from "Amniotic Pulmonary Embolism" by HR Arnold, JE Gardner, and PH Goodman, *Radiology* (1961;77:629–634), Copyright ©1961, Radiological Society of North America Inc.

10. Gotway MB, Marder SR, Hanks DK, et al. Thoracic complications of illicit drug use: an organ system approach. *RadioGraphics* 2002;22:S119–S135.

11. Restrepo CS, Carrillo JA, Martinez S, et al. Pulmonary complications from cocaine and cocaine-based substances: imaging manifstations. *RadioGraphics* 2007;27:941–956.

12. Reprinted with permission from "An Exercise in Radiologic-Pathologic Correlation" by EG Theros, MM Reeder, and JF Eckert, *Radiology* (1968;90:784–791), Copyright ©1968, Radiological Society of North America Inc.

13. Reprinted with permission from "Unilateral Pulmonary Edema" by L Calenoff, GD Kruglik, and A Woodruff, *Radiology* (1978;126:19–24), Copyright ©1978, Radiological Society of North America Inc.

14. Reprinted with permission from "Pulmonary Complications of Drug Therapy" by A Brettner, RE Heitzman, and WG Woodin, *Radiology* (1970;96:31–38), Copyright ©1970, Radiological Society of North America Inc.

15. Leatherwood DL, Heitkamp DE, Emerson RE. Pulmonary langerhans cell histiocytosis. *RadioGraphics* 2007;27:265–268.

16. Meyer CA, White CS. Cartilaginous disorders of the chest. *RadioGraphics* 1998;18:1109–1125.

17. Chong S, Lee KS, Chung MJ, et al. Neuroendocrine tumors of the lung: clinical, pathologic, and imaging findings. *RadioGraphics* 2006;26:21–58.

18. Reprinted with permission from "Bilateral Pulmonary Sequestration: CT Appearance" by KJ Wimbish, FP Agha, and TM Brady, *American Journal of Roentgenology* (1983;140:689–690), Copyright ©1983, American Roentgen Ray Society.

19. Cole TJ, Henry DA, Jolles H, et al. Normal and abnormal vascular structures that simulate neoplasms on chest radiographs: clues to the diagnosis. *RadioGraphics* 1995;15:867–891.

20. Wagner AL, Szabunio M, Hazlett KS, Wagner SG. Radiologic manifestations of round pneumonia in adults. *AJR Am J Roentgenol* 1998;170:723.

21. Seo JB, Im J-G, Goo JM, et al. Atypical pulmonary metastases: spectrum of radiologic findings. *RadioGraphics* 2001;21:403–417.

22. Erasmus JJ, Connolly JE, McAdams HP, Roggli VL. Solitary pulmonary nodules: Part 1. Morphologic evaluation for differentiation of benign and malignant lesions. *RadioGraphics* 2000;20:43–58.

23. Fang W, Washington L, Kumar. Imaging manifestations of blastomycosis: a pulmonary infection with potential dissemination. *RadioGraphics* 2007;27:641–655.

24. Jeung M-Y, Gasser B, Gangi A, et al. Bronchial carcinoid tumor of the thorax: spectrum of radiologic findings. *RadioGraphics* 2002;22:351–365.

25. Gimenez A, Franquet T, Prats R, et al. Unusual primary lung tumors: a radiologic-pathologic overview. *RadioGraphics* 2002;22:601–619.

26. Oh YW, Effman EL, Godwin JD. Pulmonary infections in immunocompromised hosts: the importance of correlating the conventional radiologic appearance with the clinical setting. *Radiology* 2000;217:647–658.

27. Reprinted from *Radiology of the Heart and Great Vessels* by RN Cooley and MH Schreiber, Williams & Wilkins Company, ©1978, with permission of JH Harris Jr.

28. Reprinted with permission from "The Ruptured Pulmonary Hydatid Cyst" by RFC Kagel and A Fatemi, *Radiology* (1961;76:60–64), Copyright ©1961, Radiological Society of North America Inc.

29. Klein JS, Carter JM. Abnormal intrathoracic gas collections: atypical appearances. *The Radiologist* 1994;1:85–94.

30. Han D, Lee KS, Franquet T, et al. Thrombotic and nonthrombotic pulmonary arterial embolism: spectrum of imaging findings. *RadioGraphics* 2003;23:1521–1539.

31. Reprinted with permission from "Eisenmenger's Syndrome" by HB Spitz, *Seminars in Roentgenology* (1968;3:373–376), Copyright ©1968, Grune & Stratton Inc.

32. Reprinted with permission from "Mediastinal Lymphadenopathy in Bubonic Plague" by VR Sites and JD Poland, *American Journal of Roentgenology* (1970;116:567–570), Copyright ©1970, American Roentgen Ray Society.

33. Reprinted with permission from "Antenatal Ultrasound Findings in Cystic Adenomatoid Malformation" by SM Donn, JN Martin, and SJ White, *Pediatric Radiology* (1981;10:180–182), Copyright ©1981, Springer-Verlag.

34. Reprinted with permission from "Bulging (Sagging) Fissure Sign in *Hemophilus influenzae* Lobar Pneumonia" by JB Francis and PB Francis, *Southern Medical Journal* (1978;71:1452–1453), Copyright ©1978, Southern Medical Association.

35. Reprinted from *Chest Roentgenology* by B Felson with permission of WB Saunders Company, ©1973.

36. Reprinted with permission from "Calcified Pulmonary Lesions: An Overview" by HT Winer-Muram and JI Sebes, *Postgraduate Radiology* (1991;11:3–21), Copyright ©1991.

37. Reprinted with permission from "Diagnosis of Chemotherapy of Lung" by HD Sostman, CE Putnam, and G Gamsu, *American Journal of Roentgenology* (1981;136:33–41), Copyright ©1981, American Roentgen Ray Society.

38. Reprinted from *Clinical Radiology in the Tropics* by WP Cockshott and H Middlemiss with permission of Churchill Livingstone Inc, ©1979.

39. Reprinted with permission from *British Journal of Radiology* (1963;36:889–901), Copyright ©1963, British Institute of Radiology.

40. Reprinted with permission from "Creeping Eruption with Transient Pulmonary Infiltration" by EH Kalmon, *Radiology* (1954;62:222–226), Copyright ©1954, Radiological Society of North America Inc.

41. Franquet T, Muller NL, Gimenez A, et al. Spectrum of pulmonary aspergillosis: histologic, clinical, and radiologic findings. *Radio Graphics* 2001;21:825.

42. Courtesy of the Armed Forces Institute of Pathology.

43. Reprinted with permission from "Computed Tomography in the Evaluation of Mediastinal Widening" by RL Baron et al, *Radiology* (1981;138:107–114), Copyright ©1981, Radiological Society of North America Inc.

44. Glazer HS, Wick MR, Anderson DJ, et al. CT of fatty thoracic masses. *AJR Am J Roentgenol* 1992;159:1181–1187.

45. Nishino M, Ashiku SK, Kocher ON, et al. The Thymus: A Comprehensive Review. *RadioGraphics* 2006;26:335–348.

46. Reprinted from *Computed Body Tomography* by JKT Lee, SS Sagel, and RJ Stanley (Eds) with permission of Raven Press, New York, ©1983.

47. Whitten CR, Khan S, Munneke GJ, Grubnic S. A diagnostic approach to mediastinal abnormalities. *RadioGraphics* 2007;27:657–671.

48. Reprinted with permission from "Parathyroid Scanning by Computed Tomography" by DD Stark et al, *Radiology* (1983;148:297–303), Copyright ©1983, Radiological Society of North America Inc.

49. Ueno T, Tanaka YO, Nagata M, et al. Spectrum of germ cell tumors: From Head to Toe. *RadioGraphics* 2004;24:387–404.

50. Rossi SE, McAdams HP, Rosado-de-Christenson ML, et al. Fibrosing Mediastinits. *RadioGraphics* 2001;21:737–757.

51. Reprinted with permission from "Laceration of the Thoracic Aorta and Brachiocephalic Arteries by Blunt Trauma" by RG Fisher, FP Hadlock, and Y Ben-Menachem, *Radiologic Clinics of North America* (1981;19:91–112), Copyright ©1981, WB Saunders Company.

52. Reprinted with permission from "The 'V' Sign in the Diagnosis of Spontaneous Rupture of the Esophagus" by NA Naclerio, *American Journal of Surgery* (1957;93:291–298), Copyright ©1957, Yorke Medical Group.

53. Reprinted with permission from "The Multiple Roentgen Manifestations of Sclerosing Mediastinitis" by DS Feigin, JC Eggleston, and FS Siegelman, *Johns Hopkins Medical Journal* (1979;144:1–8), Copyright ©1979, Johns Hopkins University Press.

54. Gaerte SC, Meyer CA, Winer-Muram, et al. Fat-containing lesions of the chest. *RadioGraphics* 2002;22:S62–S78.

55. Jeung M-Y, Gasser B, Gangi A, et al. Imaging of cystic masses of the mediastinum. *RadioGraphics* 2002;22:S79–S93.

56. Reprinted from *Computed Tomography of the Body* by AA Moss, G Gamsu, and HK Genant (Eds) with permission of WB Saunders Company, ©1983.

57. Gibbs JM, Chandrasekhar CA, Ferguson EC, Oldham SAA. Lines and Stripes: Where Did They Go? – From Conventional Radiography to CT. *RadioGraphics* 2007;27:33–48.

58. Koyama T, Ueda H, Togashi, et al. Radiologic manifestations of sarcoidosis in various organs. *RadioGraphics* 2004;24:87–104.

59. Reprinted with permission from "CT of Posterior Mediastinal Masses" by A Kawashima, EK Fishman et al, *RadioGraphics* (1991;11:1045–1067), Copyright ©1991, Radiological Society of America Inc.

60. Reprinted with permission from "Abnormalities of the Azygoesophageal Recess at Computed Tomography" by G Lund and HH Lien, *Acta Radiologica: Diagnosis* (1983;24:3–10), Copyright ©1983, Acta Radiologica.

61. Reprinted with permission from "The Lateral Decubitus Film: An Aid in Determining Air-Trapping in Children" by MA Capitanio and JA Kirkpatrick, *Radiology* (1972;103:460–461), Copyright ©1972, Radiological Society of North America Inc.

62. Reprinted with permission from "The Continuous Diaphragm Sign: A Newly Recognized Sign of Pneumomediastinum" by B Levin, *Clinical Radiology* (1973;24:337–338), Copyright ©1973, Royal College of Radiologists.

63. Reprinted with permission from "Mesotheliomas and Secondary Tumors of the Pleura" by K Ellis and M Wolff, *Seminars in Roentgenology* (1977;12:303–311), Copyright ©1977, Grune & Stratton Inc.

64. Dynes MC, White EM, Fry WA, et al. Imaging manifestations of pleural tumors. *RadioGraphics* 1992;12:1191–1201.

65. Reprinted with permission from "Roentgen Manifestations of Pleural Disease" by VA Vix, *Seminars in Roentgenology* (1977;12:277–286), Copyright ©1977, Grune & Stratton Inc.

66. Reprinted with permission from "Pleural Plaques: A Signpost of Asbestos Dust Inhalation" by EN Sargent, G Jacobson, and JS Gordonson, *Seminars in Roentgenology* (1977;12:287–297), Copyright ©1977, Grune & Stratton Inc.

67. Reprinted with permission from "Radiologic Appearance of Compromised Thoracic Catheters, Tubes, and Wires" by RD Dunbar, *Radiologic Clinics of North America* (1984;22:699–722), Copyright ©1984, WB Saunders Company.

68. Reprinted with permission from "Pneumothorax as a Complication of Feeding Tube Placement" by GL Balogh et al, *American Journal of Roentgenology* (1983;141:1275–1277), Copyright ©1983, American Roentgen Ray Society.

69. Reprinted with permission from "Distribution of Pneumothorax in the Supine and Semirecumbent Critically Ill Adult" by IM Tocino, MH Miller, and WR Fairfax, *American Journal of Roentgenology* (1985;144:901–905), Copyright ©1985, American Roentgen Ray Society.

70. Reprinted with permission from "Plasmacytoma of the Head and Neck" by RC Gromer and AJ Duvall, *Journal of Laryngology and Otology* (1973;87:861–872), Copyright ©1973, Headley Brothers, Ltd.

71. Marom EM, Goodman PC, McAdams HP. Focal abnormalities of the trachea and main bronchi. *AJR* 2001;176:707–711.

72. Prince JS, Duhamel DR, Levin DL, et al. Nonneoplastic lesions of the Tracheobronchial Wall: Radiologic Findings with Bronchoscopic Correlation. *RadioGraphics* 2002;22:S215–S230.

73. Reprinted with permission from "Tracheal Stenosis: An Analysis of 151 Cases" by AL Weber and HC Grillo, *Radiologic Clinics of North America* (1978;16:291–308), Copyright ©1978, WB Saunders Company.

74. Reprinted with permission from "Diffuse Lesions of the Trachea" by RH Choplin, WD Wehunt, and EG Theros, *Seminars in Roentgenology* (1983;18:38–50), Copyright ©1983, Grune & Stratton Inc.

75. Reprinted with permission from "'Saber Sheath' Trachea: A Clinical and Functional Study of Marked Coronal Narrowing of Intrathoracic Trachea" by R Greene and GL Lechner, *Radiology* (1975;15:255–268), Copyright ©1975, Radiological Society of North America Inc.

76. Marom EM, Goodman PC, McAdams HP. Focal abnormalities of the trachea and main bronchi. *AJR* 2001;176:707–711.

77. Marom EM, Goodman PC, McAdams HP. Diffuse abnormalities of the trachea and main bronchi. *AJR* 2001;176:713–717.

78. Chong S, Lee KS, Chung MJ, et al. Neuroendocrine tumors of the lung: Clinical, pathologic, and imaging findings. *RadioGraphics* 2006;26:41–58.

79. Seo JB, Song K-S, Lee JS, et al. Broncholithiasis: Review of the causes with radiologic-pathologic correlation. *RadioGraphics* 2002;22:S199–S213.

80. Seo JB, Lee JW, Ha SY, et al. Primary endobronchial actinomycosis associated with broncholithiasis. *Respiration* 2003;70:110–113.

81. Kim HY, Im JG, Song KS, et al. Localized amyloidosis of the respiratory system: CT features. *J Comput Assist Tomogr* 1999;23:627–631.

82. Song JW, Im JG, Shim YS, et al. Hypertrophied bronchial artery at thin-section CT in patients with bronchiectasis: correlation with CT angiographic findings. *Radiology* 1998;208:187–191.

83. Franquet T, Erasmus JJ, Gimenez A, etal. The retrotracheal space: normal anatomic and pathologic appearances. *RadioGraphics* 2002;22:S231–S246.

84. Reprinted with permission from "The 'Thumb Sign' and 'Little Finger Sign' in Acute Epiglottitis" by JK Podgore and JW Bass,

Journal of Pediatrics (1976;88:154–155), Copyright ©1976, The CV Mosby Company, St. Louis.

85. John SD, Swischuk LE. Stridor and upper airway obstruction in infants and children. *RadioGraphics* 1992;12:625–643.

86. Reprinted with permission from "The Right Paratracheal Stripe in Blunt Chest Trauma" by JH Woodring, CM Pulmano, and RK Stevens, *Radiology* (1982;143:605–608), Copyright ©1982, Radiological Society of North America Inc.

87. Reprinted with permission from "Differential Diagnosis of Chronic Diffuse Infiltrative Lung Disease on High-Resolution Computed Tomography" by NL Müller, *Seminars in Roentgenology* (1991; 26:132–142), Copyright ©1991, WB Saunders Company.

88. Reprinted with permission from Webb WR, Muller NL, Naidich DP: *High-Resolution CT of the Lung* (3rd ed.). Philadelphia, Lippincott Williams & Wilkins, 2001 (pages 259–353).

89. Reprinted with permission from "High-Resolution Computed Tomography of Asbestos-Related Diseases" by DR Aberle, *Seminars in Roentgenology* (1991;26:118–131), Copyright ©1991, WB Saunders Company.

90. Swensen SJ, Aughenbaugh GL, Douglas WW, et al. High-resolution CT of the lungs: findings in various pulmonary diseases. *AJR Am J Roentgenol* 1992;158:971–979.

91. Rossi SE, Franquet T, Valpacchio M, et al. Tree-in-Bud Pattern at Thin-Section CT of the Lungs: Radiologic-Pathologic Overview. *RadioGraphics* 2005;25:789–801.

92. Collins J, Stern EJ. Normal anatomy of the chest. In: Collins J, Stern EJ, eds. *Chest Radiology: The Essentials*. Philadelphia: Lippincott Williams & Wilkins, 1999.

93. Collins J, Blankenbaker D, Stern EJ. CT patterns of bronchiolar disease: what is "tree-in-bud"? *AJR Am J Roentgenol* 1998;171:365.

94. Reprinted with permission from "Computed Tomography of Air-Space Diseases" by SH Hommeyer et al, *Radiologic Clinics of North America* (1991;29:1065–1083), Copyright ©1991, WB Saunders Company.

95. Gervais DA, Whitman GJ, Chew FS. *Pneumocystis carinii* pneumonia. *AJR Am J Roentgenol* 1995;164:1098.

96. Reprinted with permission from "High-Resolution Computed Tomography of Focal Lung Disease" by PA Templeton and EA Zerhouni, *Seminars in Roentgenology* (1991;26:143–150), Copyright ©1991, WB Saunders Company.

97. Reprinted with permission from "Pulmonary Alveolar Proteinosis: CT Findings" by JD Godwin et al, *Radiology* (1988;169:609–613), Copyright ©1988, Radiological Society of North America.

98. Reprinted with permission from "High-Resolution Computed Tomography of Cystic Lung Disease" by DP Naidich, *Seminars in Roentgenology* (1991;26:151–174), Copyright ©1991, WB Saunders Company.

99. Reprinted from Stern EJ, Swensen SJ, Hartman TE, Frank MS. CT mosaic pattern of lung attenuation: distinguishing different causes. *AJR Am J Roentgenol* 1995;165:813.

100. Rossi SE, Erasmus JJ, Volpacchio M, et al. "Crazy-Paving" Pattern at Thin-Section CT of the Lungs: Radiologic-Pathologic Overview. *RadioGraphics* 2003;23:1509–1519.

101. Collins J, Stern EJ. Ground-glass opacity at CT: the ABCs. *AJR* 1997;169:355–367.

102. Stern EJ, Swensen SJ, Collins J, et al. *High-Resolution CT of the Chest*, 2nd ed. Philadelphia: Lippincott Williams & Wilkins, 2000, p. 33.

103. Wong KT, Antonio GE, Hui DSC, et al. Thin-section CT of severe acute respiratory syndrome: evaluation of 73 patients exposed to or with the disease. *Radiology* 2003;228:395–400.

104. Abbott GF, Rosado-de-Christenson ML, Franks TJ, et al. Pulmonary Langerhans cell histiocytosis. *RadioGraphics* 2004;24:821–841.

105. Chong S, Lee KS, Chung MJ, et al. Pneumoconiosis: comparison of imaging and pathologic findings. *RadioGraphics* 2006;26:59–77.

106. Jeong YJ, Kim K-I, Seo IJ, et al. Eosinophilic lung diseases: a clinical, radiological, and pathological overview. *RadioGraphics* 2007;27:617–637.

107. Helbich TH, Heinz-Peer G, Eichler I, et al. Cystic fibrosis: CT assessment of lung involvement in children and adults. *Radiology* 1999;213:537.

108. Gluecker T, Capasso P, Schnyder P, et al. Clinical and radiological features of pulmonary edema. *RadioGraphics* 1999;19:1507–1531.

109. Mayberry JP, Primack SL, Müller NL. Thoracic manifestations of systemic autoimmune diseases: radiographic and high-resolution CT findings. *RadioGraphics* 2000;20:1623–1635.

110. Mueller-Mang C, Grosse C, Schmid K, et al. What every radiologist should know about idiopathic interstitial pneumonias. *RadioGraphics* 2007;27:595–615.

111. Kim EA, Lee KS, Johkoh T, et al. Interstitial lung diseases associated with collagen vascular diseases: radiologic and histopathologic findings. *RadioGraphics* 2002;22:S151–S165.

112. Rossi SE, Erasmus JJ, McAdams HP, et al. Pulmonary drug toxicity: radiologic and pathologic manifestations. *Radiographics* 2000;20:1245–1259.

113. Wittram C, Maher MM, Yoo AJ. CT angiography of pulmonary embolism: diagnostic criteria and causes of misdiagnosis. *RadioGraphics* 2004;24:1219–1238.

114. Gladdish GW, Sabloff BM, Munden RF, et al. Primary thoracic sarcomas. *RadioGraphics* 2002;22:621–637.

115. Reprinted from Van Hise ML, Primack SL, Israel RS, Muller NL. CT in blunt chest trauma: indications and limitations. *RadioGraphics* 1998;18:1071.

116. Reprinted from Kuhlman JE, Pozniak MA, Collins J, Knisely BL. Radiographic and CT findings of blunt chest trauma: aortic injuries and looking beyond them. *RadioGraphics* 1998;18:1085.

117. Pineda V, Andreu J, Caceres J, et al. Lesions of the cardiophrenic space: findings at cross-sectional imaging. *RadioGraphics* 207; 27:19–32.

118. Reprinted with permission from "CT of the Axilla: Normal Anatomy and Pathology" by EK Fishman et al, *RadioGraphics* (1986;6:475–502), Copyright ©1986, Radiological Society of North America Inc.

119. Ly JQ, Sanders TG. Case 65: Hemangioma of the Chest Wall. *Radiology* 2003;229:726–729.

120. Kuhlman JE, Bouchandy L, Fishman EK, Zerhouni EA. CT and MR imaging evaluation of chest wall disorders. *RadioGraphics* 1994;14:571–595.

121. Guttentag AR, Salwen JK. Keep your eyes on the ribs: the spectrum of normal variants and diseases that involve the ribs. *Radio Graphics* 1999;19:1125–1142.

122. Weisbrod GL, Towers MJ, Chamberlain DW, et al. Thin-walled cystic lesions in bronchioalveolar carcinoma. *Radiology* 1992;185:401.

123. Haramati LB, Schulman LL, Austin JH. Lung nodules and masses after cardiac transplantation. *Radiology* 1993;188:491.

124. Remy-Jardin M, Remy J, Cortet B, et al. Lung changes in rheumatoid arthritis: CT findings. *Radiology* 1994;193:375–382.

125. Nishimura K, Itoh H, Kitaichi M, et al. Pulmonary sarcoidosis: correlation of CT and histopatholigc findings. *Radiology* 1993; 189:105–109.

126. Kim KI, Kim CW, Lee MK, et al. Imaging of occupational lung disease. *RadioGraphics* 2001;21:1371–1391.

2

Cardiovascular Patterns

Right Atrial Enlargement

Condition	Imaging Findings	Comments
Left-to-right shunt	Enlarged right atrium if this chamber is the end point of a shunt.	Atrial septal defect; endocardial cushion defect; anomalous pulmonary venous return; ruptured sinus of Valsalva aneurysm into the right atrium; left ventricular–right atrial shunt.
Right ventricular enlargement/failure	Various patterns, depending on the underlying cause.	Cor pulmonale; chronic left heart failure; mitral stenosis; tetralogy of Fallot.
Tricuspid valve disease (Fig CA 1-1)	Right atrial enlargement (may be extreme); often dilatation of the superior vena cava; right ventricular enlargement in tricuspid insufficiency.	Most commonly the result of rheumatic heart disease. Rarely an isolated lesion and generally associated with mitral or aortic valve disease. Tricuspid insufficiency is usually functional and secondary to marked dilatation of the failing right ventricle. Rare causes of isolated tricuspid valve disease include carcinoid syndrome, endomyocardial fibrosis, and right atrial myxoma.
Pulmonary stenosis or atresia (Fig CA 1-2)	Enlargement of the right atrium and right ventricle; decreased pulmonary vascularity.	Right atrial enlargement secondary to enlargement of the right ventricle.
Hypoplastic left heart syndrome (Fig CA 1-3)	Enlargement of the right atrium and right ventricle produces progressive globular cardiomegaly. Severe pulmonary venous congestion.	Consists of several conditions in which underdevelopment of left side of the heart is related to an obstructive lesion (stenosis or atresia of the mitral valve, aortic valve, or aortic arch). Causes heart failure in the first week of life.

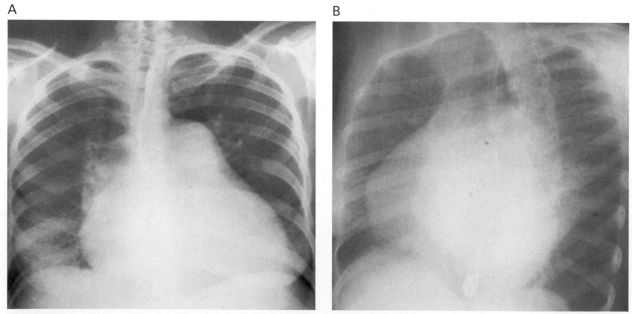

A   B

Fig CA 1-1
Tricuspid insufficiency. (A) Frontal and (B) left anterior oblique projections show striking right atrial enlargement.[1]

Condition	Imaging Findings	Comments
Tricuspid atresia	Enlargement of the right atrium and left ventricle; small right ventricle; decreased pulmonary vascularity (usually some degree of pulmonary stenosis).	Right-to-left shunt at the atrial level (patent foramen ovale or true atrial septal defect). Usually a ventricular septal defect or patent ductus arteriosus. Hypoplasia of the right ventricle and the pulmonary outflow tract. The smaller the shunt, the more marked the elevation of right atrial pressure and more striking the enlargement of this chamber.
Ebstein's anomaly (see Fig CA 6-5)	Enlargement of the right atrium causes a characteristic squared or boxed appearance of the heart. Decreased pulmonary vascularity; flat or concave pulmonary outflow tract; narrow vascular pedicle and small aortic arch.	Downward displacement of an incompetent tricuspid valve into the right ventricle so that the upper portion of the right ventricle is effectively incorporated into the right atrium. Functional obstruction to right atrial emptying produces increased pressure and a right-to-left atrial shunt (usually through a patent foramen ovale).
Uhl's disease	Radiographic pattern identical to that in Ebstein's anomaly.	Focal or complete absence of the right ventricular myocardium (the right ventricle becomes a thin-walled fibroelastic bag that contracts poorly and cannot effectively empty blood from the right side of the heart).

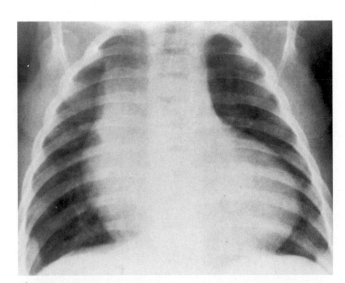

Fig CA 1-2
Pulmonary atresia. Marked right atrial enlargement associated with decreased pulmonary vascularity.

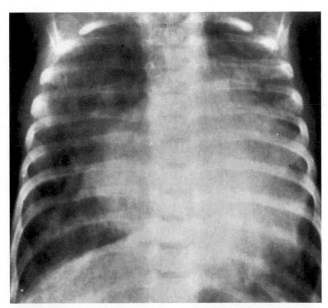

Fig CA 1-3
Hypoplastic left heart syndrome. Globular cardiomegaly with severe pulmonary venous congestion.

Right Ventricular Enlargement

Condition	Imaging Findings	Comments
Tetralogy of Fallot (Fig CA 2-1)	Enlargement of the right ventricle (though overall cardiac size is often normal); decreased pulmonary vascularity; flat or concave pulmonary outflow tract; right aortic arch in approximately 25% of patients.	Consists of (1) high ventricular septal defect, (2) obstruction to right ventricular outflow (usually infundibular pulmonary stenosis), (3) overriding of the aortic orifice above the ventricular defect, and (4) right ventricular hypertrophy. Most common cause of cyanotic congenital heart disease beyond the immediate neonatal period. If there is severe pulmonary stenosis, blood flow from both ventricles is effectively forced into the aorta, causing pronounced bulging of the ascending aorta and prominence of the aortic knob.
Pulmonary stenosis (Fig CA 2-2)	Initially normal heart size; right ventricular enlargement if severe stenosis causes systolic overloading of this chamber; poststenotic dilatation of the pulmonary artery.	Common anomaly found in isolated form or in combination with other abnormalities. The stenosis is most common at the level of the pulmonary valve (supravalvular or infundibular stenosis can occur).
Mitral stenosis (Fig CA 2-3)	Enlargement of the right ventricle (also the pulmonary outflow tract and central pulmonary arteries) reflects pulmonary arterial hypertension from transmitted increased pressure in the left atrium and the pulmonary veins.	Most common rheumatic valvular lesion (results from diffuse thickening of the valve by fibrous tissue or calcific deposits). Decreased left ventricular output causes a small aortic knob. Calcification of the mitral valve (best demonstrated by fluoroscopy) and pulmonary hemosiderosis may develop.

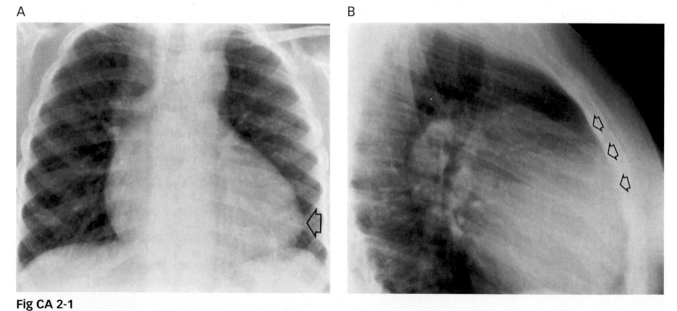

Fig CA 2-1
Tetralogy of Fallot. (A) Frontal view shows right ventricular enlargement as a lateral and upward displacement of the radiographic cardiac apex (arrow). (B) On the lateral view, the enlarged right ventricle fills most of the retrosternal space (arrows).

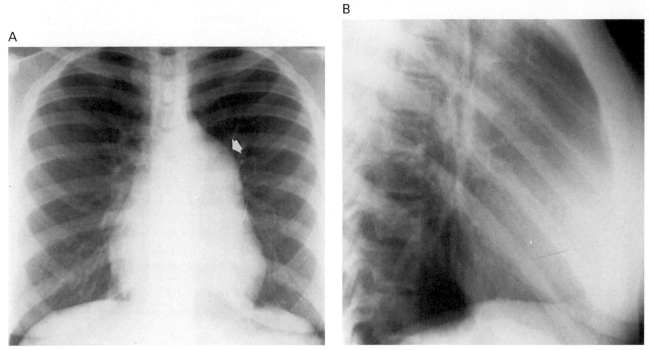

Fig CA 2-2
Pulmonary stenosis. (A) Frontal and (B) lateral views show striking poststenotic dilatation of the pulmonary artery (arrow) in addition to filling of the retrosternal air space, indicating right ventricular enlargement.

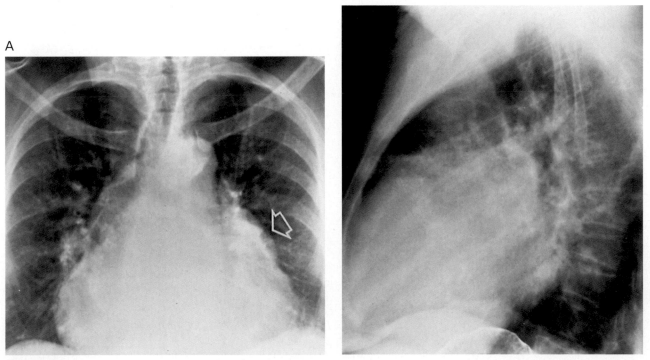

Fig CA 2-3
Mitral stenosis. (A) Frontal and (B) lateral views of the chest demonstrate cardiomegaly with enlargement of the right ventricle and left atrium. The right ventricular enlargement causes obliteration of the retrosternal air space, whereas left atrial enlargement produces a convexity of the upper left border of the heart (arrow, A).

Condition	Imaging Findings	Comments
Cor pulmonale (Fig CA 2-4)	Right ventricular enlargement associated with enlarged central pulmonary vessels, rapid tapering, and small peripheral vessels.	Primary or secondary to such conditions as chronic obstructive emphysema, diffuse interstitial fibrosis, widespread peripheral pulmonary emboli, and Eisenmenger physiology (reversed left-to-right shunt). Rare causes include metastases from trophoblastic neoplasms, immunologic disease, schistosomiasis, multiple pulmonary artery stenoses or coarctations, and vasoconstrictive diseases.
Chronic left heart failure	Enlarged right ventricle associated with left ventricular enlargement and pulmonary venous congestion.	May reflect a myocardiopathy or mitral insufficiency. The transmission of increased pressure from the left side of the heart eventually leads to the development of pulmonary arterial hypertension and enlargement of the right side of the heart.
Left-to-right shunts (see Fig CA 7-1)	Enlarged right ventricle and pulmonary outflow tract with increased pulmonary vascularity. The size of other structures varies depending on the specific underlying lesion.	Most commonly atrial septal defect, ventricular septal defect, or patent ductus arteriosus.
Tricuspid insufficiency	Right ventricular enlargement that may be obscured by the often extreme enlargement of the right atrium.	Usually functional and secondary to marked dilatation of the failing right ventricle.

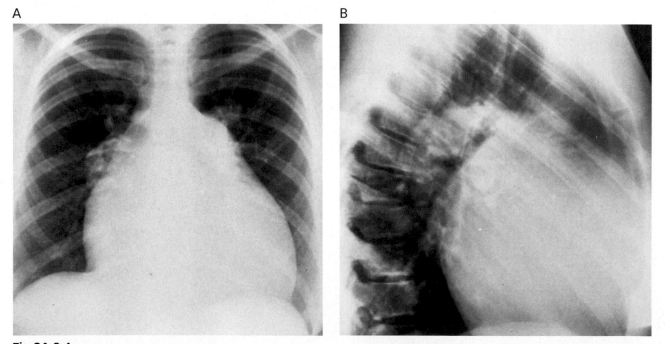

A   B

Fig CA 2-4
Cor pulmonale. (A) Frontal and (B) lateral views of the chest in a patient with primary pulmonary hypertension show marked globular cardiomegaly with prominence of the pulmonary trunk and central pulmonary arteries. The peripheral pulmonary vascularity is strikingly reduced. Right ventricular enlargement has obliterated the retrosternal air space on the lateral view.

Condition	Imaging Findings	Comments
Right-to-left shunts and admixture lesions	Various patterns, depending on the underlying cardiac anomaly.	Transposition of great vessels, trilogy of Fallot, Ebstein's anomaly, Uhl's anomaly, persistent truncus arteriosus.
Pseudotruncus arteriosus	Enlargement of the right ventricle; decreased pulmonary vascularity; flat or concave pulmonary outflow tract; right aortic arch in approximately 40% of patients.	Single vessel arising from the heart that is accompanied by a remnant of the atretic pulmonary artery (essentially the same as tetralogy of Fallot with pulmonary atresia).
Hypoplastic left heart syndrome	Right ventricular and right atrial enlargement causes progressive globular cardiomegaly. Severe pulmonary venous congestion.	Consists of several conditions in which underdevelopment of the left side of the heart is related to an obstructive lesion (stenosis or atresia of the mitral valve, aortic valve, or aortic arch). Causes heart failure in the first week of life.
Malformations obstructing pulmonary venous flow	Right ventricular enlargement associated with severe pulmonary venous congestion (increased pressure transmitted to the right side of the heart).	Congenital mitral stenosis; cor triatriatum (incomplete fibromuscular diaphragm dividing the left atrium); congenital pulmonary vein stenosis or atresia.
Pulmonary atresia (with tricuspid insufficiency)	Right ventricular enlargement associated with decreased pulmonary vascularity and a shallow or concave pulmonary artery segment.	May be an isolated anomaly or associated with transposition, atrial septal defect, or common ventricle.

Left Atrial Enlargement

Condition	Imaging Findings	Comments
Mitral stenosis (Figs CA 3-1 and CA 3-2)	Left atrial enlargement; pulmonary venous congestion; enlargement of the right ventricle, pulmonary outflow tract, and central pulmonary arteries; normal-sized left ventricle; small aortic knob (decreased left ventricular output).	Most common rheumatic valvular lesion (results from diffuse thickening of the valve by fibrous tissue or calcific deposits). Obstruction of blood flow from the left atrium into the left ventricle during diastole causes increased left atrial pressure that is transmitted to the pulmonary veins and eventually to the pulmonary arteries and the right side of the heart. Calcification of the mitral valve (best demonstrated by fluoroscopy) and pulmonary hemosiderosis may develop.

A
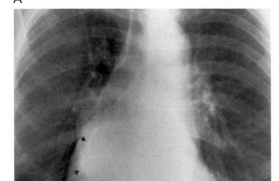

B
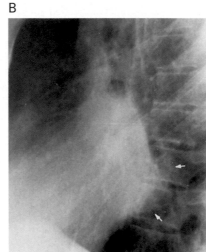

Fig CA 3-1
Mitral stenosis. (A) Frontal chest radiograph demonstrates a double contour (arrows) representing the increased density of the enlarged left atrium. (B) Lateral view confirms the left atrial enlargement (arrows) in this patient with rheumatic heart disease.

A
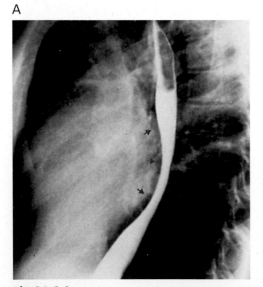

B
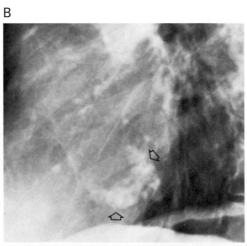

Fig CA 3-2
Mitral stenosis. (A) On a lateral view, the enlarged chamber produces a discrete posterior indentation (arrows) on the barium-filled esophagus. (B) In another patient, there is associated calcification of the mitral valve annulus (arrows).

Condition	Imaging Findings	Comments
Mitral insufficiency (Fig CA 3-3)	Left atrial enlargement (sometimes enormous); enlargement of the left ventricle; normal-sized aortic knob.	Most often caused by rheumatic heart disease. Also rupture of chordae tendineae, papillary muscle dysfunction, or severe left ventricular dilatation that distorts the mitral annulus (congestive heart failure, aortic valve disease, coarctation of the aorta). In mitral insufficiency, the left atrium is usually considerably larger than in mitral stenosis, and pulmonary venous congestion is less frequent and less prominent.
Left-to-right shunts (see Fig CA 7-3)	Left atrial enlargement, increased pulmonary vascularity, and pulmonary outflow tract. The appearance of the right atrium, right ventricle, and aorta depends on the specific lesion.	Ventricular septal defect, patent ductus arteriosus, and aorticopulmonary window are the most common causes. Also coronary artery fistula, persistent truncus arteriosus, and atrial septal defect with reversal of the shunt.
Myxoma of left atrium	Normal heart size and pulmonary vascularity until the tumor causes dysfunction of the mitral valve (radiographic pattern of mitral stenosis). Pathognomonic calcification is seen on fluoroscopy in approximately 10% of cases.	Most common primary cardiac tumor. Almost all arise in an atrium (particularly the left). The tumor is usually pedunculated and causes intermittent obstruction or traumatic injury to the mitral (or tricuspid) valve. A similar ball-valve mechanism may be produced by a left atrial thrombus. Fragmentation of the tumor may produce showers of systemic or pulmonary emboli.
Right-to-left shunts and admixture lesions	Various patterns, depending on the precise intracardiac anomaly. Left atrial enlargement may develop, though other radiographic changes are more diagnostic.	Tricuspid atresia, trilogy of Fallot, transposition of great vessels.
Endocardial fibroelastosis	Striking globular enlargement of the heart. There may be dramatic left atrial enlargement due to often-associated mitral insufficiency. Small aortic knob (decreased left ventricular output). Normal pulmonary vascularity until congestive heart failure supervenes.	Common cause of cardiac failure during the first year of life. Characterized by diffuse thickening of the left ventricular endocardium with collagen and elastic tissue.

A

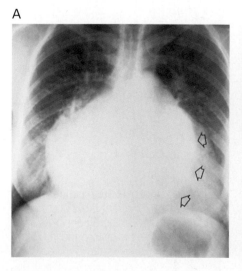

B

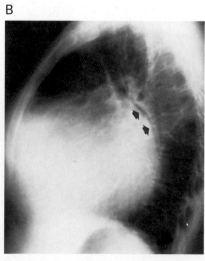

Fig CA 3-3
Mitral insufficiency. (A) Frontal and (B) lateral views of the chest demonstrate gross cardiomegaly with enlargement of the left atrium and left ventricle. Note the striking double-contour configuration (open arrows, A) and elevation of the left main bronchus (closed arrows, B), characteristic signs of left atrial enlargement. The aortic knob is normal in size, and there is no evidence of pulmonary venous congestion.

Left Ventricular Enlargement

Condition	Imaging Findings	Comments
Congestive heart failure	Left ventricular enlargement with pulmonary venous congestion. Pleural effusion is common (bilateral or right sided; unilateral left-sided effusion is rare and suggests another cause).	Precise type and degree of cardiac enlargement depend on the underlying heart disease
High-output heart disease (see figures in Section CA 17)	Left ventricular enlargement associated with prominent pulmonary vascularity (both arteries and veins) and dilatation of the main pulmonary artery.	Causes include anemia, thyrotoxicosis, beriberi, hypervolemia, arteriovenous fistulas, Paget's disease, Pickwickian obesity, polycythemia vera, and pregnancy.
Arteriosclerotic heart disease (myocardial ischemia) (Fig CA 4-1)	Plain chest radiograph is often normal. Left ventricular enlargement is a nonspecific finding that usually reflects the presence of a large quantity of infarcted myocardium.	Coronary artery calcification (see Fig CA 19-5) strongly suggests hemodynamically significant disease. The calcification primarily involves the circumflex and anterior descending branches of the left coronary artery. Best seen with cardiac fluoroscopy (infrequently visualized on routine chest radiographs).
Acute myocardial infarction (Fig CA 4-2)	Generally normal appearance. Left ventricular dilatation is usually related to superimposed pulmonary venous congestion.	Weakening of the myocardial wall at the site of an infarct may permit the development of a ventricular aneurysm, which causes focal bulging or diffuse prominence along the lower left border of the heart near the apex (located anteriorly on lateral view). Characteristic curvilinear calcification in the aneurysm wall and paradoxical or extremely limited pulsation on fluoroscopy.
Hypertension (see figures in Section CA 18)	Initially, increased workload causes left ventricular hypertrophy that produces no radiographic change or only rounding of the left heart border. Eventually, continued strain leads to dilatation and enlargement of the left ventricle. Aortic tortuosity with prominence of the ascending portion often occurs.	Widened superior mediastinum (increased fat deposition) and vertebral compression suggest Cushing's syndrome; figure-3 sign and rib notching indicate coarctation; paravertebral mass suggests pheochromocytoma; erosion of the distal clavicle suggests secondary hyperparathyroidism (renal disease).

A

B

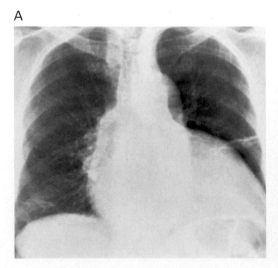
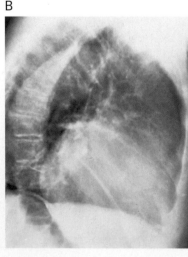

Fig CA 4-1
Arteriosclerotic heart disease. (A) Frontal and (B) lateral views of the chest show marked enlargement of the left ventricle. There is also tortuosity of the aorta and bilateral streaks of fibrosis.

Condition	Imaging Findings	Comments
Aortic insufficiency (Fig CA 4-3)	Left ventricular enlargement (dilatation and hypertrophy). Dilatation of the ascending aorta and aortic knob. As the left ventricle fails, pulmonary venous congestion develops along with left atrial enlargement (due to relative mitral insufficiency).	Most commonly caused by rheumatic heart disease; also caused by infective endocarditis, syphilis, dissecting aneurysm, and Marfan's syndrome. Congenital aortic insufficiency is usually due to a bicuspid valve.
Aortic stenosis (Fig CA 4-4)	Initially, concentric left ventricular hypertrophy produces only some rounding of the cardiac apex (overall heart size is normal). Left ventricular failure and dilatation develop late and are often accompanied by left atrial enlargement, pulmonary venous congestion, and prominence of the right ventricle and pulmonary artery. Poststenotic dilatation of the ascending aorta occurs with valvular stenosis.	May be due to rheumatic heart disease or a congenital valvular deformity (especially a bicuspid valve), or may represent a degenerative process of aging (idiopathic calcific stenosis). An aortic valve disorder due to rheumatic heart disease is rarely isolated and is most commonly associated with a significant lesion of the mitral valve. Aortic valve calcification (best seen with fluoroscopy) is common and indicates severe aortic stenosis.

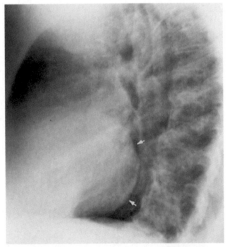

Fig CA 4-2
Acute myocardial infarction. Lateral view of the chest shows marked prominence of the left ventricle (arrows).

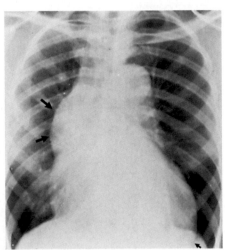

Fig CA 4-3
Aortic insufficiency. Frontal chest radiograph shows left ventricular enlargement with downward and lateral displacement of the cardiac apex. Note that the cardiac shadow extends below the dome of the left hemidiaphragm. The ascending aorta is strikingly dilated (arrows), suggesting some underlying aortic stenosis.

A

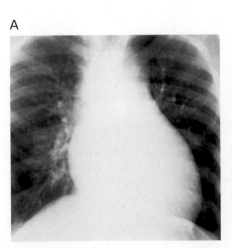

B

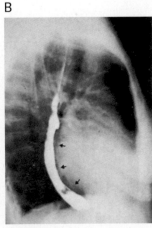

Fig CA 4-4
Aortic stenosis. (A) Frontal view shows downward displacement of the cardiac apex. (B) On a lateral view, the bulging of the lower half of the posterior cardiac silhouette causes a broad indentation on the barium-filled esophagus (arrows).

Condition	Imaging Findings	Comments
Coarctation of aorta (see Fig CA 8-1)	Enlargement of the left ventricle with a characteristic double bulge in the region of the aortic knob (figure-3 sign on plain chest radiographs and reverse figure-3, or figure-E, sign on the barium-filled esophagus). There may be rib notching (usually involving the posterior fourth to eighth ribs) but rarely developing before the age of 6 years.	In the more common "adult" type, aortic narrowing occurs at or just distal to the level of the ductus arteriosus (double bulge represents prestenotic and poststenotic dilatation). In the "infantile" variety, there is a long segment of narrowing lying proximal to the ductus (obligatory right-to-left shunt and early congestive heart failure). There is a relatively high incidence of coarctation in women with Turner's syndrome.
Mitral insufficiency (Fig CA 4-5)	Enlargement (sometimes enormous) of the left ventricle and left atrium. Small or normal aortic knob. Generally normal pulmonary vascularity (there may be pulmonary venous congestion, but it is less frequent and less prominent than in mitral stenosis).	Most often caused by rheumatic heart disease; also may be due to rupture of chordae tendineae, papillary muscle dysfunction, or severe left ventricular dilatation (aortic valve disease, congestive heart failure) distorting the mitral annulus. Coexistent mitral stenosis may produce a bizarre pattern.
Myocardiopathy (Figs CA 4-6 and CA 4-7)	Generalized cardiac enlargement, often with left ventricular predominance. May mimic pericardial effusion. The development of left ventricular failure produces pulmonary venous congestion.	Causes include inflammation (rheumatic, septic, viral, toxoplasmic); infiltration (amyloidosis, glycogen storage disease, leukemia); endocrine imbalance (thyrotoxicosis, myxedema, acromegaly); ischemia; nutritional deficiency (beriberi, alcoholism, potassium or magnesium depletion); toxicity (drugs, chemicals, cobalt); collagen diseases; and postpartum heart disease.

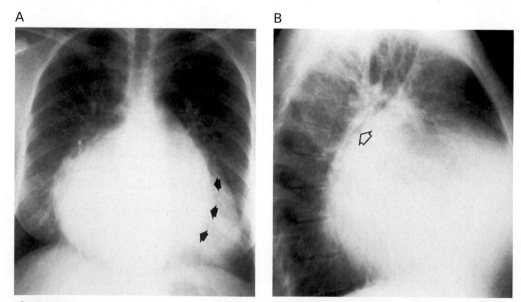

A   B

Fig CA 4-5
Mitral insufficiency. (A) Frontal and (B) lateral views of the chest demonstrate cardiomegaly with enlargement of the left ventricle and left atrium. Note the striking double-contour configuration (closed arrows) and elevation of the left main-stem bronchus (open arrow), characteristic signs of left atrial enlargement.

Condition	Imaging Findings	Comments
Left-to-right shunt (see Figs CA 7-3 and CA 7-5)	Various patterns of abnormal heart size with increased pulmonary vascularity.	Ventricular septal defect (not atrial septal defect), patent ductus arteriosus, endocardial cushion defect, aorticopulmonary window, and, infrequently, persistent truncus arteriosus.
Right-to-left shunt or admixture lesion	Various patterns of abnormal heart size and pulmonary vascularity.	Transposition of great vessels; tricuspid atresia; pulmonary stenosis with intact ventricular septum.
Endocardial fibroelastosis (Fig CA 4-8)	Generalized cardiac enlargement with hypertrophy and dilatation of the left ventricle and often dramatic left atrial enlargement (due to associated mitral insufficiency).	Diffuse thickening of the left ventricular endocardium with collagen and elastic tissue. A common cause of cardiac failure in the first year of life.

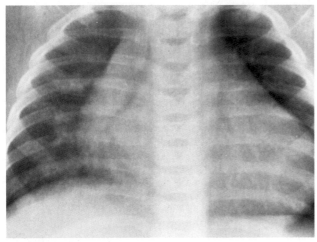

Fig CA 4-6
Glycogen storage disease. Generalized globular cardiac enlargement with a left ventricular prominence.

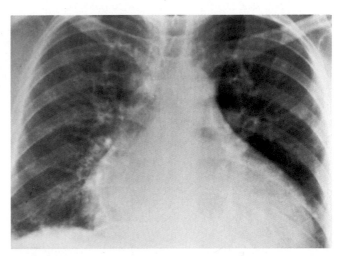

Fig CA 4-7
Alcoholic cardiomyopathy. Generalized cardiac enlargement that involves all chambers but has a left ventricular predominance. There is pulmonary vascular congestion and a right pleural effusion.

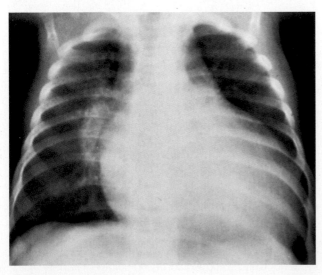

Fig CA 4-8
Endocardial fibroelastosis. Generalized cardiomegaly with prominence of the left ventricle.

Cyanotic Congenital Heart Disease with Increased Pulmonary Vascularity

Condition	Imaging Findings	Comments
Persistent truncus arteriosus (types I, II, and III) (Fig CA 5-1)	Increased pulmonary vascularity; concave pulmonary outflow tract; striking enlargement of the right ventricle, and eventual enlargement of the left atrium and left ventricle.	Failure of the common truncus arteriosus to divide normally into the aorta and the pulmonary artery. Results in a single large arterial trunk that receives the outflow of blood from both ventricles. Variable degree of cyanosis (more profound cyanosis if low pulmonary blood flow).
Transposition of great arteries (Figs CA 5-2 and CA 5-3)	Increased pulmonary vascularity (unless prominent pulmonary stenosis). Various patterns depending on the precise intracardiac anomalies (generally biventricular enlargement with an oval or egg-shaped configuration).	Reversal of the normal relation of the aorta and the pulmonary artery (the aorta arises anteriorly from the right ventricle, whereas the pulmonary artery originates posteriorly from the left ventricle). An intracardiac or extracardiac shunt (atrial and ventricular septal defects, patent ductus arteriosus) must be present to connect the two separate circulations. The shunts are bidirectional and permit mixing of oxygenated and unoxygenated blood (leading to cyanosis).
Taussig-Bing anomaly (Fig CA 5-4)	Increased pulmonary vascularity; generalized cardiomegaly.	Aorta arises from the right ventricle, whereas the pulmonary artery overrides the ventricular septum and receives blood from both ventricles. The pulmonary artery lies to the left of and slightly posterior to the aorta. Also a high ventricular septal defect.
Double-outlet right ventricle (Figs CA 5-5 and CA 5-6)	Increased pulmonary vascularity; generalized cardiomegaly; cardiac waist wider than in other types of transpositions (the aorta and pulmonary artery have a more side-to-side configuration).	Both the aorta and the pulmonary artery arise from the right ventricle. A left-to-right ventricular septal defect permits oxygenated blood from the left ventricle to pass to the right ventricle and then on to the systemic circulation.

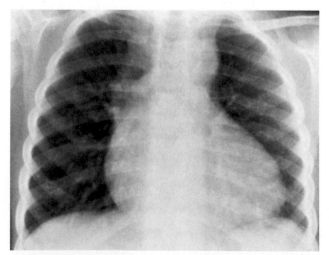

Fig CA 5-1
Persistent truncus arteriosus. Increased pulmonary vascularity, yet typical concave appearance of the pulmonary outflow tract.

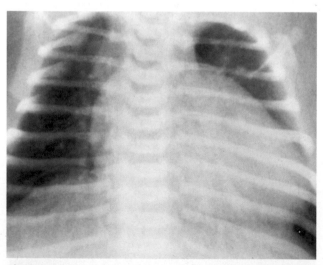

Fig CA 5-2
Transposition of the great arteries. Biventricular enlargement produces a typical oval or egg-shaped heart. Note the narrowing of the vascular pedicle due to superimposition of the abnormally positioned aorta and pulmonary artery.

Condition	Imaging Findings	Comments
Common ventricle (Fig CA 5-7)	Increased or decreased pulmonary vascularity (depending on the presence and degree of associated pulmonary stenosis); marked nonspecific globular enlargement of the heart.	Extremely large septal defect produces a functional "single ventricle." If there is associated severe pulmonary stenosis, the blood flow through the lungs is scanty, and the patient develops profound cyanosis.
Complete endocardial cushion defect (Fig CA 5-8)	Increased pulmonary vascularity; nonspecific globular enlargement of the heart (enlargement of all cardiac chambers).	Low atrial septal defect combined with a large ventricular septal defect plus a contiguous cleft in both the mitral and the tricuspid valves (common atrioventricular canal). Bidirectional shunting with right-to-left components is responsible for producing the cyanosis.

A

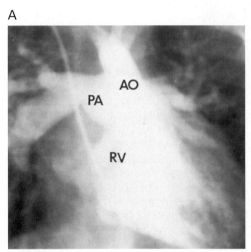

B

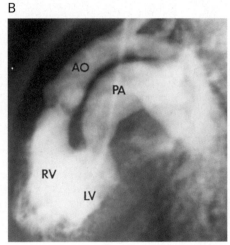

Fig CA 5-3
Transposition of the great arteries. (A) Frontal and (B) lateral views from an angiocardiogram demonstrate contrast material in the right ventricle (RV), which is situated anteriorly and to the right. It communicates through a large ventricular septal defect with the left ventricle (LV), which is located posteriorly and to the left. The transposed aorta (AO) originates from the right ventricular infundibulum directly in front of the pulmonary artery (PA), which arises from the left ventricle.[2]

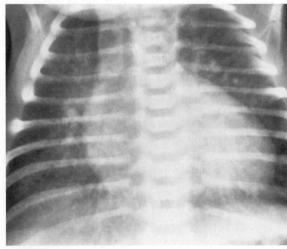

Fig CA 5-4
Taussig-Bing anomaly. Engorged pulmonary vasculature, oval cardiomegaly, and a laterally pointing apex.

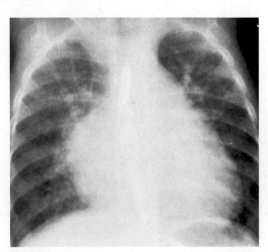

Fig CA 5-5
Double-outlet right ventricle. Generalized cardiomegaly with increased pulmonary vascularity. Because the aorta and the pulmonary artery have a more side-to-side configuration, the cardiac waist is relatively wider than in other types of transpositions.

Condition	Imaging Findings	Comments
Total anomalous pulmonary venous return (Fig CA 5-9)	Increased pulmonary vascularity; "snowman" or figure-8 configuration in types I and II; characteristic indentation on the lower esophagus by the anomalous vein as it descends through the diaphragm in type III.	Pulmonary veins connect to the right atrium directly or to the systemic veins or their tributaries. Because all the pulmonary venous blood returns to the right atrium, a right-to-left shunt through an interatrial communication is necessary for blood to reach the left side of the heart and the systemic circulation (producing cyanosis).
Reversal of left-to-right shunt (Eisenmenger physiology) (Fig CA 5-10)	Increased fullness of the central pulmonary arteries with abrupt narrowing and pruning of peripheral vessels.	Development of pulmonary hypertension causes reversal of the shunt leading to unoxygenated blood entering the systemic circulation (cyanosis). Most commonly develops with atrial and ventricular septal defects and patent ductus arteriosus.

A

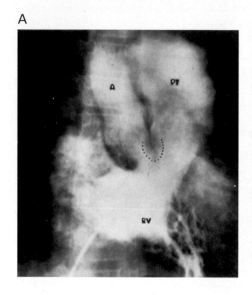

B

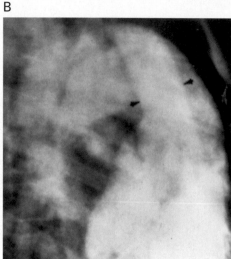

Fig CA 5-6
Double-outlet right ventricle. (A) Frontal view from a selective right ventriculogram shows simultaneous and equal opacification of both great vessels from the right ventricle (RV). The ventricular septal defect was immediately beneath the crista supraventricularis (dotted line). (B) A lateral view shows the aorta (arrows) superimposed over the posterior two-thirds of the pulmonary trunk. (A, aorta; PT, pulmonary trunk.)[3]

A

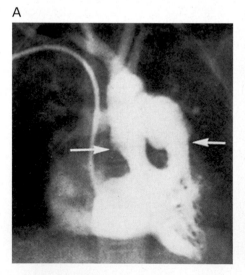

B

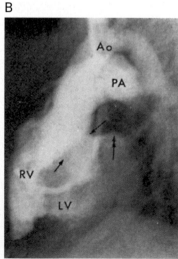

Fig CA 5-7
Single ventricle. (A) Frontal view from a right ventriculogram shows muscular tracts leading from the right ventricle to both great arteries, the valves of which (arrows) are at the same horizontal level. (B) A lateral view shows the anteriorly situated right ventricle (RV) communicating with the left ventricle (LV) via a ventricular septal defect (single arrows). (PA, pulmonary artery; Ao, aorta.)[4]

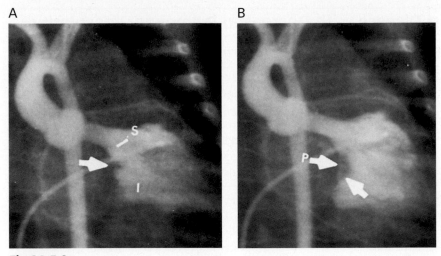

Fig CA 5-8
Common atrioventricular canal. (A) Left ventricular angiogram (frontal view) in early systole shows the cleft (arrow) between the superior (S) and inferior (I) segments of the anterior mitral leaflet located along the right contour of the ventricle. There is no evidence of mitral insufficiency or an interventricular shunt. (B) In diastole, the ventricular outflow tract is narrowed and lies in a more horizontal position than normal. The right border of the ventricle can be followed directly into the scooped-out margin (arrows) of the interventricular septum. The attachment of the posterior mitral leaflet (P) is also visible because of a thin layer of contrast material trapped between the leaflet and the posterior ventricular wall.[5]

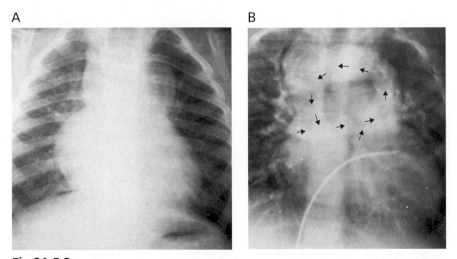

Fig CA 5-9
Total anomalous pulmonary venous return (type I). (A) Frontal chest radiograph demonstrates a snowman, or figure-8, heart with right atrial and right ventricular enlargement. The widening of the superior mediastinum is due to the large, anomalous inverted-U–shaped vein. The pulmonary vascularity is greatly increased. The large pulmonary artery is hidden in the superior mediastinal silhouette. (B) Angiocardiogram demonstrates that all the pulmonary veins drain into the inverted-U–shaped vessel that eventually empties into the superior vena cava (arrows). The widening of the mediastinum produced by this vessel causes the snowman heart.[6]

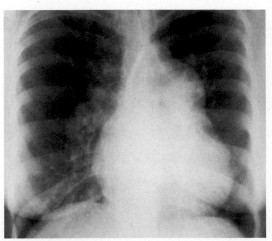

Fig CA 5-10
Eisenmenger physiology in patent ductus arteriosus. There is an increased fullness of the central pulmonary arteries with an abrupt narrowing and paucity of peripheral vessels.

Cyanotic Congenital Heart Disease with Decreased Pulmonary Vascularity

Condition	Imaging Findings	Comments
Tetralogy of Fallot (Fig CA 6-1)	Decreased pulmonary vascularity; flat or concave pulmonary outflow tract; enlargement of the right ventricle; right aortic arch in approximately 25% of cases.	Most common cause of cyanotic congenital heart disease beyond the immediate neonatal period includes (1) high ventricular septal defect, (2) obstruction to right ventricular outflow (usually infundibular stenosis), (3) overriding of the aortic orifice above the ventricular defect, and (4) right ventricular hypertrophy.
Pseudotruncus arteriosus (truncus arteriosus type IV) (Fig CA 6-2)	Decreased pulmonary vascularity; flat or concave pulmonary outflow tract; enlargement of the right ventricle; right aortic arch in approximately 40% of cases.	Single large arterial trunk receives the outflow of blood from both ventricles. The pulmonary arteries are absent, so the pulmonary circulation is supplied by bronchial or other collateral vessels.
Trilogy of Fallot (Fig CA 6-3)	Decreased pulmonary vascularity; poststenotic dilatation of pulmonary artery; heart size often normal (usually some evidence of right ventricular hypertrophy).	Combination of pulmonary valvular stenosis with an intact ventricular septum and an interatrial shunt (patent foramen ovale or true atrial septal defect). Increased pressure on the right side of the heart due to pulmonary stenosis causes the interatrial shunt to be right to left.
Tricuspid atresia/stenosis (Fig CA 6-4)	Decreased pulmonary vascularity (usually some degree of pulmonary stenosis); striking enlargement of the right atrium if small atrial shunt; large left ventricle; small right ventricle.	Right-to-left shunt at the atrial level (patent foramen ovale or true atrial septal defect). Usually there is also a ventricular septal defect or a patent ductus arteriosus. Hypoplasia of the right ventricle and pulmonary outflow tract is evident. The smaller the shunt, the more marked the elevation of right atrial pressure and more striking the enlargement of this chamber. Tricuspid atresia without pulmonary stenosis produces marked cardiomegaly and increased pulmonary vascularity.

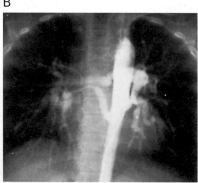

Fig CA 6-1
Tetralogy of Fallot. Plain chest radiograph demonstrates decreased pulmonary vascularity and a flat pulmonary outflow tract. Note the characteristic lateral displacement and upward tilting of the prominent left cardiac apex (*coeur en sabot* appearance).

A

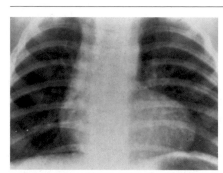

B

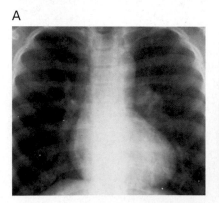

Fig CA 6-2
Pseudotruncus arteriosus. (A) Plain chest radiograph shows the pulmonary vascularity to be strikingly diminished. (B) Angiogram shows that most of the blood supply to the lungs originates from two large arteries arising from the descending aorta.[1]

Condition	Imaging Findings	Comments
Ebstein's anomaly (Fig CA 6-5)	Decreased pulmonary vascularity; flat or concave pulmonary outflow tract; characteristic squared or boxed appearance of the heart (bulging of the right heart border by the enlarged right atrium); narrow vascular pedicle; and small aortic arch.	Downward displacement of an incompetent tricuspid valve into the right ventricle so that the upper portion of the right ventricle is effectively incorporated into the right atrium. The functional obstruction to right atrial emptying produces increased pressure and a right-to-left atrial shunt (usually through a patent foramen ovale).
Uhl's disease	Radiographic pattern identical to that in Ebstein's anomaly.	Focal or complete absence of the right ventricular myocardium (the right ventricle becomes a thin-walled fibroelastic bag that contracts poorly and cannot effectively empty blood from the right side of the heart).
Pulmonary atresia or severe pulmonary stenosis (Fig CA 6-6)	Decreased pulmonary vascularity; shallow or concave pulmonary artery segment; variable cardiomegaly.	May be an isolated anomaly or associated with transposition, atrial septal defect, or common ventricle.

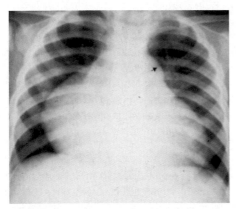

Fig CA 6-3
Trilogy of Fallot. Decreased pulmonary vascularity with prominent poststenotic dilatation (arrow) of the pulmonary artery. There is enormous right atrial and moderate right ventricular enlargement.[6]

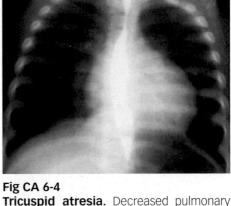

Fig CA 6-4
Tricuspid atresia. Decreased pulmonary vascularity with elongation and rounding of the left border of the heart.

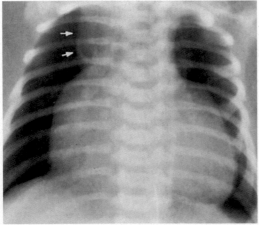

Fig CA 6-5
Ebstein's anomaly. In addition to decreased pulmonary vascularity, there is enlargement of the right atrium, causing upward and outward bulging of the right border of the heart (squared appearance). Widening of the right side of the superior portion of the mediastinum (arrows) reflects marked dilatation of the superior vena cava due to right ventricular failure.

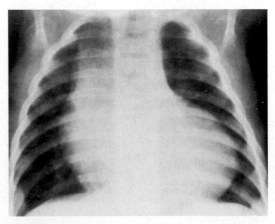

Fig CA 6-6
Pulmonary atresia. Decreased pulmonary vascularity with a concave outflow tract and moderate cardiomegaly.

Acyanotic Congenital Heart Disease with Increased Pulmonary Blood Flow

Condition	Imaging Findings	Comments
Atrial septal defect (Fig CA 7-1)	Increased pulmonary vascularity; enlarged right atrium, right ventricle, and pulmonary outflow tract; normal left atrium and left ventricle; small aorta.	Most common congenital cardiac lesion. The magnitude of the shunt depends on the size of the defect, the relative compliance of the ventricles, and the difference in atrial pressure. May be combined with mitral stenosis (Lutembacher's syndrome) and cause a substantial increase in the workload of the right ventricle.
Ventricular septal defect (Fig CA 7-2)	Increased pulmonary vascularity; enlarged right ventricle, pulmonary outflow tract, left atrium, and sometimes left ventricle (may be normal); normal right atrium; normal or small aorta.	Common congenital cardiac anomaly. The magnitude of the shunt depends on the size of the defect and the difference in ventricular pressure. There may also be a shunt from the left ventricle to the right atrium.
Patent ductus arteriosus (Fig CA 7-3)	Increased pulmonary vascularity; enlargement of the left atrium, left ventricle, aorta, and pulmonary outflow tract; normal right atrium; enlarged or normal right ventricle.	Ductus extends from the bifurcation of the pulmonary artery to join the aorta just distal to the left subclavian artery (shunts blood from the pulmonary artery into the systemic circulation during intrauterine life). The aortic end of the ductus (infundibulum) is often dilated to produce a convex bulge on the left border of the aorta just below the knob.
Endocardial cushion defect (Fig CA 7-4)	Increased pulmonary vascularity; nonspecific globular enlargement of the heart (enlargement of all cardiac chambers).	Low atrial septal defect combined with a high ventricular septal defect. Most often occurs in children with Down's syndrome.

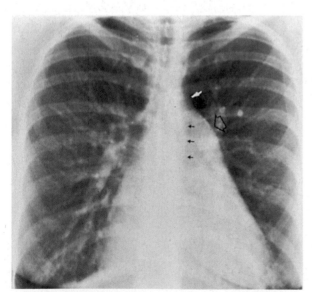

Fig CA 7-1
Atrial septal defect. Frontal view of the chest demonstrates cardiomegaly along with an increase in pulmonary vascularity reflecting the left-to-right shunt. Filling of the retrosternal space indicates enlargement of the right ventricle. The small aortic knob (white arrow) and descending aorta (small black arrows) are dwarfed by the enlarged pulmonary outflow tract (large open arrow).

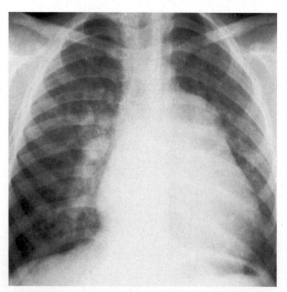

Fig CA 7-2
Ventricular septal defect. The heart is enlarged and somewhat triangular, and there is an increase in pulmonary vascular volume. The pulmonary trunk is very large and over-shadows the normal-sized aorta, which seems small by comparison.[1]

Condition	Imaging Findings	Comments
Aortic valvular stenosis (Fig CA 9-3)	Bulging of the ascending aorta (poststenotic dilatation). Aortic valve calcification (best seen on fluoroscopy) is common and indicates severe stenosis.	May be congenital (usually bicuspid valve) or acquired (generally on a rheumatic basis). Increased prominence of the left heart border (overall heart size is often normal). Substantial cardiomegaly reflects left ventricular failure and dilatation.
Aortic insufficiency (Fig CA 9-4)	Moderate dilatation of the ascending aorta and aortic knob (marked dilatation, especially of the ascending aorta, suggests underlying aortic stenosis). Enlargement of the left ventricle.	Most commonly due to rheumatic heart disease. Other causes include syphilis, infective endo-carditis, dissecting aneurysm, and Marfan's syndrome. Left ventricular failure leads to pulmonary venous congestion and left atrial enlargement (relative mitral insufficiency).
Syphilitic aortitis (Fig CA 9-5)	Dilatation of the ascending aorta, frequently with mural calcification.	May cause inflammation of the aortic valvular ring that results in aortic insufficiency. Approximately one-third of patients develop narrowing of the coronary ostia that may lead to symptoms of ischemic heart disease.
Takayasu's disease ("pulseless" disease)	Widening and contour irregularity of the aorta (especially the arch). May also involve major aortic branches. Linear calcifications frequently occur.	Nonspecific obstructive arteritis, primarily affecting young women, in which granulation tissue destroys the media of large vessels. The resulting mural scarring causes luminal narrowing and occlusion. There is usually fever and constitutional symptoms. Characteristic smooth and tapering arterial narrowing on angiography.

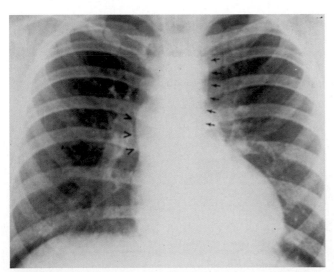

Fig CA 9-3
Aortic valvular stenosis. There is prominence of the left ventricle with poststenotic dilatation of the ascending aorta (arrowheads). The aortic knob and descending aorta (arrows) are normal.[10]

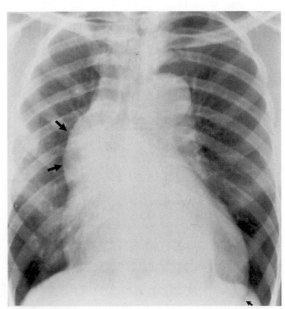

Fig CA 9-4
Aortic insufficiency. Marked dilatation of the ascending aorta (arrows), suggesting some underlying aortic stenosis. The left ventricle is enlarged with downward and lateral displacement of the cardiac apex. Note that the cardiac shadow extends below the dome of the left hemidiaphragm (small arrow).

Condition	Imaging Findings	Comments
Coarctation of aorta (see Fig CA 8-1)	Prominence of the ascending aorta. Characteristic double bulge in the region of the aortic knob (figure-3 sign on plain chest radiographs and reverse figure-3, or figure-E, sign on the barium-filled esophagus). There may be rib notching (usually involving the posterior fourth to eighth ribs but rarely developing before the age of 6 years) and dilated internal mammary arteries (soft-tissue density on lateral films).	In the more common "adult" type, the aortic narrowing occurs at or just distal to the level of the ductus arteriosus. The double bulge represents prestenotic and poststenotic dilatation.
Pseudocoarctation of aorta (Fig CA 9-6)	Two bulges in the region of the aortic knob mimic true coarctation. No rib notching or internal mammary collaterals (as no obstruction or hemodynamic abnormality).	Buckling or kinking of the aortic arch in the region of the ligamentum arteriosum. The bulges represent dilated portions of the aorta just proximal and distal to the kink. The upper bulge is usually higher than the normal aortic knob and can simulate a left superior mediastinal tumor.
Patent ductus arteriosus (Fig CA 9-7)	Prominent aortic knob; increased pulmonary vascularity; enlargement of the left atrium, left ventricle, and pulmonary outflow tract. The aortic end of the ductus (infundibulum) is often dilated to produce a convex bulge on the left border of the aorta just below the knob.	Ductus extends from the bifurcation of the pulmonary artery to join the aorta just distal to the left subclavian artery (shunts blood from the pulmonary artery into the systemic circulation during intrauterine life). Aortic prominence is a differential point from other major left-to-right shunts (atrial and ventricular septal defects).

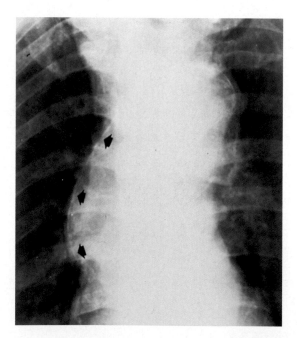

Fig CA 9-5
Syphilitic aortitis. Aneurysmal dilatation of the ascending aorta with extensive linear calcification of the wall (arrows). Some calcification is also seen in the distal aortic arch.

Condition	Imaging Findings	Comments
Tetralogy of Fallot with severe pulmonary stenosis	Pronounced bulging of the ascending aorta and prominence of the aortic knob.	Severe pulmonary stenosis effectively forces the aorta to drain both ventricles. A similar appearance occurs in pseudotruncus arteriosus (essentially tetralogy of Fallot with pulmonary atresia).
Aneurysm of sinus of Valsalva (see Fig CA 7-6)	Large aneurysm produces a smooth local bulge in the right anterolateral cardiac contour (a small aneurysm is undetectable). Curvilinear calcification often occurs in the aneurysm wall.	Primarily involves the sinus above the right cusp of the aortic valve. An acute rupture (usually into the right ventricle) causes a sudden large left-to-right shunt.
Corrected transposition (Fig CA 9-8)	Smooth bulging of the upper left border of the heart replaces the normal double bulge of the aortic knob and the pulmonary artery segment.	Combination of transposition of the origins of the aorta and the pulmonary artery and inversion of the ventricles and their accompanying atrioventricular valves. A single bulge represents the displaced ascending aorta and right ventricular outflow tract.

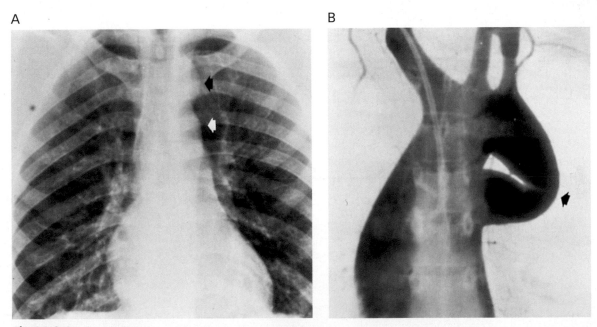

A   B

Fig CA 9-6
Pseudocoarctation of the aorta. (A) Frontal view of the chest demonstrates two bulges (arrows) producing a well-demarcated figure-3 sign in the region of the aortic knob. The upper bulge (black arrow) is higher than the normal aortic knob and simulates a mediastinal mass. Because there is no hemodynamic abnormality, the heart is normal in size, and there is no rib notching. (B) In another patient, an aortogram demonstrates extreme kinking of the descending aorta (arrow) without an area of true coarctation.

Condition	Imaging Findings	Comments
Persistent truncus arteriosus	Bulge in the region of the ascending aorta (represents the large single arterial trunk).	Failure of the common truncus arteriosus to divide normally into the aorta and the pulmonary artery, resulting in a single large arterial trunk that receives the outflow of blood from both ventricles.
Connective tissue disorders (Fig CA 9-9)	Generalized dilatation of the aorta. Increased incidence of aneurysm and dissection.	Conditions include Ehlers-Danlos syndrome, Marfan's syndrome, osteogenesis imperfecta, and pseudoxanthoma elasticum.

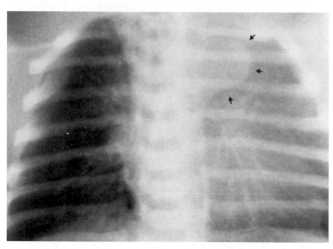

Fig CA 9-7
Patent ductus arteriosus. A convex bulge (arrows) on the left side of the superior mediastinum represents dilatation of the aortic end of the ductus ("ductus bump").

A
B

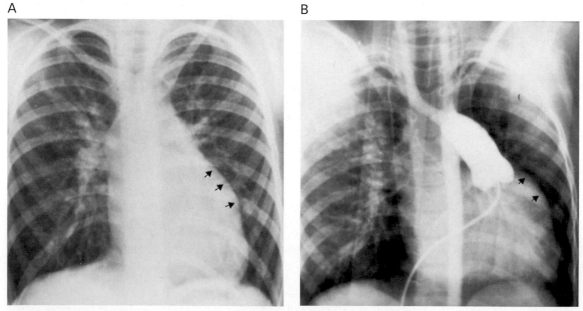

Fig CA 9-8
Corrected transposition with ventricular septal defect. (A) There is fullness of the upper left border of the heart (arrows). Because of the left-to-right ventricular shunt, the pulmonary vasculature is engorged. (B) A film from an angiocardiogram demonstrates the inverted aorta and right ventricular outflow tract (arrows).[6]

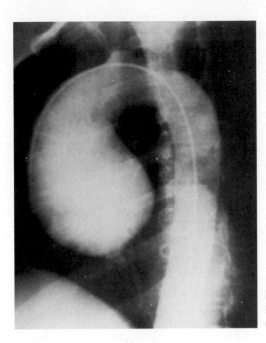

Fig CA 9-9
Marfan's syndrome. Arteriogram shows enormous dilatation of the aneurysmal ascending aorta.

Small Ascending Aorta or Aortic Arch

Condition	Imaging Findings	Comments
Atrial septal defect (see Fig CA 7-1)	Small aorta; increased pulmonary vascularity; enlarged right atrium, right ventricle, and pulmonary outflow tract.	Shunting of blood away from the left side of the heart into the pulmonary circulation causes decreased flow through the aorta.
Ventricular septal defect (see Fig CA 7-2)	Small (or normal) aorta; increased pulmonary vascularity; enlarged right ventricle, pulmonary outflow tract, and left atrium.	Shunting of blood away from the left side of the heart into the pulmonary circulation causes decreased flow through the aorta.
Infantile type of coarctation of aorta	Small (or normal) aorta; pulmonary venous congestion; cardiomegaly (biventricular but more prominent on the right).	Narrowing of a long segment of aorta proximal to the ductus arteriosus. Always a patent ductus arteriosus and often a ventricular septal defect to deliver blood from the pulmonary artery to the descending aorta and the systemic circulation. No rib notching, internal mammary collaterals, or figure-3 or figure-E signs.
Mitral stenosis	Small aorta; enlarged left atrium and increased pulmonary venous congestion; eventual enlargement of the right ventricle, pulmonary outflow tract, and central pulmonary arteries.	Decreased left ventricular output causes diminished aortic blood flow.
Decreased cardiac output	Small aorta; various patterns of heart size; usually pulmonary venous congestion, pleural effusion, and prominence of the superior vena cava.	Gross cardiomegaly in endocardial fibroelastosis and the cardiomyopathies. Normal-sized or small heart with characteristic calcification in chronic constrictive pericarditis.
Endocardial cushion defect	Nonspecific globular enlargement of the heart with increased pulmonary vascularity.	Atrial and ventricular septal defects cause shunting of blood away from the left side of the heart into the pulmonary circulation and thus decreased flow through the aorta.
Hypoplastic left heart syndrome	Small aorta; globular cardiomegaly with severe pulmonary venous congestion.	Underdevelopment of the left side of the heart is related to an obstructive lesion that causes decreased aortic blood flow.
Supravalvular aortic stenosis (Fig CA 10-1)	Aortic knob is often small.	Underdevelopment and stenosis of the supravalvular portion of the aorta. Different from the poststenotic aortic dilation that occurs with valvular aortic stenosis.
Transposition of great vessels (Fig CA 10-2)	Narrowing of the vascular pedicle on frontal projection.	Caused by superimposition of the abnormally positioned aorta and pulmonary artery combined with absence of the normal thymic tissue because of stress atrophy. Widening of the vascular pedicle on lateral projection (due to the anterior position of the aorta with reference to the pulmonary artery).

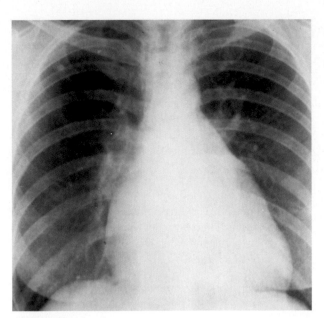

Fig CA 10-1
Congenital aortic stenosis. Small aortic arch with moderate enlargement of the left ventricle.[9]

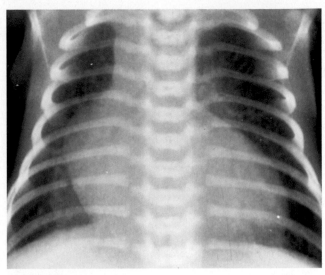

Fig CA 10-2
Transposition of great vessels. Typical oval or egg-shaped heart with a small aortic arch due to narrowing of the vascular pedicle resulting from superimposition of the abnormally positioned aorta and pulmonary artery.

Major Anomalies of the Aortic Arch and Pulmonary Artery

Condition	Imaging Findings	Comments
Right aortic arch		
Mirror-image pattern (see Fig CA 12-1)	No indentation on the barium-filled esophagus on lateral projection.	No vessel crosses the mediastinum posterior to the esophagus. Frequently associated with congenital heart disease (tetralogy of Fallot, truncus and pseudotruncus, tricuspid atresia, and transposition).
Aberrant left subclavian artery (Fig CA 11-1)	Characteristic oblique posterior indentation on the barium-filled esophagus.	Left subclavian artery arises as the most distal branch of the aorta and courses across the mediastinum posterior to the esophagus to reach the left upper extremity. No associated congenital heart disease.
Isolated left subclavian artery	No esophageal impression.	Left subclavian artery is atretic at its base (totally isolated from the aorta) and receives its blood supply from the left pulmonary artery or via the ipsilateral vertebral artery (congenital subclavian steal syndrome).
Right aortic arch with left descending aorta	Prominent indentation on the posterior wall of the barium-filled esophagus.	Transverse portion of the aorta must cross the mediastinum (posterior to the esophagus) so that the aorta descends on the left.
Cervical aortic arch (Fig CA 11-2)	Posterior impression on the esophagus (caused by the distal arch or the proximal descending aorta).	Ascending aorta extends higher than usual so that the aortic arch is in the neck. Pulsatile mass above the clavicle simulates an aneurysm. No associated congenital heart disease.

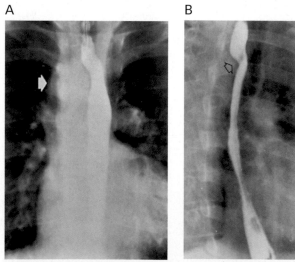

Fig CA 11-1
Right aortic arch with aberrant left subclavian artery.
(A) Frontal view from an esophagram demonstrates the right aortic arch (arrow). (B) Oblique posterior impression on the esophagus (arrow) represents the aberrant left subclavian artery as it courses to reach the left upper extremity.

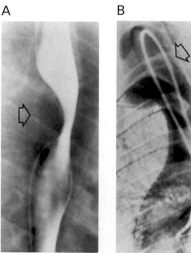
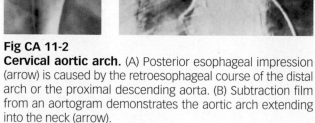

Fig CA 11-2
Cervical aortic arch. (A) Posterior esophageal impression (arrow) is caused by the retroesophageal course of the distal arch or the proximal descending aorta. (B) Subtraction film from an aortogram demonstrates the aortic arch extending into the neck (arrow).

Condition	Imaging Findings	Comments
Double aortic arch (Fig CA 11-3)	Bulges on both sides of the superior mediastinum (the right is usually larger and higher than the left). Reverse S-shaped indentation on the barium-filled esophagus.	In most patients, the aorta ascends on the right, branches, and finally reunites on the left. The two limbs of the aorta completely encircle the trachea and the esophagus, forming a ring.
Aberrant right subclavian artery (Fig CA 11-4)	Posterior esophageal indentation on lateral views. On frontal views, characteristic impression running obliquely upward and to the right.	Arises as the last major vessel of the aortic arch (just distal to the left subclavian) and must course across the mediastinum behind the esophagus to reach the right upper extremity. No associated congenital heart disease.
Aberrant left pulmonary artery (pulmonary sling) (Fig CA 11-5)	Typical impression on the posterior aspect of the trachea just above the carina and a corresponding indentation on the anterior wall of the barium-filled esophagus.	Aberrant left pulmonary artery arises from the right pulmonary artery and must cross the mediastinum (between the trachea and the esophagus) to reach the left lung.

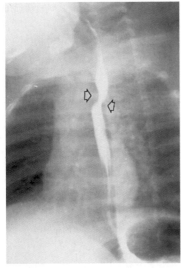

Fig CA 11-3
Double aortic arch. Characteristic reverse S-shaped indentation on the esophagus (arrows). As usual, the right (posterior) arch is higher and larger than the left (anterior) arch.[6]

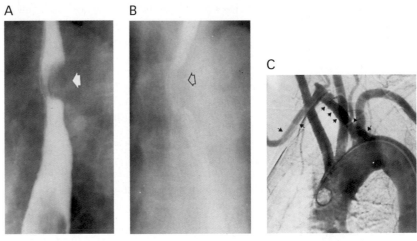

Fig CA 11-4
Aberrant right subclavian artery. (A) Lateral view from an esophagram demonstrates a posterior esophageal impression (arrow). (B) On a frontal view, the esophageal impression (arrow) runs obliquely upward and to the right. (C) Subtraction film from an arteriogram shows the aberrant vessel (arrows) arising distal to the left subclavian artery.

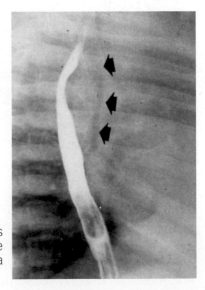

Fig CA 11-5
Aberrant left pulmonary artery. Lateral esophagram demonstrates the characteristic indentation of the anterior wall of the esophagus. Note the posterior impression and anterior displacement of the trachea (arrows) caused by the aberrant artery.[11]

Congenital Heart Disease Associated with the Right Aortic Arch (Mirror-Image Branching)

Condition	Imaging Findings	Comments
Pseudotruncus arteriosus	Decreased pulmonary vascularity; flat or concave pulmonary outflow tract; enlargement of the right ventricle.	Right aortic arch in approximately 40% of cases. Single vessel arising from the heart is accompanied by a remnant of the atretic pulmonary artery (essentially the same as tetralogy of Fallot with pulmonary atresia).
Tetralogy of Fallot	Decreased pulmonary vascularity; flat or concave pulmonary outflow tract; enlargement of the right ventricle.	Right aortic arch in approximately 25% of cases. Consists of (1) high ventricular septal defect, (2) obstruction to right ventricular outflow (usually infundibular pulmonary stenosis), (3) overriding of the aortic orifice above the ventricular defect, and (4) right ventricular hypertrophy.
Persistent truncus arteriosus (Fig CA 12-1)	Increased pulmonary vascularity; concave pulmonary outflow tract; striking enlargement of the right ventricle and eventual enlargement of the left atrium and left ventricle.	Right aortic arch in approximately 25% of cases. Failure of the common truncus arteriosus to divide normally into the aorta and the pulmonary artery results in a single large arterial trunk that receives the outflow from both ventricles.
Tricuspid atresia	Decreased pulmonary vascularity; striking enlargement of the right atrium if small atrial shunt; large left ventricle; small right ventricle.	Right aortic arch in approximately 5% of cases. An obligatory right-to-left shunt at the atrial level (there may also be a ventricular septal defect or patent ductus arteriosus). Hypoplasia of the right ventricle and pulmonary outflow tract.
Transposition of great vessels	Increased pulmonary vascularity; generally biventricular enlargement (oval or egg-shaped configuration); narrowed vascular pedicle.	Right aortic arch in approximately 5% of cases. Reverse of the normal relation of the aorta and the pulmonary artery (the aorta arises anteriorly from the right ventricle and the pulmonary artery originates posteriorly from the left ventricle).

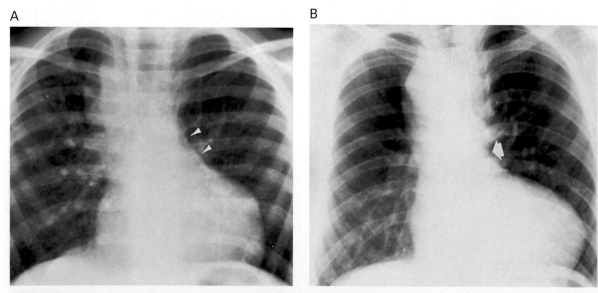

A   B

Fig CA 12-1
Persistent truncus arteriosus. Two patients with the characteristic concave appearance of the pulmonary outflow tract (arrowheads, arrow) associated with a right aortic arch.

Dilatation of the Main Pulmonary Artery

Condition	Imaging Findings	Comments
Normal variant (Fig CA 13-1)	Isolated prominence of pulmonary artery segment; normal pulmonary vascularity; no associated cardiac abnormality.	Common appearance in adolescents and adults younger than 30 years of age (especially women).
Congestive heart failure	Cardiomegaly with evidence of pulmonary venous congestion. Often pleural effusion and Kerley's lines.	Failure of the left side of the heart leads to increased blood volume in the pulmonary circulation.
High-output heart disease (Fig CA 13-2)	Cardiomegaly with prominent pulmonary vascularity (both arteries and veins).	Anemia; thyrotoxicosis; beriberi; hypovolemia (fluid overload, overtransfusion); peripheral arteriovenous fistulas; Paget's disease; Pickwickian obesity; polycythemia vera; pregnancy.
Cor pulmonale (Figs CA 13-3 and CA 13-4)	Enlargement of the main and hilar pulmonary arteries with rapid tapering and small peripheral vessels. Initially normal heart size, then right ventricular enlargement, and eventually distention of the superior vena cava.	Caused by diffuse lung disease (obstructive emphysema, interstitial fibrosis); diffuse pulmonary arterial disease (thromboembolism, arteritis, primary pulmonary hypertension); chronic heart disease (reversed left-to-right shunt, left ventricular failure, mitral valve disease); and chronic hypoxia (chest deformity, neuromuscular disease, Pickwickian obesity, high-altitude dwelling).

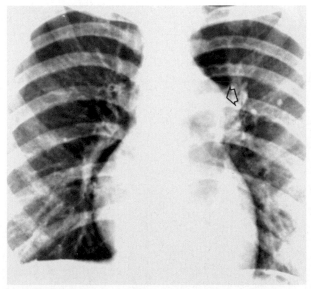

Fig CA 13-1
Idiopathic dilatation of the pulmonary artery. Plain chest radiograph in a normal young woman demonstrates prominence of the pulmonary artery (arrow) that simulates the poststenotic dilatation associated with pulmonary valvular stenosis.

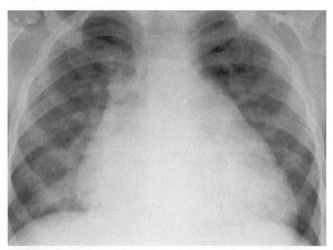

Fig CA 13-2
Thyrotoxicosis. Generalized cardiomegaly with increased pulmonary vascularity.

A

B

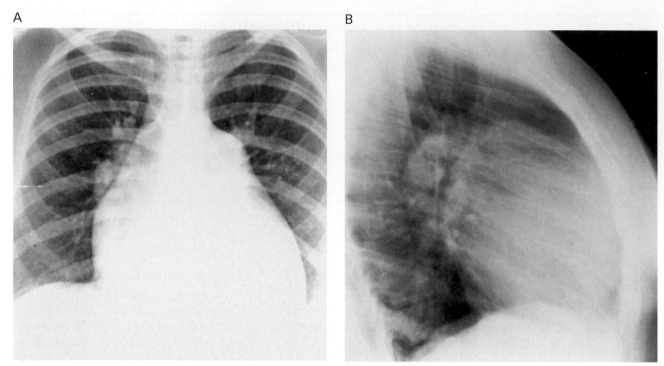

Fig CA 13-3
Cor pulmonale (primary pulmonary hypertension). (A) Frontal and (B) lateral views of the chest show prominence of the pulmonary outflow tract and markedly dilated central pulmonary vessels. The lateral displacement of the cardiac apex and filling of the retrosternal air space indicate right ventricular enlargement.

A

B

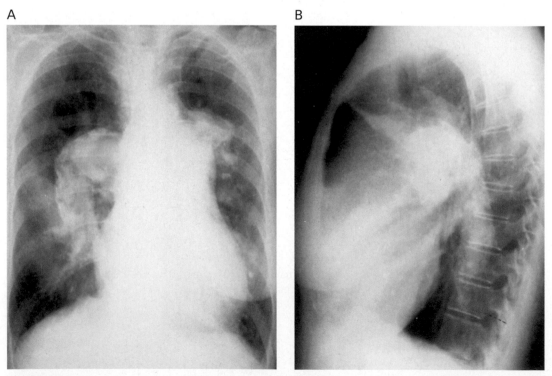

Fig CA 13-4
Eisenmenger syndrome in atrial septal defect. (A) Frontal and (B) lateral films demonstrate slight but definite cardiomegaly and a great increase in the size of the pulmonary trunk. The right and left pulmonary artery branches are huge, but the peripheral pulmonary vasculature is relatively sparse. Long-standing pulmonary hypertension has produced degenerative intimal changes in the pulmonary arteries, which have become densely calcified.[1]

Condition	Imaging Findings	Comments
Left-to-right shunt (Fig CA 13-5)	Various patterns, depending on the level and extent of the shunt.	Most commonly atrial septal defect, ventricular septal defect, or patent ductus arteriosus.
Pulmonary thromboembolic disease (see Fig C 10-4)	Enlargement of the main pulmonary artery segment.	Caused by pulmonary hypertension or distention of the vessel by bulk thrombus. This sign is primarily of value when serial radiographs demonstrate progressive enlargement.
Pulmonary valvular stenosis (Fig CA 13-6)	Prominence of the main pulmonary artery segment.	Common anomaly with poststenotic dilatation of the left pulmonary artery (central dilatation of the right pulmonary artery, but the dilated segment is hidden in the mediastinum).
Mitral stenosis or insufficiency	Enlargement of the left atrium and right ventricle; normal-sized left ventricle and small aortic arch; pulmonary vascular congestion.	Obstruction of flow from the left atrium to the left ventricle during diastole results in increased pressure and enlargement of the left atrium. The increased pressure is transmitted to the pulmonary veins and eventually to the pulmonary arteries and the right side of the heart. Usually caused by rheumatic valvular lesion; also by congenital mitral stenosis and the parachute deformity (all chordae tendineae originating from a single papillary muscle). There is a similar mechanism in the hypoplastic left heart syndrome and a large left atrial myxoma.

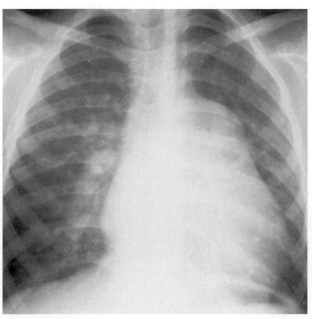

Fig CA 13-5
Ventricular septal defect. The pulmonary trunk is very large and overshadows the normal-sized aorta, which seems small by comparison. The pulmonary artery branches in the hilum and in the periphery of the lung are enlarged, and the pulmonary vascular volume is increased. The heart is enlarged and somewhat triangular.[1]

Condition	Imaging Findings	Comments
Partial anomalous pulmonary venous return (see Fig CA 7-8)	Increased pulmonary vascularity; enlarged right atrium, right ventricle, and main pulmonary artery segment; normal left atrium and left ventricle; small aorta.	One or more pulmonary veins connected to the right atrium or its tributaries. Virtually indistinguishable from an atrial septal defect radiographically. Scimitar sign (crescent-shaped anomalous venous channel) on the right if associated with hypoplasia of the right lung.
Trilogy of Fallot (Fig CA 13-7)	Poststenotic dilatation of the pulmonary artery; decreased pulmonary vascularity; heart size often normal (usually some evidence of right ventricular hypertrophy).	Combination of pulmonary valvular stenosis with an intact ventricular septum and an interatrial shunt (patent foramen ovale or true atrial septal defect). Increased pressure on the right side of the heart due to pulmonary stenosis causes the interatrial shunt to be right to left (patient is cyanotic).
Tricuspid atresia without pulmonary stenosis	Marked cardiomegaly and increased pulmonary vascularity.	May be associated with transposition of the great vessels.
Total anomalous pulmonary venous return (see Fig CA 5-9)	Increased pulmonary vascularity and enlarged main pulmonary artery segment; various patterns and characteristic "snowman," or figure-8, sign.	All pulmonary veins connect to the right atrium directly or to the systemic veins or their tributaries. Because all pulmonary venous blood returns to the right atrium, a right-to-left shunt through an interatrial communication is necessary for blood to reach the left side of the heart and the systemic circulation.

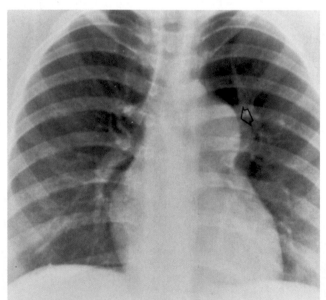

Fig CA 13-6
Pulmonary valvular stenosis. Severe poststenotic dilatation of the pulmonary outflow tract (arrow). The heart size and pulmonary vascularity remain within normal limits.

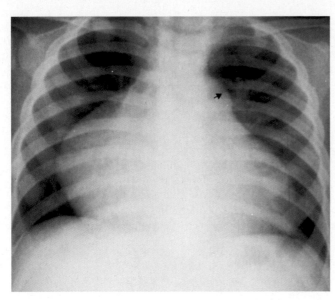

Fig CA 13-7
Trilogy of Fallot. Marked poststenotic dilatation (arrow) of the pulmonary artery with decrease in overall pulmonary vascularity. There is enormous right atrial and moderate right ventricular enlargement.[6]

Dilatation of the Superior Vena Cava*

Condition	Comments
Increased central venous pressure (Fig CA 14-1)	In the great majority of cases, this pattern is caused by congestive heart failure or by cardiac tamponade due to pericardial effusion or constrictive pericarditis.
Intrathoracic neoplasm (Figs CA 14-2 to CA 14-4)	There is often an associated soft-tissue mass. Primarily bronchogenic carcinoma (especially oat cell carcinoma), but also tumors of the esophagus and the mediastinum.

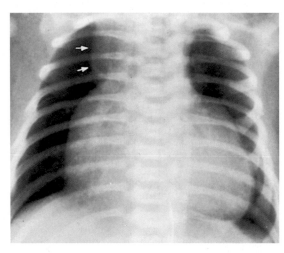

Fig CA 14-1
Right ventricular failure. Plain chest radiograph in a patient with Ebstein's anomaly shows widening of the right side of the superior portion of the mediastinum (arrows), reflecting marked dilatation of the superior vena cava. There is enlargement of the right atrium, causing upward and outward bulging of the right border of the heart (squared appearance).

A   B

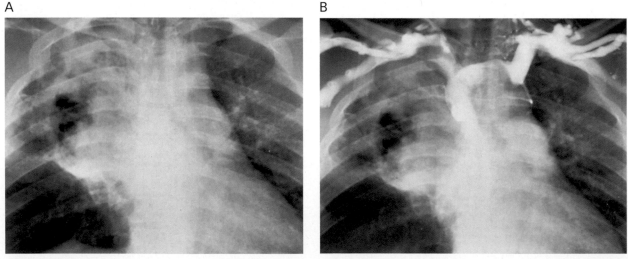

Fig CA 14-2
Bronchogenic carcinoma. (A) Frontal view of the chest shows a bulky, irregular mass filling much of the right upper lobe. (B) Bilateral upper extremity venograms show almost complete occlusion of the superior vena cava by the large malignant neoplasm.

*Pattern: Smooth, well-defined widening of the right side of the upper half of the mediastinum.

Condition	Comments
Renal artery stenosis (Fig CA 18-2)	Most commonly due to arteriosclerotic narrowing that tends to occur in the proximal portion of the vessel close to its origin from the aorta. Poststenotic dilatation is common. Bilateral renal artery stenoses are noted in up to one-third of the patients. At times, renal artery stenosis may be detected only on oblique projections that demonstrate the vessel origins in profile.
Fibromuscular hyperplasia (Fig CA 18-3)	Characteristic "string-of-beads" pattern, in which there are alternating areas of narrowing and dilatation (representing microaneurysms). Smooth, concentric stenoses occur less frequently. Most commonly affects young women and is often bilateral.
Perirenal hematoma (Page kidney)	Dense fibrous encasement of the kidney after healing of a subcapsular or perirenal hematoma compresses the renal parenchyma and causes an alteration of the intrarenal hemodynamics that produces ischemia and hypertension. The kidney is often enlarged and demonstrates a mass effect with distortion of the collecting system. Arteriography reveals splaying and stretching of the intrarenal arteries and often irregular staining in the healing portion of the hematoma. Removal of the kidney or evacuation of the offending mass may result in clearing of the hypertension.
Renal parenchymal disease	Causes include glomerulonephritis, chronic pyelonephritis, polycystic kidney, renal tumor, and renal agenesis or hypoplasia.

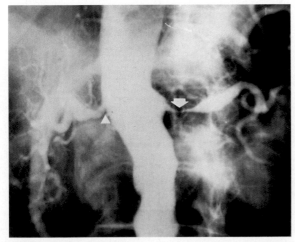

Fig CA 18-2
Renovascular hypertension. Bilateral arteriosclerotic renal artery stenoses (arrowhead, arrow).

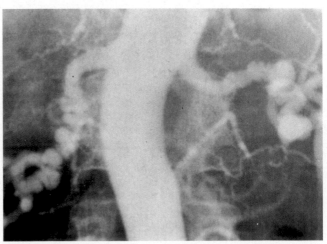

Fig CA 18-3
Renovascular hypertension. String-of-beads pattern of fibromuscular dysplasia bilaterally.

Condition	Comments
Coarctation of aorta (see Fig CA 8-1)	Suggestive radiographic findings include inordinate dilatation of the ascending aorta, widening of the left superior mediastinum, the figure-E or figure-3 sign, and rib notching.
Adrenal disease	Causes include Cushing's syndrome (suggested by widening of the superior mediastinum due to increased fat deposition associated with osteoporosis and compression changes in the dorsal vertebrae), pheochromocytoma (may produce a paravertebral mass), adrenocortical adenoma, carcinoma, primary aldosteronism, and the adrenogenital syndrome.
Other endocrine disorders	Hyperthyroidism, acromegaly, and the use of estrogen-containing oral contraceptives (this may be the most common form of secondary hypertension).
Collagen disease	Systemic lupus erythematosus; polyarteritis nodosa.
Neurogenic	Dysautonomia (familial autonomic dysfunction; Riley-Day syndrome); psychogenic.

Cardiovascular Calcification

Condition	Comments
Aortic wall Arteriosclerosis (Fig CA 19-1)	Elongation and tortuosity of the aorta with linear plaques of calcification that most commonly occur in the aortic knob and transverse arch. In severe disease, the entire aorta may be outlined by extensive calcification in its wall.
Aneurysm	An increased diameter of the aorta indicates an aneurysm, whereas an increased distance between intimal calcification and the outer wall of the aorta suggests a dissection.
Aortitis (Fig CA 19-2)	Dilatation and prominence of the ascending aorta with thin, curvilinear streaks of calcification (often extensive) is characteristic of syphilitic aortitis; linear calcification also frequently occurs in patients with Takayasu's aortitis ("pulseless" disease), a nonspecific obstructive arteritis that primarily affects young women.
Valvular/annulus Aortic annulus or valve (Fig CA 19-3)	Calcification of the annulus tends to be heavy and distinct, unlike valvular calcification, which is usually stippled and often not detected on plain radiographs (best demonstrated on fluoroscopic examination). Causes include arteriosclerosis, rheumatic aortic valve disease, infective endocarditis, and a congenital defect of the aortic valve.

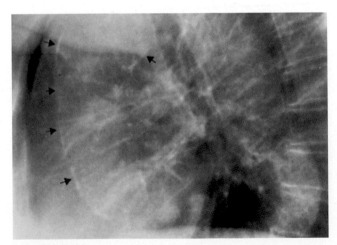

Fig CA 19-1
Arteriosclerosis. Lateral view of the chest demonstrates calcification of the anterior and posterior walls of the ascending aorta (arrows). The descending thoracic aorta is tortuous.

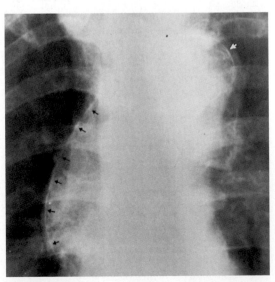

Fig CA 19-2
Syphilitic aortitis. Aneurysmal dilatation of the ascending aorta with extensive linear calcification of the wall (black arrows). Some calcification is also seen in the distal aortic arch (white arrow).

Condition	Comments
Mitral valve	Develops in patients with long-standing severe mitral stenosis and is often indistinct and easily missed on plain radiographs (best demonstrated by fluoroscopy). The amount of calcification does not reflect the degree of functional disturbance. Multiple calcific or ossific nodules throughout the lower portions of the lungs may develop in areas of chronic interstitial edema.
Mitral annulus (Fig CA 19-4)	Dense curved or annular calcified band around the mitral valve that usually reflects underlying arteriosclerosis. Although usually insignificant, a rigid annulus may cause functional insufficiency of the mitral valve.

A

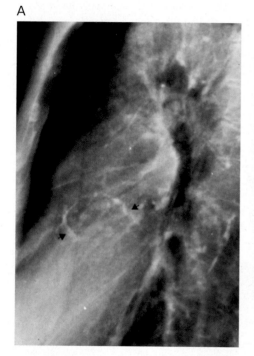

B

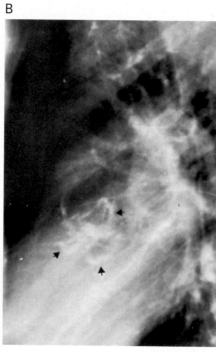

Fig CA 19-3
Aortic stenosis. Calcification in (A) the aortic annulus (arrows) and (B) the three leaflets of the aortic valve (arrows).

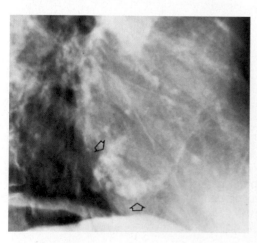

Fig CA 19-4
Mitral annulus calcification (arrows) in mitral stenosis.

Condition	Comments
Coronary artery (Fig CA 19-5)	Punctate, patchy, or tubular densities that primarily involve the circumflex and anterior descending branches of the left coronary artery and are most commonly seen along the left margin of the heart below the pulmonary artery segment. Although infrequently visualized on routine chest radiographs, calcification of a coronary artery strongly suggests the presence of hemodynamically significant arteriosclerotic coronary artery disease. Cardiac fluoroscopy is far more sensitive than plain chest radiography in demonstrating coronary artery calcification, though there is controversy about the prognostic significance of fluoroscopically identified coronary artery calcification in patients with ischemic heart disease. In patients younger than 50 years of age, coronary artery calcification is a strong predictor of major narrowing in women and a moderate predictor in men. In older patients, calcification has less predictive value.
Sinus of Valsalva	Calcification primarily involves the wall of an aortic sinus aneurysm and is usually best seen on the lateral view.
Left atrium (Figs CA 19-6 and CA 19-7)	Calcification of the left atrial wall usually reflects long-standing severe mitral stenosis and appears as a thin curvilinear rim. Atrial myxomas calcify in approximately 10% of cases and are best seen by fluoroscopy (may present the pathognomonic appearance of a calcified mass prolapsing into the ventricle during systole). Calcification in the left atrial appendage represents a calcified thrombus.
Ventricular aneurysm (Fig CA 19-8)	Complication of myocardial infarction in which weakening of the myocardial wall permits the development of a local bulge at the site of the infarct. Curvilinear calcification in the wall of an aneurysm is an infrequent but important finding.

A   B

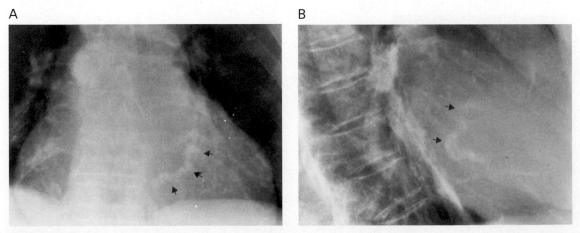

Fig CA 19-5
Coronary artery calcification (arrows) in ischemic heart disease. (A) Frontal and (B) lateral views of the chest.

Condition	Comments
Myocardium	Most commonly a manifestation of an old myocardial infarct. Rare causes include myocardial damage (trauma, myocarditis, and rheumatic fever), hyperparathyroidism, and vitamin D toxicity.
Pericardium (Fig CA 19-9)	Calcific plaques in a thickened pericardium are present in approximately half of patients with constrictive pericarditis. Though the heaviest deposits of calcium are located anteriorly, posterior calcification and calcification of the pericardium adjacent to the diaphragm can often be seen. At times, the heart appears to be encased in a virtually pathognomonic calcific shell.
Ductus arteriosus (Fig CA 19-10)	Calcification mimicking involvement of the aortic wall may rarely occur in patients with a patent or a closed ductus arteriosus.

A

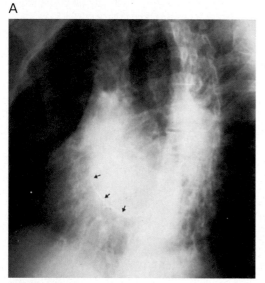

B

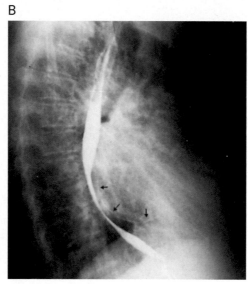

Fig CA 19-6
Left atrial calcification. (A) Overpenetrated film in the left anterior oblique position and (B) lateral view with barium in the esophagus show enlargement of the left atrium and calcification of the wall of this chamber (arrows) in a patient with mitral stenosis.[12]

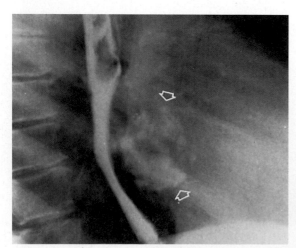

Fig CA 19-7
Left atrial myxoma. The arrows point to calcification in the tumor. The myxoma has led to destruction of the mitral valve with resulting left atrial enlargement that causes an impression on the barium-filled esophagus.

A

B

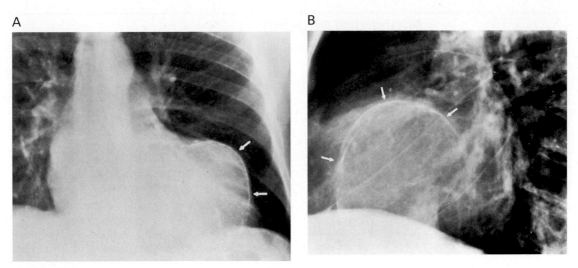

Fig CA 19-8
Ventricular aneurysm. (A) Frontal and (B) lateral views of the chest demonstrate bulging and curvilinear peripheral calcification (arrows) along the lower left border of the heart near the apex. Note the relatively anterior position of the aneurysm on the lateral view.

A

B

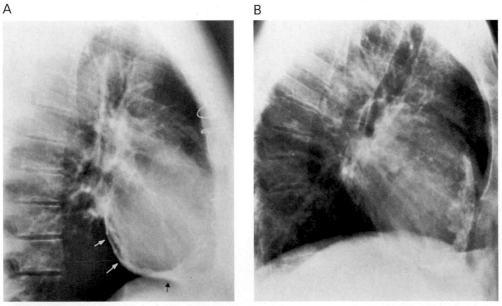

Fig CA 19-9
Pericardial calcification (A and B). Lateral views of the chest demonstrate dense plaques of pericardial calcification (arrows) in two patients with chronic constrictive pericarditis due to tuberculosis.

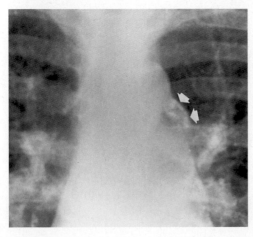

Fig CA 19-10
Ductus arteriosus calcification (arrows).

Pericardial Effusion

Condition	Comments
Congestive heart failure	Evidence of pulmonary venous congestion. An associated pleural effusion is common (frequently unilateral on the right, rarely on the left; may be bilateral).
Collagen disease (see Fig CA 34-9)	Systemic lupus erythematosus; scleroderma; polyarteritis nodosa; rheumatoid disease. There may be unilateral or bilateral pleural effusion (especially in lupus). Generalized reticulonodular disease (more prominent in the lung bases) may occur.
Infectious pericarditis (Fig CA 20-1)	Most commonly coxsackievirus. Also other infections (eg, bacterial, tuberculous, histoplasmic, amebic, toxoplasmic).
Postcardiac surgery	Accumulation of fluid after pericardiotomy. Evidence of surgical clips and sutures.
Postmyocardial infarction syndrome (Dressler's syndrome) (Fig CA 20-2)	Autoimmune phenomenon characterized by fever and pleuropericardial chest pain beginning 1 to 6 weeks after an acute myocardial infarction. Other manifestations include pleural effusion that is bilateral in 50% of patients (usually greater on the left) and an ill-defined pneumonia (often with atelectatic streaks) that may be bilateral or involve only the left base.

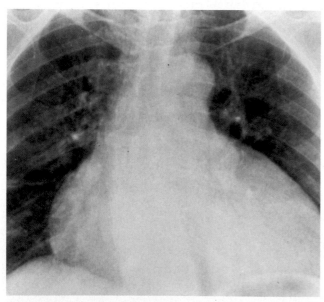

Fig CA 20-1
Infectious pericarditis. Globular enlargement of the cardiac silhouette reflects a combination of pericarditis and pericardial effusion in a patient with coxsackievirus infection. There are small pleural effusions bilaterally.

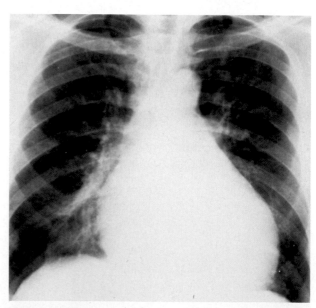

Fig CA 20-2
Dressler's syndrome. Chest film obtained 3 weeks after an acute myocardial infarction demonstrates a large pericardial effusion appearing as a rapid increase in heart size in comparison with an essentially normal-sized heart 1 week earlier.

Condition	Comments
Trauma	Rapid development of a pericardial effusion may produce severe alteration of cardiac function with minimal change in the radiographic cardiac silhouette.
Tumor of pericardium or heart	Direct invasion from carcinoma of the lung or mediastinal lymphoma, or metastases from melanoma or tumors of the lung or breast. Radiation therapy may produce complete (but usually temporary) resolution of the fluid.
Uremia (Fig CA 20-3)	Develops in approximately 15% of patients on prolonged hemodialysis. May collect rapidly and be life threatening.

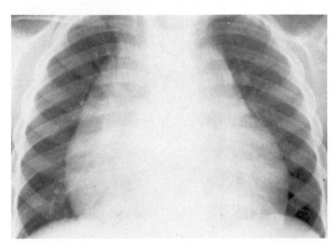

Fig CA 20-3
Uremia. Globular enlargement of the cardiac silhouette in a child on prolonged hemodialysis.

A   B

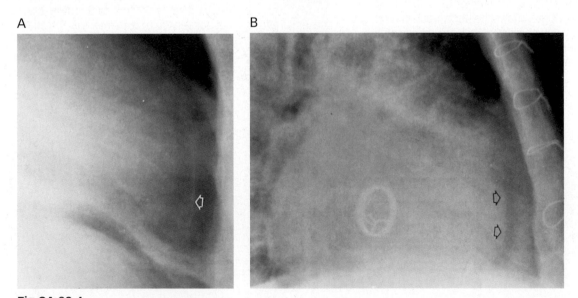

Fig CA 20-4
Epicardial fat pad sign in pericardial effusion. (A) In a normal person, a thin, relatively dense line (arrow) representing the normal pericardium lies between the anterior mediastinal and subepicardial fat. (B) Lateral chest radiograph demonstrates a wide soft-tissue density separating the subepicardial fat stripe (arrows) from the anterior mediastinal fat. This is a virtually pathognomonic sign of pericardial effusion or thickening.

Condition	Comments
Radiation therapy	May follow the use of moderately high doses (4000 rads in 4 to 5 weeks, as in the treatment of Hodgkin's disease or breast carcinoma).
Myxedema	May cause massive chronic pericardial effusion (rarely tamponade).
Bleeding diathesis	Severe chronic anemia; erythroblastosis fetalis; excessive anticoagulant therapy.
Idiopathic	Diagnosis of exclusion for acute pericardial effusion.

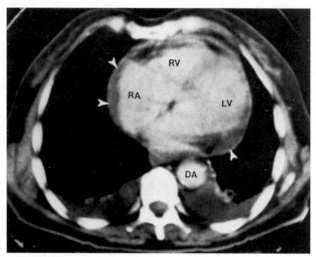

Fig CA 20-5
Pericardial effusion. CT scan made after the injection of intravenous contrast material shows the pericardial effusion as a low-density area (arrowheads) that is clearly demarcated from the contrast-enhanced blood in the intracardiac chambers and descending aorta. Note the bilateral pleural effusions posteriorly. (DA, descending aorta; LV, left ventricle; RA, right atrium; RV, right ventricle.)[13]

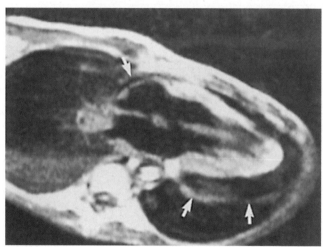

Fig CA 20-6
Pericardial effusion. MRI scan shows the pericardium (arrows) to be displaced away from the heart by a huge pericardial effusion that has very little signal intensity. The effect of gravity is seen in the posterior location of both the pericardial and the right pleural effusions.[14]

Constrictive Pericarditis

Condition	Comments
Tuberculosis (Figs CA 21-1 and CA 21-2)	Etiologic agent in up to one-third of older series. Now an infrequent cause.
Other infections	Pyogenic (especially staphylococcal or pneumococcal); histoplasmosis; viral (especially coxsackie B).
Radiation therapy	May follow the use of moderately high doses (4000 rads in 4 to 5 weeks, as for the treatment of Hodgkin's disease or carcinoma of the breast).
Uremia	Relatively high incidence in patients on prolonged hemodialysis.
Trauma	Hemopericardium leading to dense fibrosis.
Idiopathic	Underlying cause of pericardial disease is often undetermined. Probably represents an asymptomatic or forgotten bout of acute pericarditis.

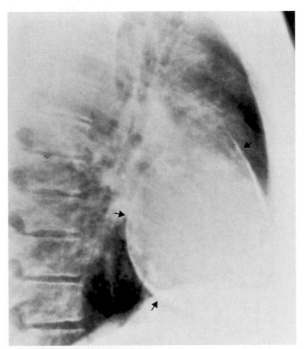

Fig CA 21-1
Chronic constrictive pericarditis. Dense calcification in the pericardium (arrows) completely surrounding a normal-sized heart.

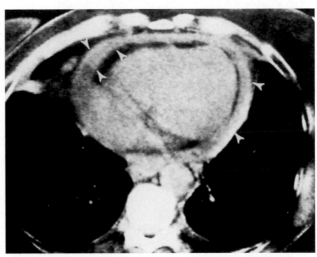

Fig CA 21-2
Chronic constrictive pericarditis. CT scan performed during an infusion of contrast material shows enhancement of the soft-tissue-density pericardium (arrowheads), which is up to 6 mm thick.[13]

Pericardial Disease on Computed Tomography and Magnetic Resonance Imaging

Condition	Imaging Findings	Comments
Pericardial effusion (Figs CA 22-1 to CA 22-4)	On CT, a simple pericardial effusion has attenuation close to that of water. A higher attenuation suggests malignancy, hemopericardium, purulent exudates, or an effusion associated with hypothyroidism. Low attenuation effusions have been reported with chylopericardium. On MRI, the intensity of nonhemorrhagic pericardial effusion is low on T1-weighted images and high on GRE images. The appearance is reversed with hemorrhagic pericardial effusions, which have high signal intensity of T1-weighted images and low intensity on GRE images. Malignant effusions may be associated with an irregularly thickened pericardium of pericardial nodularity.	Develops from obstruction of the venous or lymphatic drainage of the heart secondary to heart failure, renal insufficiency, infection (bacterial, viral, or tuberculosis), neoplasm (carcinoma of lung or breast, or lymphoma), or injury (trauma or myocardial infarction). Although echocardiography is considered the primary imaging modality, both CT and MRI can help characterize the underlying abnormality as well as provide a wider field of view that enables detection of associated abnormalities in the mediastinum and lungs.

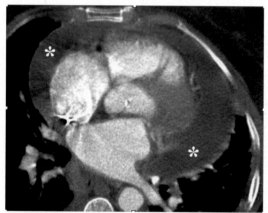

Fig CA 22-1
Pericardial effusion (simple). Contrast CT scan shows an effusion (*) with the same attenuation as water.[15]

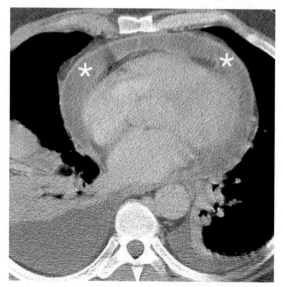

Fig CA 22-2
Pericardial effusion (serosanguinous). Contrast CT scan shows a moderate-sized enhancing effusion (*).[15]

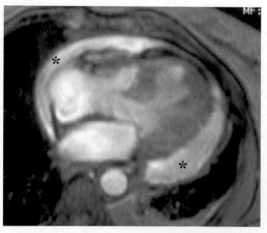

Fig CA 22-3
Pericardial effusion (nonhemorrhagic). Cine GRE image shows a high-signal-intensity effusion (*), consistent with nonhemorrhagic fluid.[15]

Condition	Imaging Findings	Comments
Constrictive pericarditis (Figs CA 22-5 to CA 22-7)	Pericardial thickness of 4 mm or more is abnormal and, when accompanied by clinical findings of heart failure, is highly suggestive of constrictive pericarditis. CT is exquisitely sensitive for detecting pericardial calcification, which is also associated with constrictive pericarditis.	Most frequent causes are cardiac surgery and radiation therapy. Less common etiologies include infection (viral or tuberculous), connective tissue disease, uremia, and neoplasm. The demonstration of pericardial thickening on CT and MRI can aid in making the critical distinction between constrictive pericarditis and restrictive cardiomyopathy, which have similar clinical manifestations and findings on cardiac catheterization and echocardiography.

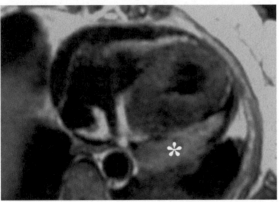

Fig CA 22-4
Pericardial effusion (hemorrhagic). Axial T1-weighted MR image shows an effusion with high signal intensity (*), suggestive of hemorrhage.[15]

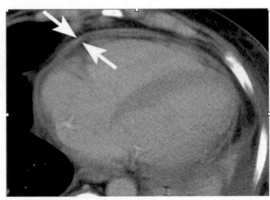

Fig CA 22-5
Constrictive pericarditis. Contrast CT scan shows pericardial thickening (arrows) in this patient, who presented with symptoms of heart failure after mediastinal irradiation for Hodgkin's lymphoma.[15]

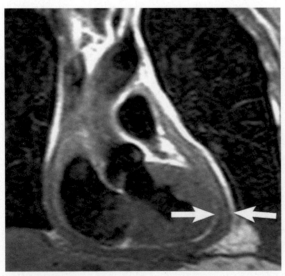

Fig CA 22-6
Constrictive pericarditis. Coronal T1-weighted MR image shows abnormally thickened pericardium (arrows) outlined by epicardial and mediastinal fat.[15]

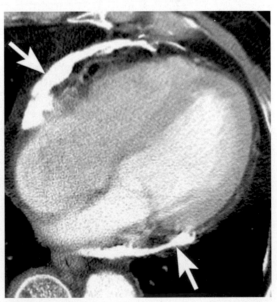

Fig CA 22-7
Constrictive pericarditis. Contrast CT shows dense pericardial calcification (arrows) in a patient with a history of hemopericardium.[15]

Condition	Imaging Findings	Comments
Pericarditis without constriction (Figs CA 22-8 and CA 22-9)	Enhancement of the thickened pericardium on CT indicates inflammation. On MRI, the normal pericardium (composed primarily of fibrous tissue), as well as the purely fibrous or calcified pericardium in chronic pericardial disease, has a low signal intensity on both T1- and T2-weighted images. Thickened pericardium with moderate-to-high signal is seen in subacute pericarditis, and contrast enhancement also is a sign of pericardial inflammation.	Pericardial thickening without clinical symptoms of constrictive pericarditis can be caused by inflammation secondary to acute pericarditis, uremia, rheumatic heart disease, rheumatoid arthritis, sarcoidoisis, and mediastinal irradiation.

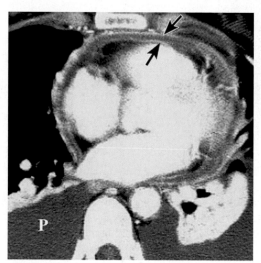

Fig CA 22-8
Infectious pericarditis. Contrast CT scan shows enhancement of the pericardium (arrows), indicative of inflammation. Note the associated small pericardial effusion and large bilateral pleural effusions (P).[15]

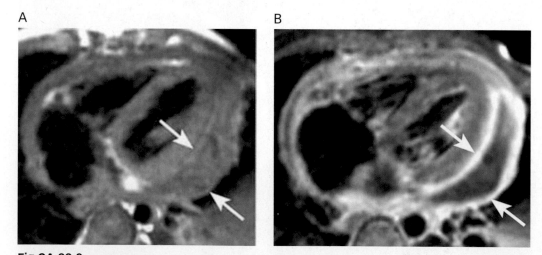

Fig CA 22-9
Infectious pericarditis. (A) T1-weighted MR image shows a crescent-shaped area of intermediate signal intensity (arrows) surrounding the ventricles, which indicates either pericardial thickening or effusion. (B) Contrast T1-weighted image with fat saturation shows marked thickening and enhancement of the pericardium (arrows), findings consistent with inflammation. There is also a moderate-sized pericardial effusion.[15]

Condition	Imaging Findings	Comments
Pericardial masses		Although pericardial masses are often detected initially with echocardiography, CT attenuation or MR signal intensity characteristics, the degree of contrast enhancement, and the presence or absence of blood flow on cine MR images can help differentiate among them.
Cysts (Figs CA 22-10 and CA 22-11)	Thin-walled structure without internal septa that typically has the attenuation and signal intensity of pure water. Occasionally, a cyst may contain highly proteinaceous fluid that produces high signal intensity on T1-weighted MR images.	Congenital pericardial cysts are formed when a portion of the pericardium is pinched off during early development. Generally found in the right cardiophrenic angle, they may occur anywhere in the mediastinum. In unusual sites, they may be indistinguishable from brochogenic or thymic cysts.

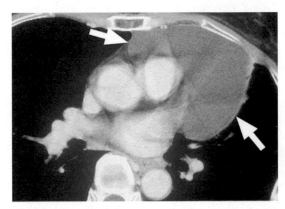

Fig CA 22-10
Pericardial cyst. Contrast CT scan shows a nonenhancing homogeneous mass (arrows) with the attenuation of water, located adjacent to the pulmonary artery.[15]

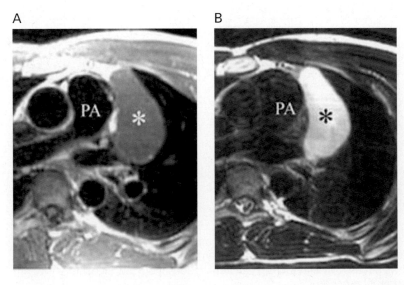

A

B

Fig CA 22-11
Pericardial cyst. (A) T1-weighted contrast MR image shows a nonenhancing mass (*) of intermediate signal intensity adjacent to the main pulmonary artery. (B) On a T2-weighted image, the mass (*) has homogeneous high signal intensity.[15]

Condition	Imaging Findings	Comments
Hematomas (Figs CA 22-12 and CA 22-13)	Acute hematomas have homogeneous high signal intensity on T1 and T2 images. Subacute hematomas (1 to 4 weeks old) typically show heterogeneous signal, with areas of hyperintensity on both these sequences. On T1-weighted and GRE images, chronic organized hematomas may show a dark peripheral rim and low-signal-intensity internal foci that may represent calcification, fibrosis, or hemosiderin deposition. High-signal areas on T1- and T2-weighted images often correspond to hemorrhagic fluid.	Coronary or ventricular pseudoaneurysms or neoplaasms may resemble hematomas on MR images. However, these entities demonstrate contrast enhancement, which is not seen with hematomas. The detection of internal flow in a pseudoaneurysm on velocity-encoded cine MR imaging also can differentiate this condition from a hematoma.

A
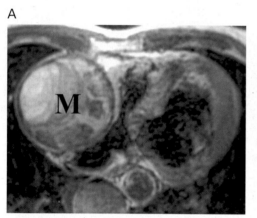

B
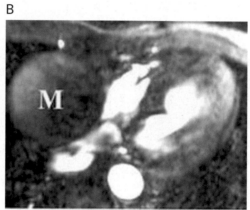

Fig CA 22-12
Pericardial hematoma. (A) T1-weighted contrast image shows a nonenhancing mass of heterogeneous signal intensity (M) in the right atrioventricular groove. (B) Phase velocity-encoded cine image shows no blood blow in the mass (M), a finding indicative of hematoma rather than pseudoaneurysm.[15]

A
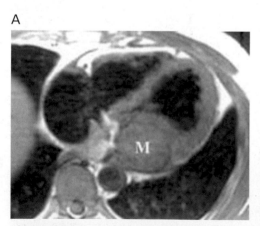

B
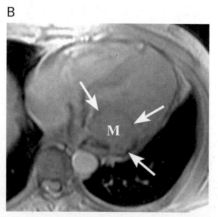

Fig CA 22-13
Pericardial hematoma (chronic, organized). (A) T1-weighted MR image in a patient who had sustained blunt chest trauma 8 years previously shows a well-circumscribed mass (M) with intermediate signal intensity in the left atrioventricular groove that compresses the left atrium and ventricle. (B) Cine GRE image shows a mass (M) with low-signal-intensity foci and a low-signal-intensity rim (arrows), which are indicative of central and peripheral calcifications.[15]

Condition	Imaging Findings	Comments
Neoplasms Metastases (Fig CA 22-14)	On CT, metastatic involvement is suggested by an irregularly thickened pericardium or pericardial mass associated with an effusion. On MRI, tumor invasion of the pericardium causes focal obliteration of the pericardial line, which remains intact if an adjacent tumor extends only up to it. Hemorrhagic pericardial effusions secondary to metastases usually have high signal intensity on all SE images. The signal intensity of most neoplasms is low on T1 and high on T2. An exception is metastatic melanoma, which may have high signal intensity on T1-weighted images because of the paramagnetic metals bound by melanin. Most metastases show significant contrast enhancement.	Pericardial metastases are much more common than primary pericardial tumors. They may seed the pericardium via the blood stream or lymphatics, or directly invade from the lung or mediastinum. Cancers of the breast and lung are the most common sources of metastases to the pericardium, followed by lymphoma and melanoma.
Primary neoplasms (Figs CA 22-15 and CA 22-16)	Lipoma typically has low attenuation on CT images and high signal intensity on T1-weighted MR images. The CT demonstration of calcium or fat in a pericardial mass suggests a teratoma. Fibroma generally has low signal intensity on T2-weighted images and shows poor or no enhancement due to poor vascularization. Mesotheliomas occasionally demonstrate pericardial nodules or plaques in addition to a pericardial effusion. Lymphoma, sarcoma, and liposarcoma typically appear as large heterogeneous masses, frequently associated with a serosanguineous effusion.	Primary pericardial neoplasms are rare. Benign tumors include lipoma, teratoma, fibroma, and hemangioma; malignant primary tumors include mesothelioma, lymphoma, sarcoma, and liposarcoma.

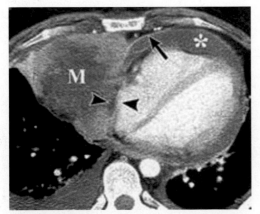

Fig CA 22-14
Metastatic lymphoma. Contrast CT scan shows a large heterogeneous anterior mediastinal mass (M) with central necrosis, which has invaded the pericardium (arrowheads). Note the moderate pericardial effusion (*) and associated enhancement of the pericardium.[15]

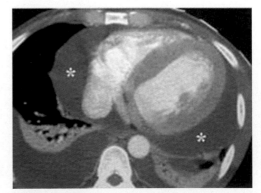

Fig CA 22-15
Primary pericardial mesothelioma. Contrast CT scan shows a large pericardial effusion (*) and no pericardial nodules (which occur in this disease but are rare).[15]

Condition	Imaging Findings	Comments
Congenital absence of the pericardium (Fig CA 22-17)	Interposition of lung tissue between the aorta and the main segment of the pulmonary artery with rotation of the heart toward the left (normally, the aorticopulmonary window is covered by pericardium and contains some fat). At times, the left atrial appendage bulges through the defect.	Congenital absence of the pericardium is rare. Most pericardial defects are partial and occur on the left.

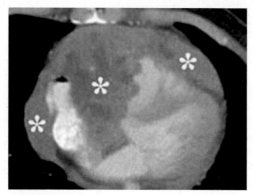

Fig CA 22-16
Primary pericardial lymphoma. Contrast CT scan shows an irregular, enhancing soft-tissue mass (*), which has infiltrated the entire pericardium.[15]

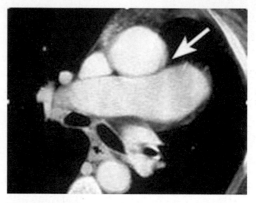

Fig CA 22-17
Congenital absence of the pericardium. Contrast CT scan shows interposition of lung tissue between the aorta and the main segment of the pulmonary artery (arrow), indicating the absence of the pericardium in this area. Note the rotation of the heart toward the left.[15]

Sources

1. Reprinted from *Radiology of the Heart and Great Vessels* by RN Cooley and MH Schreiber, Williams & Wilkins Company, ©1978, with permission of JH Harris Jr.

2. Reprinted with permission from "Transposition of the Great Arteries" by A Barcia et al, *American Journal of Roentgenology* (1967;100:249–261), Copyright ©1967, American Roentgen Ray Society.

3. Reprinted with permission from "Roentgenographic Features in a Case with Origin of Both Great Vessels from the Right Ventricle without Pulmonary Stenosis" by LS Carey and JE Edwards, *American Journal of Roentgenology* (1965;93:268–287), Copyright ©1965, American Roentgen Ray Society.

4. Reprinted with permission from "Angiocardiographic and Anatomic Findings in Origin of Both Great Arteries from the Right Ventricle" by FJ Hallerman et al, *American Journal of Roentgenology* (1970;109:51–66), Copyright ©1970, American Roentgen Ray Society.

5. Reprinted with permission from "Endocardial Cushion Defects" by MG Baron, *Radiologic Clinics of North America* (1968;6:43–52), Copyright ©1968, WB Saunders Company.

6. Reprinted from *Plain Film Interpretation in Congenital Heart Disease* by LE Swischuk with permission of Williams & Wilkins Company, ©1979.

7. Reprinted with permission from "Other Forms of Left-to-Right Shunt" by LP Elliott, *Seminars in Roentgenology* (1966;1:120–136); Copyright ©1966, Grune & Stratton Inc.

8. Reprinted with permission from "Coronary Arteriovenous Fistula" by I Steinberg and GR Holswade, *American Journal of Roentgenology* (1972;116:82–90), Copyright ©1972, American Roentgen Ray Society.

9. Reprinted with permission from "Congenital Aortic Stenosis" by FB Takekawa et al, *American Journal of Roentgenology* (1966;98:800–821), Copyright ©1966, American Roentgen Ray Society.

10. Reprinted from *Diagnostic Imaging in Internal Medicine* by RL Eisenberg with permission of McGraw-Hill Book Company, ©1985. Courtesy of Marvin Belasco, MD.

11. Reprinted with permission from "Anomalous Origin of the Left Pulmonary Artery from the Right Pulmonary Artery" by KL Jue et al, *American Journal of Roentgenology* (1965;95:598–610), Copyright ©1965, American Roentgen Ray Society.

12. Reprinted with permission from "Left Atrial Calcification" by SCW Vickers et al, *Radiology* (1959;72:569–575), Copyright ©1959, Radiological Society of North America Inc.

13. Reprinted from *Computed Body Tomography* by JKT Lee, SS Sagel, and RJ Stanley (Eds) with permission of Raven Press, New York, ©1989.

14. Reprinted with permission from "Cardiac Magnetic Resonance Imaging" by SW Miller et al, *Radiological Clinics of North America* (1985;23:745–764), Copyright ©1985, WB Saunders Company.

15. Wang ZJ, Reddy GP, Gotway MB, et al. CT and MR Imaging of Pericardial Disease. *RadioGraphics* 2003;23:S167–S180.

3

Gastrointestinal Patterns

Esophageal Motility Disorders

Condition	Imaging Findings	Comments
Cricopharyngeal achalasia (Fig GI 1-1)	Hemispherical or horizontal, shelf-like protrusion on the posterior aspect of the esophagus at approximately the C5-C6 level.	Failure of the upper esophageal sphincter to relax. Can result in dysphagia by obstructing the passage of a swallowed bolus. In severe disease, can cause aspiration and pneumonia.
Total laryngectomy (pseudodefect)	Appearance identical to that of cricopharyngeal achalasia.	Clinically, the patient complains of dysphagia on the way down and dysphonia with esophageal speech on the way up.
Scleroderma (Fig GI 1-2)	Dilated, atonic esophagus involving only the smooth muscle portion (from the aortic arch down). Normal stripping wave in the upper third of the esophagus (which is composed primarily of striated muscle). Patulous lower esophageal sphincter with gastroesophageal reflux. In the upright position, barium flows rapidly into the stomach.	Atrophy of smooth muscle with replacement by fibrosis. Often asymptomatic, though the patient may be required to eat or drink in a sitting or an erect position. High incidence of gastroesophageal reflux leading to peptic esophagitis and stricture formation.

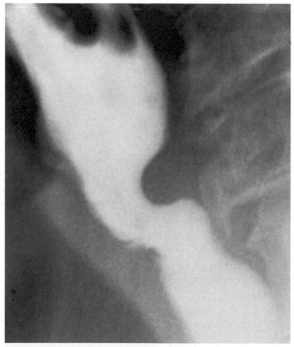

Fig GI 1-1
Cricopharyngeal achalasia.

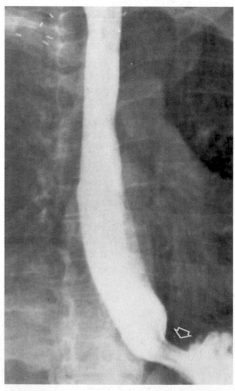

Fig GI 1-2
Scleroderma. Note the patulous esophagogastric junction (arrow).

Condition	Imaging Findings	Comments
Achalasia (Figs GI 1-3 to GI 1-5)	Dilatation and tortuosity of the esophagus that can produce a widened mediastinum (often with an air-fluid level) primarily on the right side adjacent to the cardiac shadow. Multiple uncoordinated tertiary contractions. Smoothly tapered, conical narrowing of the distal esophagus (beak sign). In the erect position, small spurts of barium enter the stomach (jet effect). Length of narrowed segment (<3.5 cm) and degree of proximal dilatation (>4 cm) suggests primary achalasia.	Incomplete relaxation of the lower esophageal sphincter related to a paucity or absence of ganglion cells in the myenteric plexuses (Auerbach's) of the distal esophageal wall. Denervation hypersensitivity response to Mecholyl (synthetic acetylcholine). A similar appearance may be produced by any generalized or localized interruption of the reflex arc controlling normal esophageal motility (eg, diseases of the medullary nuclei, abnormality of the vagus nerve, destruction of myenteric ganglion cells by inflammatory disease, or carcinoma of the distal esophagus or the gastric cardia).

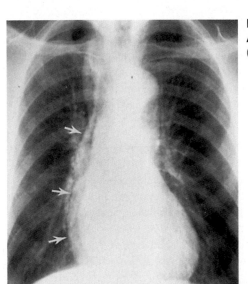

Fig GI 1-3
Achalasia. The margin of the dilated, tortuous esophagus (arrows) parallels the right border of the heart.

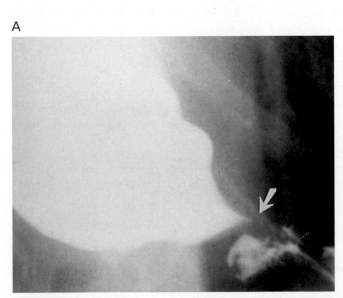

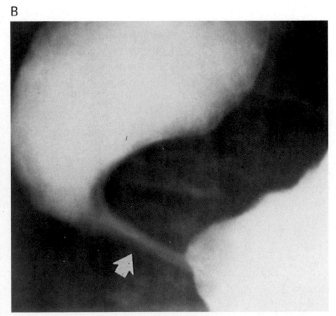

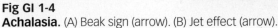

Fig GI 1-4
Achalasia. (A) Beak sign (arrow). (B) Jet effect (arrow).

Condition	Imaging Findings	Comments
Chagas' disease	Pattern identical to that of achalasia.	Destruction of the myenteric plexuses by the protozoan *Trypanosoma cruzi*, which also causes megacolon with chronic constipation, ureteral dilatation, and myocarditis.
Diffuse esophageal spasm (Fig GI 1-6)	Tertiary contractions of abnormally high amplitude that can obliterate the lumen. Corkscrew pattern of transient sacculations or pseudodiverticular (rosary bead esophagus).	Classic clinical triad of massive uncoordinated esophageal contractions, chest pain, and increased intramural pressure. Symptoms are frequently caused or aggravated by eating, but can occur spontaneously and even awaken the patient at night.
Presbyesophagus	Nonpropulsive tertiary contractions that are usually occasional and mild but may become frequent and strong.	Condition of aging that may be the result of a minor cerebrovascular accident affecting the central nuclei. Usually asymptomatic but can cause moderate dysphagia.
Esophagitis (Fig GI 1-7)	Initially, repetitive nonperistaltic tertiary contractions that occur distal to the point of disruption of the primary wave. If severe, can result in complete aperistalsis.	Disordered esophageal motility is the earliest and most frequent radiographic abnormality in esophageal inflammation, whether secondary to reflux, corrosive agents, infection, amyloidosis, or radiation injury.
Primary muscle disorders (Fig GI 1-8)	Disordered peristalsis involving the upper third of the esophagus (containing striated muscle). In myasthenia gravis, the initial swallow is often normal, but peristalsis weakens on repeated swallows. In myotonic dystrophy, there is reflux across the cricopharyngeus muscle (continuous column of barium extending from the hypopharynx to the cervical esophagus even when the patient is not swallowing).	Patient unable to develop a good pharyngeal peristaltic wave. In myasthenia gravis, muscular fatigue results from failure of neural transmission between the motor end plate and the muscle fiber. In myotonic dystrophy, an anatomic abnormality of the motor end plate leads to atrophy and an inability of the contracted muscle to relax. Other primary muscle disorders include polymyositis, dermatomyositis, amyotrophic lateral sclerosis, myopathies secondary to steroids and abnormal thyroid function, and oculopharyngeal myopathy.
Primary neural disorders	Various patterns of abnormal motility, including profound motor incoordination of the pharynx and the upper esophageal sphincter, diffuse tertiary contractions, and an achalasia pattern.	Causes include peripheral or central cranial nerve palsy, cerebrovascular occlusive disease affecting the brainstem, high unilateral cervical vagotomy, bulbar poliomyelitis, syringomyelia, multiple sclerosis, and familial dysautonomia (Riley-Day syndrome).
Diabetes mellitus	Various patterns of abnormal motility, including tertiary contractions and esophageal dilatation with a substantial delay in esophageal emptying when the patient is recumbent.	Markedly decreased amplitude of pharyngeal and peristaltic contractions. Primarily involves diabetics with a neuropathy of long duration.
Alcoholism	Diminished peristalsis, most pronounced in the distal portion.	Probably reflects a combination of alcoholic myopathy and neuropathy.
Drugs	Aperistalsis and dilatation of the esophagus (mimics scleroderma).	Anticholinergic agents (atropine, Pro-Banthine).
Obstructive lesions	Initially, tertiary contractions are produced in an attempt to pass the obstruction. Eventually, there may be a dilated and virtually aperistaltic esophagus.	Lesions that may cause esophageal obstruction include tumors, foreign bodies, webs, strictures, and Schatzki's rings.

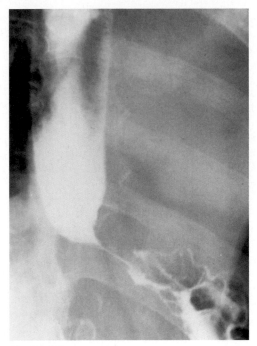

Fig GI 1-5
Achalasia pattern caused by the proximal extension of carcinoma of the fundus of the stomach.

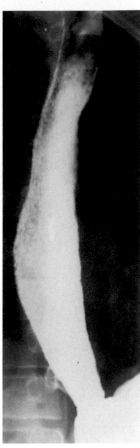

Fig GI 1-6
Diffuse esophageal spasm.

Fig GI 1-7
Candidiasis. Aperistalsis and esophageal dilatation are associated with diffuse ulceration.

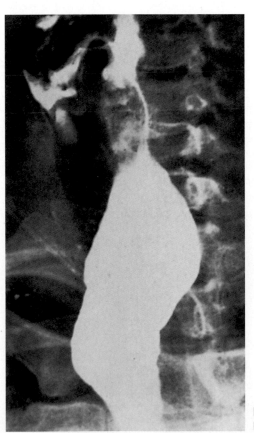

Fig GI 1-8
Myotonic dystrophy.[1]

Extrinsic Impressions on the Cervical Esophagus

Condition	Imaging Findings	Comments
Cricopharyngeus muscle (Fig GI 2-1)	Relatively constant posterior impression on the esophagus at approximately the C5-C6 level.	Caused by failure of the cricopharyngeus muscle to relax. A similar posterior impression can often be observed after total laryngectomy.
Pharyngeal venous plexus (Fig GI 2-1)	Anterior impression on the esophagus at about the C6 level. Appearance varies from swallow to swallow.	Caused by prolapse of lax mucosal folds over the rich central submucosal pharyngeal venous plexus. Occurs in 70% to 90% of adults and is thus considered a normal finding.
Esophageal web (Figs GI 2-1 through GI 2-3)	Smooth, thin lucent band (occasionally multiple) arising from the anterior wall of the esophagus near the pharyngoesophageal junction.	Usually an incidental finding of no clinical importance, but can be associated with epidermolysis bullosa, benign mucous membrane pemphigus, or the "Plummer-Vinson syndrome."
Anterior marginal osteophyte (Fig GI 2-4)	Smooth, regular indentation on the posterior wall of the esophagus at the level of an intervertebral disk space.	Usually asymptomatic but may produce pain or difficulty in swallowing (especially with profuse osteophytosis and diffuse idiopathic skeletal hyperostosis).
Thyroid enlargement or mass (Fig GI 2-5)	Smooth impression on and displacement of the lateral wall of the esophagus, usually with parallel displacement of the trachea.	Caused by localized or generalized hypertrophy of the gland, inflammatory disease, or thyroid malignancy.
Parathyroid mass	Impression on and displacement of the lateral wall of the esophagus.	Can aid in determining the site of the lesion in a patient with symptoms of hyperparathyroidism due to a functioning parathyroid tumor.
Lymphadenopathy	Smooth impression on and displacement of the esophagus.	May be calcified.
Soft-tissue abscess or hematoma	Impression on and displacement of the esophagus.	Abscess may contain gas.
Spinal neoplasm or inflammation	Posterior impression on the esophagus (may be irregular).	Suggested if there is associated destruction of a vertebral body.
Ectopic gastric mucosal rest (Fig GI 2-6)	Persistent ring-like narrowing of the upper esophagus.	Congenital condition that is almost always asymptomatic but rarely can produce dysphagia.
Narrow thoracic inlet	Extrinsic compression of esophagus at the cervicodorsal junction.	Rare anatomic variant. CT is required to exclude a mass and permit measurement of the thoracic inlet.

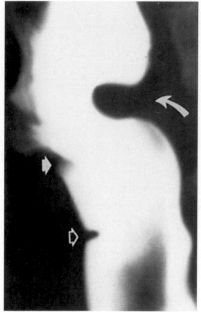

Fig GI 2-1
Three impressions on the cervical esophagus: **cricopharyngeal impression** (curved arrow), **pharyngeal venous plexus** (short closed arrow), and **esophageal web** (short open arrow).[2]

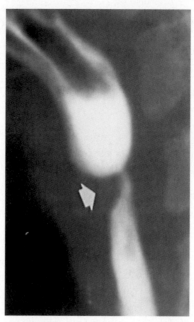

Fig GI 2-2
Epidermolysis bullosa. A stenotic web (arrow) results from the healing of subepidermal blisters involving the mucous membranes.

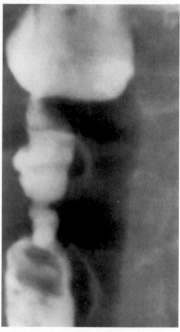

Fig GI 2-3
Benign mucous membrane pemphigus. Postinflammatory scarring causes a long, irregular area of narrowing suggestive of a malignant process.

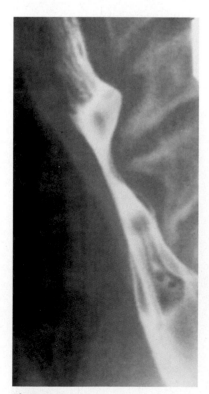

Fig GI 2-4
Anterior marginal osteophytes.

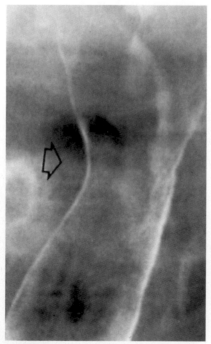

Fig GI 2-5
Enlargement of the thyroid gland. Smooth impression in the cervical esophagus (arrow).

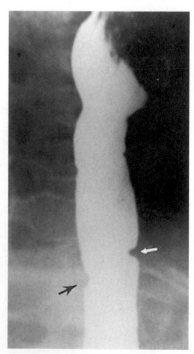

Fig GI 2-6
Ectopic gastric mucosa. Persistent ring-like narrowing (arrows) in the upper esophagus at the level of the thoracic inlet.[3]

Extrinsic Impressions on the Thoracic Esophagus

Condition	Imaging Findings	Comments
Normal structures		
Aortic knob (Fig GI 3-1)	Broad impression on the esophagus at the level of the transverse arch.	More prominent as the aorta becomes increasingly dilated and tortuous with age.
Left main-stem bronchus (Fig GI 3-1)	Narrower impression on the esophagus at the level of the carina.	
Left inferior pulmonary vein/confluence of left pulmonary veins	Impression on the anterior aspect of the left wall of the esophagus 4 to 5 cm below the carina.	Seen in approximately 10% of patients (especially in a steep left posterior oblique [LPO] projection). The vascular nature of the indentation can be confirmed by the Valsalva and Mueller maneuvers (the impression becomes smaller and more prominent, respectively).
Right inferior supra-azygous recess	Smooth extrinsic impression on the right posterolateral wall of the upper thoracic esophagus between the thoracic inlet and the aortic arch.	Seen in approximately 10% of individuals, this impression should not be mistaken for lymphadenopathy or other mediastinal mass.
Vascular abnormalities		
Right aortic arch (Fig GI 3-2)	Impression on the right lateral wall of the esophagus at a level slightly higher than the normal left aortic knob. Deviation of the trachea to the left.	If no posterior esophageal impression (mirror-image pattern), congenital heart disease (especially tetralogy of Fallot) is frequently associated. If there is an oblique posterior indentation on the esophagus (aberrant left subclavian artery), congenital heart disease is rarely associated.
Cervical aortic arch (see Fig CA 11-2)	Pulsatile mass causing a posterior impression on the esophagus above the clavicle.	Caused by the retroesophageal course of the distal arch or the proximal descending aorta. No coexistent intracardiac congenital heart disease.

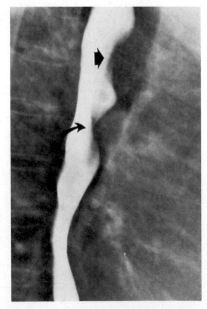

Fig GI 3-1
Normal esophageal impressions caused by the aorta (short arrow) and left main-stem bronchus (long arrow).

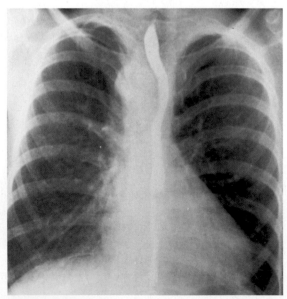

Fig GI 3-2
Right aortic arch.

Condition	Imaging Findings	Comments
Barrett esophagus (Fig GI 4-4)	Ulceration can occur anywhere along the columnar epithelium and tends to be deep and penetrating like peptic gastric ulcers. Postinflammatory stricture of the esophagus often develops.	Often associated with hiatal hernia and reflux, though the ulcer is generally separated from the hernia by a variable length of normal-appearing esophagus. High propensity for developing adenocarcinoma in the columnar-lined portion of the esophagus.
Infectious esophagitis *Candida* (Fig GI 4-5)	Multiple ulcerations of various sizes that can involve the entire thoracic esophagus. Irregular nodular mucosal pattern with marginal serrations. May be a single large ulcer in patients with AIDS.	Most frequently develops in patients with chronic debilitating diseases or undergoing immunosuppressive therapy. Disordered esophageal motility (dilated, atonic esophagus) is often an early finding.
Herpetic (Fig GI 4-6)	Similar to candidiasis, though the background mucosa is often otherwise normal.	Self-limited viral inflammation that predominantly affects patients with disseminated malignancy or abnormal immune systems.

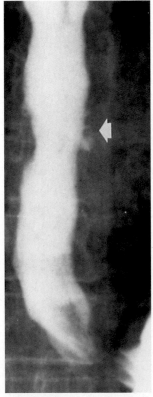

Fig GI 4-4
Barrett esophagus. Ulcerations (arrow) have developed at a distance from the esophagogastric junction.

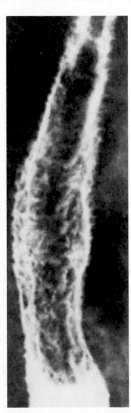

Fig GI 4-5
***Candida* esophagitis.** Multiple ulcers and nodular plaques produce the grossly irregular contour of a shaggy esophagus. This manifestation of far-advanced candidiasis is now infrequent because of earlier and better treatment of the disease.[7]

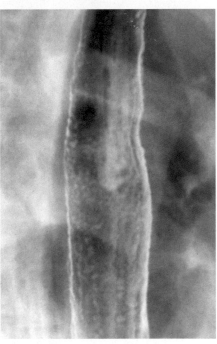

Fig GI 4-6
Herpes simplex esophagitis. Innumerable punctate and linear areas of ulceration.[8]

Condition	Imaging Findings	Comments
Cytomegalovirus (Fig GI 4-7)	Diffuse or segmental ulcerating colitis, primarily affecting the distal half of the esophagus with extension into the gastric fundus. Often solitary, large, relatively flat ulcer.	Most frequently develops in patients with AIDS or other cause of compromised immune system. Widely distributed organism that usually causes only a subclinical infection in a normal adult host.
Tuberculous (Fig GI 4-8)	Single or multiple ulcers that may mimic malignancy. Sinuses and fistulous tracts are common.	Intense fibrotic response often narrows the esophageal lumen. Numerous miliary granulomas can produce multiple nodules.
Human immunodeficiency virus (Fig GI 4-9)	Giant, relatively flat, ovoid or irregular lesions that typically involve the middle third of the esophagus.	Causes odynophagia in patients with acute or chronic HIV infection who have no evidence of the usual opportunistic fungal or viral organisms. Ulcers heal spontaneously or respond to oral steroids (thus must be distinguished from giant ulcers of cytomegalovirus, which require treatment with potentially toxic antiviral agents).

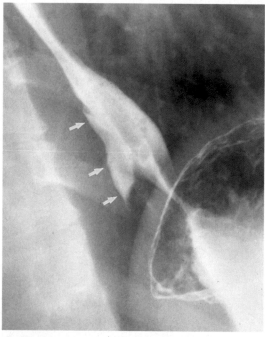

Fig GI 4-7
Cytomegalovirus. Deep focal ulcer in the distal esophagus (arrows).[9]

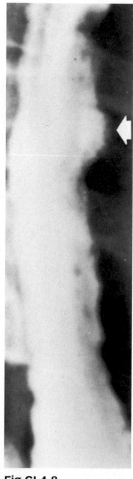

Fig GI 4-8
Tuberculosis. Diffuse mucosal irregularity of the esophagus associated with sinus tracts extending anteriorly into the mediastinum (arrow).[10]

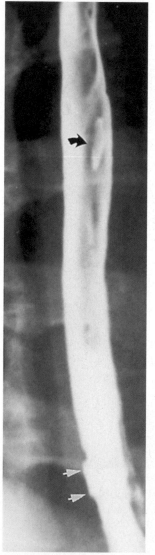

Fig GI 4-9
Human immunodeficiency virus. Long, ovoid lesion seen en face in the upper esophagus (black arrow). Note the more distal lesion (white arrows) seen in profile.

Condition	Imaging Findings	Comments
Other organisms	Various patterns of ulceration, nodularity, and fistulous tracts.	Rare manifestation of syphilis and histoplasmosis.
Carcinoma of the esophagus (Figs GI 4-10 and GI 4-11)	Ulcer crater (often irregular) surrounded by an unchanging bulging mass projecting into the esophageal lumen.	In the relatively uncommon primary ulcerative esophageal carcinoma, virtually all of an eccentric, flat mass is ulcerated. Ulceration is an infrequent manifestation of esophageal lymphoma.
Corrosive esophagitis (Fig GI 4-12)	Diffuse superficial or deep ulceration involves a long portion of the esophagus.	Most severe corrosive injuries are caused by alkali. Fibrous healing results in gradual esophageal narrowing.
Radiation injury	Multiple ulcerations of various sizes that can involve the entire thoracic esophagus. Irregular nodular mucosal pattern with marginal serrations.	Appearance indistinguishable from that of *Candida* esophagitis (which is far more common in patients undergoing chemotherapy or radiation therapy for malignant disease). Develops after relatively low radiation doses in patients who simultaneously or sequentially receive Adriamycin or actinomycin D.
Crohn's disease/ eosinophilic esophagitis (Fig GI 4-13)	Various patterns of ulceration, nodularity, and fistulous tracts.	Infrequent esophageal involvement.

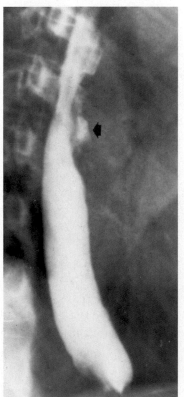

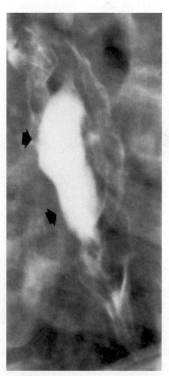

Fig GI 4-10
Squamous carcinoma of the esophagus. On a profile view, the lesion appears as an ulcer crater (arrow) surrounded by a bulging mass projecting into the esophageal lumen.

Fig GI 4-11
Primary ulcerative carcinoma. Characteristic meniscoid ulceration (arrows) surrounded by a tumor mass.

Condition	Imaging Findings	Comments
Drug-induced esophagitis (Fig GI 4-14)	Various patterns of superficial or deep esophageal ulcerations.	Primarily occurs in patients who have delayed esophageal transit time (abnormal peristalsis, hiatal hernia with reflux, or relative obstruction). Most commonly associated with potassium chloride tablets; other causes include tetracycline, emperonium bromide, quinidine, and ascorbic acid.
Sclerotherapy of esophageal varices (Fig GI 4-15)	Focal or diffuse ulceration that varies in size, shape, and depth.	Most frequent cause of rebleeding. The degree of ulceration is directly related to the amount of sclerosant solution used, the number of injections, and the number of columns of varices injected.
Intramural esophageal pseudodiverticulosis (Fig GI 4-16)	Multiple, small (1–3 mm), ulcer-like projections arising from the esophageal wall. There is frequently an associated smooth stricture in the upper esophagus.	Rare disorder in which the pseudodiverticula represent the dilated ducts of submucosal glands. *Candida albicans* can be cultured from approximately half the patients, though there is no evidence suggesting the fungus as a causative agent.

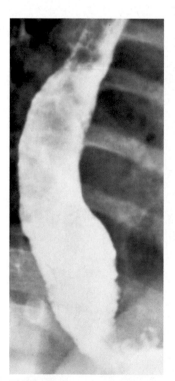
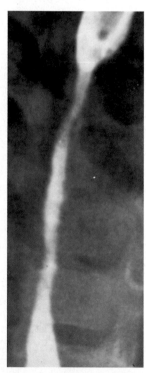

Fig GI 4-12
Corrosive esophagitis. (A) Dilated, boggy esophagus with ulceration 8 days after the ingestion of a caustic agent. (B) Stricture formation is evident on an esophagram obtained 3 months after the caustic injury.

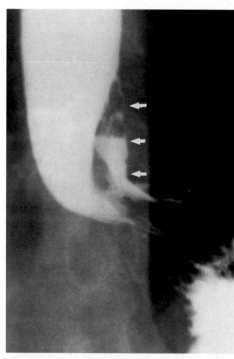

Fig GI 4-13
Crohn's esophagitis. Long intramural sinus tract (arrows).[11]

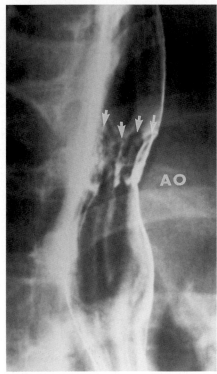

Fig GI 4-14
Drug-induced esophagitis. Several focal and linear ulcers (arrows) coalescing in the proximal thoracic esophagus at the level of the aortic arch (AO), related to the ingestion of penicillin tablets for pharyngitis.[12]

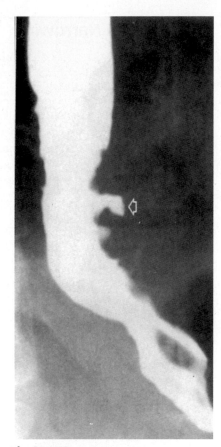

Fig GI 4-15
Variceal sclerotherapy. Barium esophagram performed 2 weeks after two courses of endoscopic injection sclerotherapy shows diffuse ulceration in the distal third of the esophagus and one intramural sinus tract (arrow).[13]

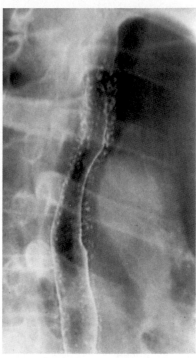

Fig GI 4-16
Intramural pseudodiverticulosis.

Esophageal Narrowing

Condition	Imaging Findings	Comments
Esophageal web (Fig GI 5-1)	Smooth, thin lucent band arising from the anterior wall of the esophagus near the pharyngo-esophageal junction. Rarely distal or multiple.	Usually an incidental finding of no clinical importance, but can be associated with epidermolysis bullosa, benign mucous membrane pemphigus, chronic graft-versus-host disease, or the Plummer-Vinson syndrome. Fluoroscopically guided balloon dilatation has been reported as an easy and highly effective technique for treating symptomatic webs.
Lower esophageal ring (Schatzki's ring) (Fig GI 5-2)	Smooth, concentric narrowing of the esophagus arising several centimeters above the diaphragm.	Can cause dysphagia if the width of the lumen is less than 12 mm.
Carcinoma of esophagus (Fig GI 5-3)	Initially, a flat plaque-like lesion on one wall of the esophagus. Later, an encircling mass with irregular luminal narrowing and overhanging margins.	Major cause of dysphagia in patients older than 40. Close association with drinking and smoking and with head and neck carcinomas. Spreads rapidly and often ulcerates.
Malignancy of fundus of the stomach (Fig GI 5-4)	Irregular narrowing and nodularity of the distal esophagus.	Develops in 10% to 15% of adenocarcinomas and in 2% to 10% of lymphomas arising in the cardia.

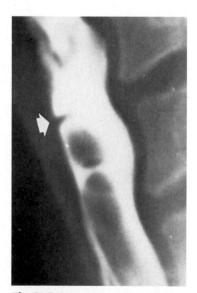

Fig GI 5-1
Esophageal web (arrow).

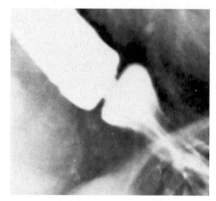

Fig GI 5-2
Lower esophageal ring.

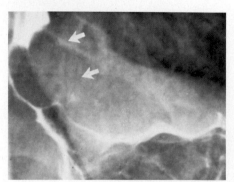

Fig GI 5-4
Adenocarcinoma of the fundus involving the esophagus. An irregular tumor of the superior aspect of the fundus extends proximally as a large mass (arrows) that almost obstructs the distal esophagus.

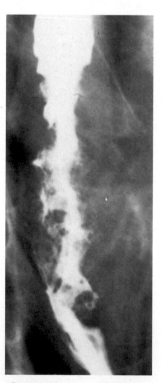

Fig GI 5-3
Esophageal carcinoma. Irregular narrowing of an extensive segment of the thoracic portion of the esophagus.

Condition	Imaging Findings	Comments
Reflux esophagitis (Figs GI 5-5 and GI 5-6)	Asymmetric, often irregular, stricture of the esophagus that usually extends to the cardio-esophageal junction.	Often, but not always, associated with a hiatal hernia.
Barrett esophagus (Fig GI 5-7)	Smooth stricture that generally involves the midportion of the thoracic esophagus.	Usually a variable length of normal-appearing esophagus separates the stricture from the cardio esophageal junction. A technetium scan can demonstrate the columnar tissue in the lower esophagus.

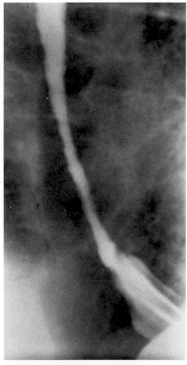

Fig GI 5-5
Reflux esophagitis. The long esophageal stricture is associated with a hiatal hernia.

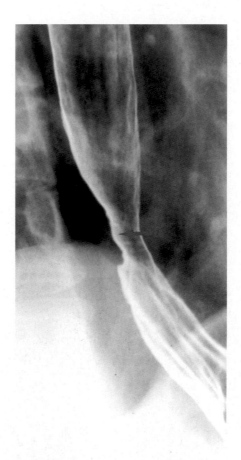

Fig GI 5-6
Reflux esophagitis. Eccentric area of narrowing in the distal esophagus (arrow), which resulted from asymmetric scarring.[14]

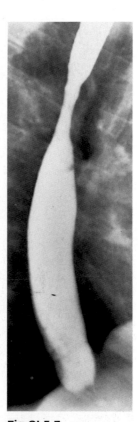

Fig GI 5-7
Barrett esophagus. Smooth stricture in the upper thoracic esophagus.

Condition	Imaging Findings	Comments
Corrosive esophagitis (Fig GI 5-8)	Long stricture that involves a large portion of the esophagus down to the cardioesophageal junction.	Most severe injuries are caused by the ingestion of alkali.
Drug ingestion (Fig GI 5-9)	Segmental area of concentric narrowing.	Drugs such as quinidine, potassium chloride, alendronate, and aspirin or other nonsteroidal anti-inflammatory agents may cause severe esophagitis with large areas of ulceration and the development of strictures. The esophagitis typically results from prolonged irritation of that mucosa caused by pills that lodge in the esophagus at sites of extrinsic compression by adjacent structures, such as the aortic arch, left main bronchus, or enlarged left chambers of the heart.
Prolonged nasogastric intubation (Fig GI 5-10)	Smooth narrowing of the distal esophagus.	Caused by reflux esophagitis (tube prevents hiatal closure) or mucosal ischemia (compression effect of the tube).

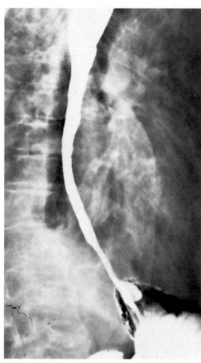

Fig GI 5-8
Extensive caustic stricture due to lye ingestion that involves almost the entire thoracic esophagus.

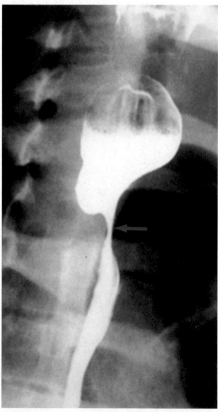

Fig GI 5-9
Drug-induced stricture. Slightly asymmetric focal area of narrowing in the upper thoracic esophagus (arrow) above the level of the aortic arch in a patient who developed dysphagia 6 months after taking potassium chloride for hypokalemia.[14]

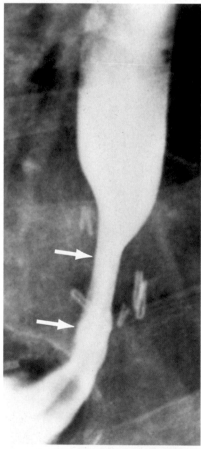

Fig GI 5-10
Nasogastric intubation stricture. Relatively long segment of narrowing in the distal esophagus (arrows), which developed 5 months after prolonged nasogastric intubation.[14]

Condition	Imaging Findings	Comments
Radiation (Fig GI 5-11)	Relatively long segment of smooth, concentric, tapered narrowing within a pre-existing radiation portal	This appearance can usually be distinguished from the more irregular narrowing, asymmetric mass effect, and ulceration associated with recurrent tumor in the mediastinum.
Infectious or granulomatous disorders (Fig GI 5-12)	Various patterns of esophageal narrowing.	Tuberculosis; histoplasmosis; syphilis; herpes simplex; Crohn's disease; eosinophilic esophagitis.
Motility disorders (see Fig GI 1-4)	Various patterns of esophageal narrowing.	Achalasia (failure of the lower esophageal sphincter to relax, beak sign); diffuse esophageal spasm (prolonged strong contractions).

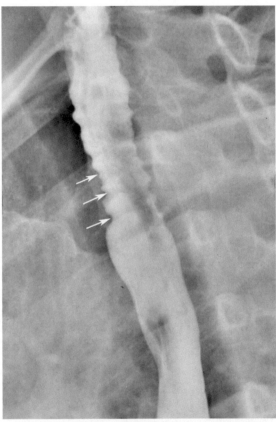

Fig GI 5-11
Radiation-induced stricture. Long segment of smooth tapered narrowing (arrows) in the upper esophagus in a patient who had undergone medistinal irradiation.[15]

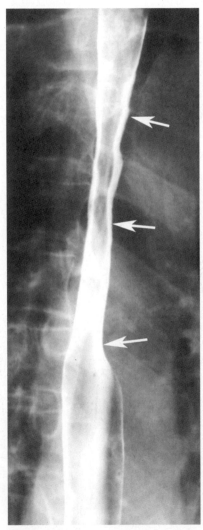

Fig GI 5-12
Eosinophilic esophagitis. Moderately long stricture in the upper thoracic esophagus. Note the multiple distinctive ring-like indentations (arrows) in the region of the stricture that are frequently seen in this condition.[16]

Condition	Imaging Findings	Comments
Intramural esophageal pseudodiverticulosis (Fig GI 5-13)	Smooth stricture in the upper third of the esophagus associated with multiple small ulcer-like projections arising from the esophageal wall.	Dilatation of the stricture generally ameliorates the symptoms of dysphagia.
Skin disease (Fig GI 5-14)	Concentric or asymmetric narrowing in the upper or mid-esophagus, sometimes with associated webs.	Epidermolysis bullosa dystrophica and benign mucous membrane pemphigoid.
Congenital esophageal stenosis (Fig GI 5-15)	Focal stricture containing ring-like indentations in the mid-esophagus.	A severe form that occurs in newborns or infants and usually requires surgery. However, a milder form is occasionally seen in young or even middle-aged adults with a lifelong history of mild, "compensated" dysphagia and recurrent food impactions.
Miscellaneous causes (Figs GI 5-16 to GI 5-17)	Various patterns of esophageal narrowing.	Endoscopic sclerotheraphy of esophageal varices, glutaraldehyde contamination at endoscopy, graft-versus-host disease, and Behcet disease.

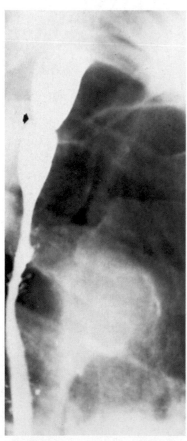

Fig GI 5-13
Intramural esophageal pseudo-diverticulosis. The arrow points to the upper esophageal stricture.

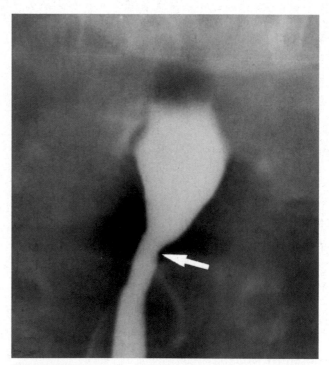

Fig GI 5-14
Benign mucous membrane pemphigoid. Focal stricture in the upper esophagus (arrow) near the thoracic inlet.[14]

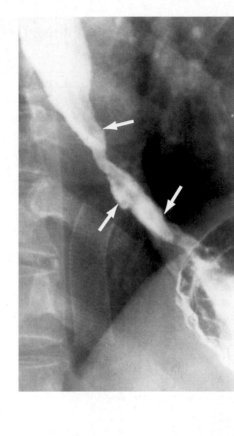

Fig GI 5-16
Endoscopic sclerotherapy. Long, irregular stricture in the distal esophagus (straight white arrows) that resulted from scarring caused by prior endoscopic sclerotherapy for esophageal varices. Note also the flat ulcer in the region of the stricture (white arrow). Black arrows indicate a transjugular intrahepatic portosystemic shunt.[14]

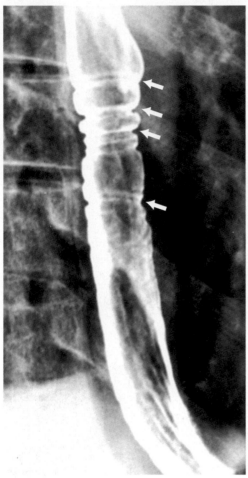

Fig GI 5-15
Congenital esophageal stenosis. Mild narrowing in the mid-esophagus with ring-like indentations (arrows) in the region of the stricture.[14]

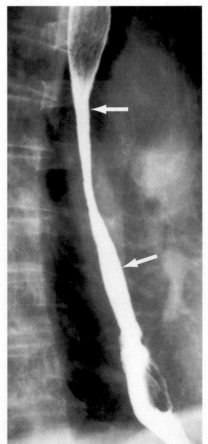

Fig GI 5-17
Glutaraldehyde-induced stricture. Long stricture involving the middle and distal esophagus (arrows). In the absence of any other predisposing factors, this stricture was presumed to be caused by toxicity from residual glutaraldehyde contamination at endoscopy.[14]

Esophageal Filling Defects

Condition	Imaging Findings	Comments
Benign tumors		
Spindle cell tumor (Fig GI 6-1)	Smooth, rounded intramural defect that is sharply demarcated from the adjacent esophageal wall. No infiltration, ulceration, or overhanging margins.	Most commonly leiomyoma, which is usually asymptomatic and rarely ulcerates, bleeds, or undergoes malignant transformation. Occasionally contains pathognomonic amorphous calcification.
Fibrovascular polyp (Fig GI 6-2)	Large, oval or elongated, sausage-like intraluminal mass.	Though rare, the second most common type of benign esophageal tumor. Large polyps can locally widen the esophagus, but do not cause complete obstruction or wall rigidity as with carcinoma.
Inflammatory esophagogastric polyp (Fig GI 6-3)	Filling defect in the region of the esophagogastric junction that is usually in continuity with a markedly thickened gastric fold.	Probably represents a stage in the evolution of chronic esophagitis (polyp reflects thickening of the proximal aspect of an inflamed gastric fold).
Villous adenoma	Filling defect with typical barium filling of the frond-like interstices.	Tumor of intermediate malignant potential.

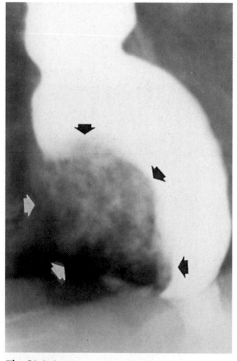

Fig GI 6-1
Leiomyoma. Note the amorphous calcifications in this smoothly lobulated intramural tumor (arrows).[17]

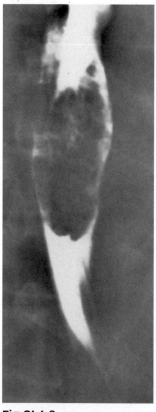

Fig GI 6-2
Fibrovascular polyp.

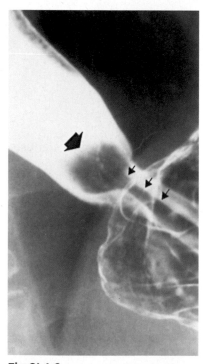

Fig GI 6-3
Inflammatory esophagogastric polyp. Distal esophageal filling defect (large arrow) in continuity with a thickened gastric fold (small arrows).

Condition	Imaging Findings	Comments
Malignant tumors		
Carcinoma of esophagus (Fig GI 6-4)	Irregular circumferential lesion with destruction of mucosal folds, overhanging margins, and abrupt transition to adjacent normal tissue.	Less frequently, carcinoma can present as a localized polypoid mass, often with deep ulceration and a fungating appearance.
Carcinoma or lymphoma of fundus of stomach (see Fig GI 5-4)	Irregular filling defect of the lower esophagus.	Continuous with malignancy of the gastric cardia.
Sarcoma (Fig GI 6-5)	Bulky mass that may ulcerate.	Rare lesions. Leiomyosarcoma; carcinosarcoma (nests of squamous epithelium surrounded by interlacing bundles of spindle-shaped cells with numerous mitoses); pseudosarcoma (low-grade nonsquamous malignancy often associated with adjacent squamous cell carcinoma).
Other malignancies (Fig GI 6-6)	Variable appearance.	Rare cases of melanoma, lymphoma, metastases, or verrucous carcinoma (exophytic, papillary, or warty tumor that rarely metastasizes and has a much better prognosis than typical squamous cell carcinoma).

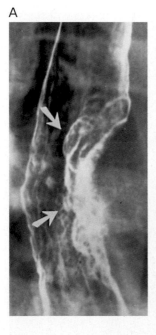

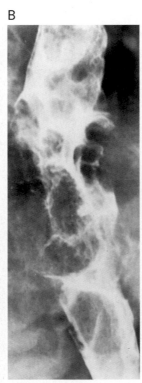

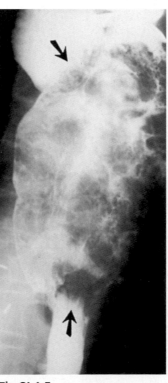

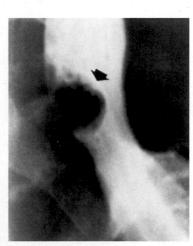

Fig GI 6-6
Verrucous squamous cell carcinoma. The smooth-surfaced filling defect in the distal esophagus (arrow) has a benign appearance.

Fig GI 6-4
Carcinoma of the esophagus. (A) Localized polypoid mass with ulceration (arrows). (B) Bulky irregular filling defect with destruction of mucosal folds.

Fig GI 6-5
Carcinosarcoma. Bulky, intraluminal, polypoid mass (arrows).

Condition	Imaging Findings	Comments
Lymph node enlargement (see Fig GI 3-5)	Extrinsic impression simulating an intramural esophageal lesion.	Usually caused by metastases or a granulomatous process (especially tuberculosis). Occasionally due to syphilis, sarcoidosis, histoplasmosis, or Crohn's disease.
Infectious esophagitis (Fig GI 6-7)	Diffuse pattern of multiple round and oval nodular defects.	Most commonly candidiasis, which is usually associated with ulceration and a shaggy contour of the esophageal wall. Rarely, herpetic esophagitis.
Esophageal varices (Fig GI 6-8)	Diffuse, round and oval filling defects reflecting serpiginous thickening of folds.	Dilated venous structures of varices change size and appearance with variations in intrathoracic pressure. Distal esophagus involved in portal hypertension. "Downhill" varices in the upper esophagus are due to superior vena cava obstruction.
Duplication cyst (Fig GI 6-9)	Eccentric impression simulating an intramural mass.	Alimentary tract duplications occur least commonly in the esophagus. They rarely communicate with the esophageal lumen.

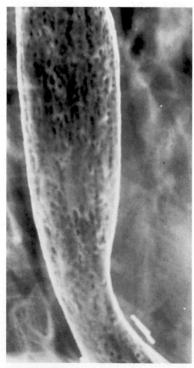

Fig GI 6-7
Candida **esophagitis.** Numerous plaque-like defects in the middle and distal esophagus. Note that the plaques have discrete margins and a predominantly longitudinal orientation.

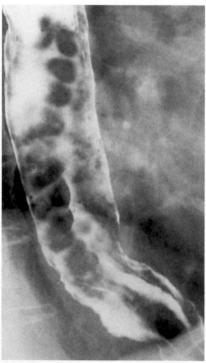

Fig GI 6-8
Esophageal varices.

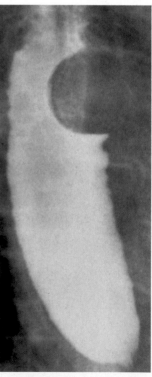

Fig GI 6-9
Duplication cyst. Eccentric impression on the barium-filled esophagus simulates an intramural mass.

Condition	Imaging Findings	Comments
Foreign bodies (Fig GI 6-10)	Various patterns depending on the material swallowed.	Usually impacted in the distal esophagus just above the level of the diaphragm. Often a distal stricture, especially if the impaction is in the cervical portion of the esophagus. Irregular margins may mimic an obstructing carcinoma.
Intramural hematoma	Soft, elongated filling defect with smooth borders.	Submucosal bleeding with intramural dissection of the esophageal wall has been described as resulting from emetics, after endoscopic instrumentation, and in patients having impaired hemostasis (hemophilia, thrombocytopenia) or receiving anticoagulant therapy.
Hirsute esophagus	Single or multiple filling defects representing a mass of hair or multiple hair follicles, respectively.	Complication of reconstructive surgery of the pharynx and esophagus in which skin flaps are mobilized and rotated to reconstruct a "skin tube esophagus" to restore anatomic continuity of the gastrointestinal tract.
Prolapsed gastric folds	Irregular filling defect in the distal esophagus.	Serial radiographs demonstrate reduction of the prolapse, return of the gastric folds below the diaphragm, and a normal distal esophagus.

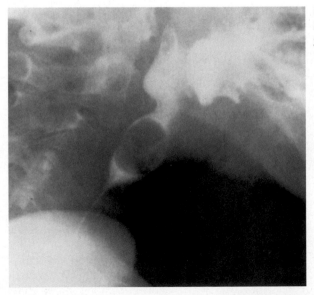

Fig GI 6-10
Foreign body. Cherry pit impacted in the cervical esophagus proximal to a caustic stricture.

Esophageal Diverticula

Condition	Imaging Findings	Comments
Zenker's diverticulum (Figs GI 7-1 and GI 7-2)	Arises from the upper esophagus with its neck lying in the midline of the posterior wall at the pharyngoesophageal junction (approximately the C5–C6 level).	Pulsion diverticulum that is apparently related to premature contraction or other motor incoordination of the cricopharyngeus muscle. May cause dysphagia or even esophageal obstruction.
Cervical traction diverticulum (Fig GI 7-3)	Variable appearance. Arises from any portion of the esophageal wall.	Rare condition resulting from fibrous healing of an inflammatory process in the neck or secondary to postsurgical changes (eg, laryngectomy).
Lateral diverticulum	Arises in a lateral or anterolateral direction at the level of the pharyngoesophageal junction (just below the transverse portion of the cricopharyngeus muscle).	Also known as Killian-Jamieson diverticula, they are considerably smaller than Zenker's diverticula and are much less likely to be associated with overflow aspiration and consequent pneumonia (because the diverticulum lies below the cricopharyngeus and allows the muscle to close above it).
Thoracic diverticulum (Fig GI 7-4)	Arises in the middle third of the thoracic esophagus opposite the bifurcation of the trachea in the region of the hilum of the lung.	Traction diverticulum that develops in response to the pull of fibrous adhesions after mediastinal lymph node infection. There are often adjacent calcified mediastinal lymph nodes from healed granulomatous disease.

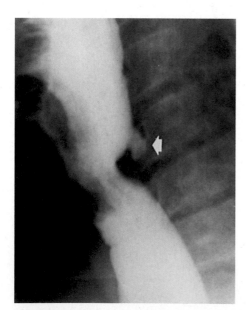

Fig GI 7-1
Small Zenker's diverticulum (arrow).

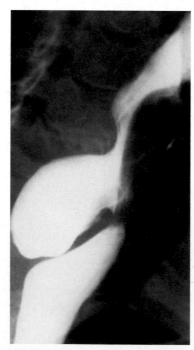

Fig GI 7-2
Large Zenker's diverticulum almost occluding the esophageal lumen.

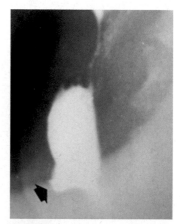

Fig GI 7-3
Cervical traction diverticulum (arrow) caused by postoperative scarring after total laryngectomy.

Condition	Imaging Findings	Comments
Epiphrenic diverticulum (Fig GI 7-5)	Occurs in the distal 10 cm of the esophagus and tends to have a broad, short neck.	Pulsion diverticulum that is probably related to incoordination of esophageal peristalsis and relaxation of the lower sphincter. If small, can simulate an esophageal ulcer (though the mucosal pattern of the adjacent esophagus is normal).
Intramural esophageal pseudodiverticulosis (Fig GI 7-6)	Multiple small (1–3 mm), ulcer-like projections arising from the esophageal wall. There is frequently an associated smooth stricture in the upper esophagus. Approximately half of the patients have diffused disease, whereas the rest have segmental disease (typically with evidence of chronic esophagitis or distal esophageal strictures).	Rare disorder with pseudodiverticula (mimicking Rokitansky-Aschoff sinuses of the gallbladder) representing dilated ducts of submucosal glands. *Candida albicans* can be cultured from approximately half the patients, though there is no evidence suggesting that the fungus is a causative agent. Intramural tracks bridging two or more pseudodiverticula and running parallel to the lumen may mimic ulceration or frank perforation.
Intraluminal diverticulum (Fig GI 7-7)	Thin radiolucent line separates the barium-filled pouch of mucosal membrane that is open proximally and closed distally.	Rare entity that usually is related to mucosal damage secondary to increased intraluminal pressure in an esophagus that has been constricted by an inflammatory process.

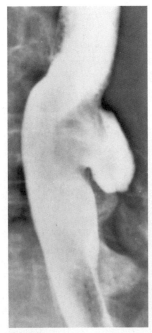

Fig GI 7-4
Thoracic diverticulum.

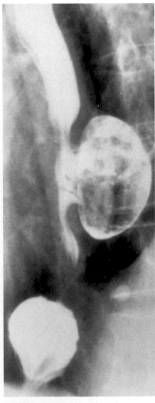

Fig GI 7-5
Epiphrenic diverticulum.

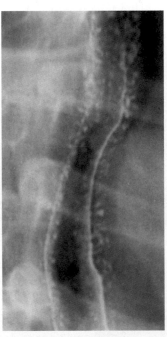

Fig GI 7-6
Intramural esophageal pseu-dodiverticulosis.

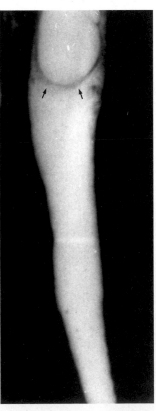

Fig GI 7-7
Intraluminal esophageal diverticulum.
The wall of the diverticulum appears as a thin radiolucent line (arrows). Note the moderate irregular stenosis of the distal esophagus secondary to the acid ingestion that resulted in the formation of the intraluminal diverticulum.[18]

Gastric Ulceration

Condition	Imaging Findings	Comments
Peptic ulcer disease (Fig GI 8-1)	Classic signs of benignancy include penetration, Hampton line, ulcer collar, ulcer mound, and radiation of smooth, slender mucosal folds to the edge of the crater.	If the ulcer crater is very shallow, a thin layer of barium coating results in a ring shadow. Irregular folds merging into a mound of polypoid tissue around the crater suggest a malignancy. Fundal ulcers above the level of the cardia are usually malignant.
Gastritis (Fig GI 8-2)	Ulcers vary from superficial erosions to deep niches.	Superficial erosions occur with gastritis due to alcohol, anti-inflammatory agents, or Crohn's disease. Frank ulcerations develop in patients with corrosive gastritis or granulomatous infiltration.
Benign tumor	Central ulceration in a mass.	Predominantly spindle cell tumors, especially leiomyoma.
Radiation injury	Discrete ulcerations identical to peptic disease.	Pain is unrelenting and has no relation to meals. High incidence of perforation and hemorrhage. Healing is minimal even with intensive medical therapy.
MALT lymphoma (Fig GI 8-3)	Discrete ulcer surrounded by a mass and associated with regional or generalized enlargement of rugal folds.	Previously termed *pseudolymphoma*, mucosa-associated lymphoid tissue lymphoma has a much more favorable prognosis than high-grade lymphoma; early diagnosis and prompt treatment may lead to cure.

A
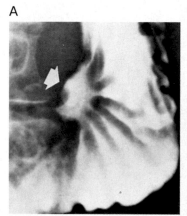

B
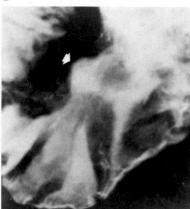

Fig GI 8-1
Fold patterns in gastric ulcers (arrow). (A) Small, slender folds radiating to the edge of a benign ulcer. (B) Thick folds radiating to an irregular mound of tissue surrounding a malignant gastric ulcer (arrow).

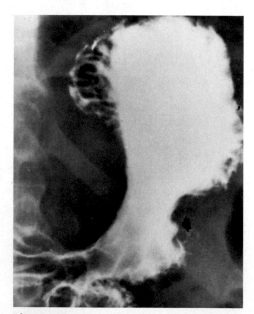

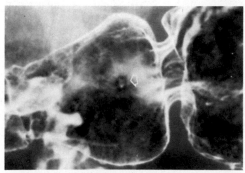

Fig GI 8-2
Gastritis. Superficial gastric erosions (arrow). Tiny flecks of barium, representing erosions, are surrounded by radiolucent halos, representing mounds of edematous mucosa.

Fig GI 8-3
MALT lymphoma. Greater curvature ulcer (arrow) surrounded by a soft-tissue mass and associated with regional enlargement of rugal folds.

Condition	Imaging Findings	Comments
Carcinoma (Fig GI 8-4)	Ulcers vary from shallow erosions in superficial mucosal lesions to huge excavations in fungating polypoid masses.	Signs of malignant ulcer include Carman's meniscus sign (and Kirklin complex) and abrupt transition between normal mucosa and abnormal, usually nodular, tissue surrounding the ulcer. The ulcer does not penetrate beyond the normal gastric lumen.
Lymphoma (Fig GI 8-5)	Irregular ulcer that often is larger than the adjacent gastric lumen. Combination of a large ulcer and an extraluminal mass may suggest extravasation of barium.	May be indistinguishable from carcinoma. Findings suggestive of lymphoma include splenomegaly and extrinsic impressions on the barium-filled stomach (due to retrogastric and other regional lymph nodes).
Sarcoma (Fig GI 8-6)	Large central ulceration in a mass that often has a prominent exophytic component.	Primarily leiomyosarcoma, which often is radiographically indistinguishable from its benign spindle cell counterpart.
Metastases (Fig GI 8-7)	Single or multiple bull's-eye lesions.	Most commonly caused by malignant melanoma. An identical appearance can be due to metastases from carcinoma of the breast or lung.

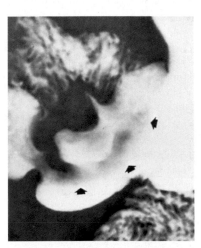

Fig GI 8-4
Carcinoma of the stomach. Carman's meniscus sign in malignant gastric ulcer. The huge ulcer has a semicircular configuration with its inner margin convex toward the lumen. The ulcer is surrounded by the radiolucent shadow of an elevated ridge of neoplastic tissue (arrows).

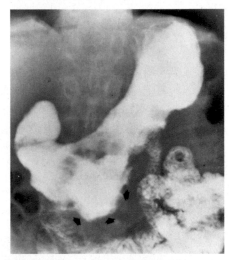

Fig GI 8-5
Gastric lymphoma. Huge, irregular ulcer (arrows) in a neoplastic gastric mass.

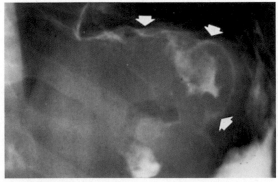

Fig GI 8-6
Leiomyosarcoma of the stomach. The large fundal mass (arrows) shows exophytic extension and ulceration.

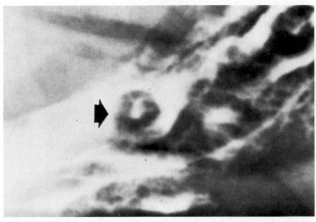

Fig GI 8-7
Gastric metastases from melanoma (arrow).

Narrowing of the Stomach

Condition	Imaging Findings	Comments
Carcinoma (Figs GI 9-1 and GI 9-2)	Thickening and fixation of the stomach wall, usually beginning near the pylorus and progressing upward.	By far the most common cause of the linitis plastica pattern. Tumor invasion of the gastric wall stimulates a strong desmoplastic response. Gastric carcinoma can also cause segmental narrowing.
Lymphoma	Luminal narrowing that primarily involves the antral region, mimicking scirrhous carcinoma.	Unlike the rigidity and fixation of scirrhous carcinoma, residual peristalsis and flexibility of the stomach wall are often preserved in Hodgkin's disease.
Metastases (Fig GI 9-3)	Circumferential narrowing of the stomach, usually with more segmental involvement than in a primary gastric malignancy.	Direct extension from carcinoma of the pancreas or transverse colon or desmoplastic hematogenous metastases (eg, carcinoma of the breast).
Peptic ulcer disease (Fig GI 9-4)	Antral narrowing and rigidity due to intense spasm.	Acute ulcer may not be seen because of the lack of antral distensibility. Peptic ulcer–induced rigidity usually heals with adequate antacid therapy. Midgastric ulcer in an elderly patient may heal with an hour-glass deformity.
Crohn's disease (Fig GI 9-5)	Smooth, tubular antrum flaring into a normal gastric body and fundus (ram's horn sign).	Often cobblestoning of antral folds with fissures and ulceration. Concomitant involvement of the adjacent duodenal bulb and proximal sweep produces the pseudo–Billroth-I pattern.
Other infiltrative disorders (Fig GI 9-6)	Mural thickening and luminal narrowing predominantly involve the antrum.	Sarcoidosis; syphilis; tuberculosis; strongyloidiasis; cytomegalovirus; toxoplasmosis; eosinophilic gastritis; polyarteritis nodosa.

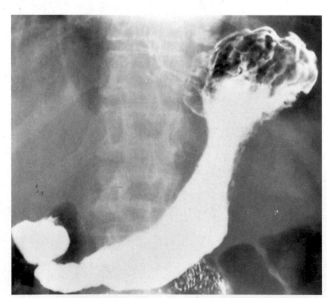

Fig GI 9-1
Scirrhous carcinoma of the stomach producing a linitis plastica pattern.

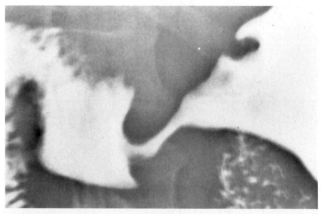

Fig GI 9-2
Adenocarcinoma of the stomach causing segmental constriction of the antrum.

Condition	Imaging Findings	Comments
Hamartoma	Multiple filling defects.	No malignant potential. Occurs in Peutz-Jeghers syndrome and Cowden's disease.
Spindle cell tumor (Fig GI 10-3)	Single intramural mass, often with central ulceration.	Most commonly, leiomyoma. A large lesion may have an intraluminal component or produce an extensive exogastric mass mimicking extrinsic gastric compression.
Malignant tumors Polypoid carcinoma (Fig GI 10-4)	Sessile mass that is usually relatively large, irregular, and ulcerated.	Increased incidence in patients with atrophic gastritis and pernicious anemia. May be difficult to distinguish from a benign gastric polyp.
Lymphoma (Fig GI 10-5)	Large, bulky polypoid lesion that is usually irregular and ulcerated.	Factors favoring lymphoma rather than carcinoma include multiple ulcerating polypoid tumors and adjacent thickening of folds (rather than the atrophic mucosal pattern often seen in carcinoma).

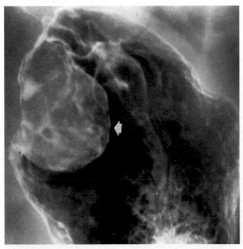

Fig GI 10-3
Leiomyoma of the fundus (arrow).

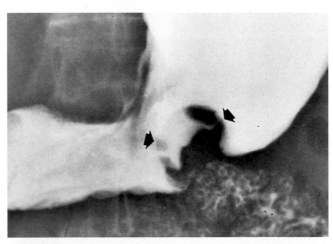

Fig GI 10-4
Carcinoma of the stomach. A huge ulcer is evident in the smooth, fungating polypoid mass (arrows).

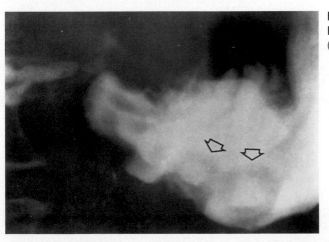

Fig GI 10-5
Lymphoma. Multiple ulcerated, polypoid gastric masses (arrows).

Condition	Imaging Findings	Comments
Metastases (see Fig GI 8-7)	Usually multiple, often ulcerated (bull's-eye appearance).	Most commonly due to malignant melanoma. Also caused by carcinomas of the breast and lung.
Sarcoma (Fig GI 10-6)	Large, bulky mass that is often ulcerated.	Most are leiomyosarcomas, which are difficult to differentiate from their benign spindle cell counterparts (large exogastric mass suggests malignancy).
Villous adenoma	Characteristic barium filling of the interstices of the tumor. Often multiple.	Rare lesion with a substantial incidence of malignancy.
Carcinoid	Broad-based mass that is often ulcerated.	Slow-growing lesion with long survivals (even in the presence of regional or hepatic dissemination).
Ectopic pancreas (Fig GI 10-7)	Smooth submucosal mass with central umbilication.	Most commonly found on the greater curvature of the distal antrum close to the pylorus. Central umbilication represents the orifice of an aberrant pancreatic duct rather than ulceration.
Enlarged gastric folds (Fig GI 10-8)	Multiple nodular filling defects (if viewed end-on).	Ménétrier's disease; gastric varices; Crohn's disease; sarcoidosis; tuberculosis; eosinophilic gastritis.

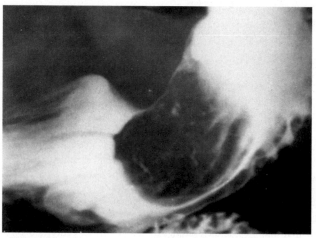

Fig GI 10-6
Leiomyosarcoma. There is scattered ulceration in this bulky tumor.

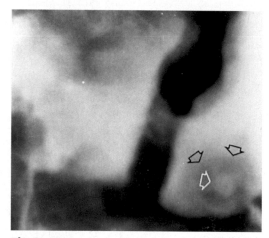

Fig GI 10-7
Ectopic pancreas. Central opacification (white arrow) of a rudimentary pancreatic duct in a soft-tissue mass (black arrows) in the distal antrum.

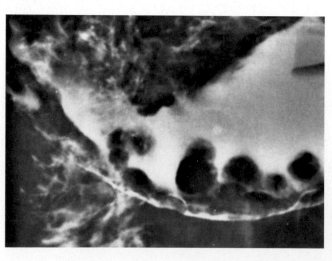

Fig GI 10-8
Alcoholic gastritis. Multiple nodular filling defects (suggesting polyps) are due to enlarged gastric folds viewed on end.

Condition	Imaging Findings	Comments
Bezoar (Fig GI 10-9)	Large mass that may fill the entire stomach. Occasionally completely smooth (simulating an enormous gas bubble).	Contrast material coating the mass and infiltrating the interstices may produce a characteristic mottled or streaked appearance. Phytobezoars (undigested vegetable material) and trichobezoars (hairballs).
Foreign body/blood clot	Single or multiple filling defects.	Variety of ingested substances and any cause of esophageal or gastric bleeding.
Peptic ulcer disease (Figs GI 10-10 and GI 10-11)	Various appearances (with or without ulceration).	Can represent a large mound of edema surrounding an acute ulcer, an incisura on the wall opposite an ulcer crater, or a double pylorus.
Langerhans cell histiocytosis (inflammatory fibroid polyp)	Sharply defined, smooth, round or oval mass (usually in the antrum).	Nonspecific inflammatory infiltrate that is usually asymptomatic (no food allergy or peripheral eosinophilia as in eosinophilic gastritis).
Duplication cyst	Filling defect or extrinsic mass impression.	Very rare. Tends to be asymptomatic, to involve the greater curvature, and to not communicate with the gastric lumen.
Fundoplication (Fig GI 10-12)	Prominent filling defect at the esophagogastric junction. The mass is generally smoothly marginated and symmetric on both sides of the distal esophagus.	Fundal pseudotumor secondary to a surgical procedure for hiatal hernia repair. In a Nissen fundoplication, the gastric fundus is wrapped around the lower esophagus to create an intra-abdominal esophageal segment with a natural valve mechanism at the esophagogastric junction.

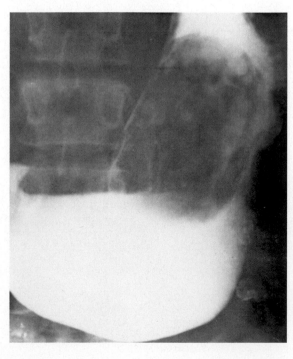

Fig GI 10-9
Glue bezoar in a young model-airplane builder. The smooth mass simulates an enormous air bubble.

Condition	Imaging Findings	Comments
MALT lymphoma	Multiple, rounded, often confluent nodules of varying size (<1 cm) that primarily involve the body and antrum of the stomach.	Appearance may mimic enlarged areae gastricae. Larger single masses are often ulcerated.

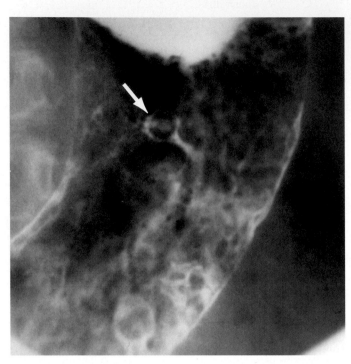

Fig GI 10-10.
Peptic ulcer disease. There are innumerable small mucosal and submucosal polypoid masses, several of which contain ulcer craters (arrow).[21]

A

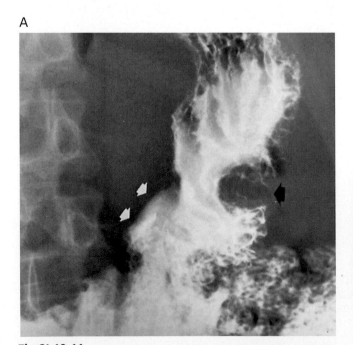

B

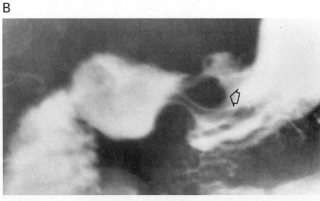

Fig GI 10-11
Peptic ulcer disease. (A) Large incisura (black arrow) simulating a filling defect on the greater curvature. The incisura is incited by a long ulcer (white arrows) on the lesser curvature. (B) Double pylorus. The true pylorus and the accessory channel along the lesser curvature are separated by a bridge, or septum, that produces the appearance of a discrete lucent filling defect (arrow).